Fundamentals of SARS-CoV-2 Biosensors

Fundamentals of SARS-CoV-2 Biosensors

Editors

Carlos Torres-Torres
Blanca Estela García-Pérez

MDPI • Basel • Beijing • Wuhan • Barcelona • Belgrade • Manchester • Tokyo • Cluj • Tianjin

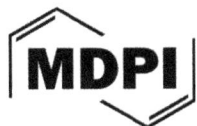

Editors
Carlos Torres-Torres
Instituto Politécnico Nacional
Laboratory of Optics
Mexico

Blanca Estela García-Pérez
Instituto Politécnico Nacional
Escuela Nacional de Ciencias Biológicas
Mexico

Editorial Office
MDPI
St. Alban-Anlage 66
4052 Basel, Switzerland

This is a reprint of articles from the Special Issue published online in the open access journal *Biosensors* (ISSN 2079-6374) (available at: https://www.mdpi.com/journal/biosensors/special_issues/SAR_BIOSEN).

For citation purposes, cite each article independently as indicated on the article page online and as indicated below:

LastName, A.A.; LastName, B.B.; LastName, C.C. Article Title. *Journal Name* **Year**, *Volume Number*, Page Range.

ISBN 978-3-0365-5767-0 (Hbk)
ISBN 978-3-0365-5768-7 (PDF)

© 2022 by the authors. Articles in this book are Open Access and distributed under the Creative Commons Attribution (CC BY) license, which allows users to download, copy and build upon published articles, as long as the author and publisher are properly credited, which ensures maximum dissemination and a wider impact of our publications.

The book as a whole is distributed by MDPI under the terms and conditions of the Creative Commons license CC BY-NC-ND.

Contents

Carlos Torres-Torres and Blanca Estela García-Pérez
Fundamentals of SARS-CoV-2 Biosensors
Reprinted from: *Biosensors* **2022**, *12*, 880, doi:10.3390/bios12100880 1

Wei Yin Lim, Boon Leong Lan and Narayanan Ramakrishnan
Emerging Biosensors to Detect Severe Acute Respiratory Syndrome Coronavirus 2 (SARS-CoV-2): A Review
Reprinted from: *Biosensors* **2021**, *11*, 434, doi:10.3390/bios11110434 5

Kseniya V. Serebrennikova, Nadezhda A. Byzova, Anatoly V. Zherdev, Nikolai G. Khlebtsov, Boris N. Khlebtsov, Sergey F. Biketov and Boris B. Dzantiev
Lateral Flow Immunoassay of SARS-CoV-2 Antigen with SERS-Based Registration: Development and Comparison with Traditional Immunoassays
Reprinted from: *Biosensors* **2021**, *11*, 510, doi:10.3390/bios11120510 31

Tao Peng, Xueshima Jiao, Zhanwei Liang, Hongwei Zhao, Yang Zhao, Jie Xie, You Jiang, Xiaoping Yu, Xiang Fang and Xinhua Dai
Lateral Flow Immunoassay Coupled with Copper Enhancement for Rapid and Sensitive SARS-CoV-2 Nucleocapsid Protein Detection
Reprinted from: *Biosensors* **2022**, *12*, 13, doi:10.3390/bios12010013 45

Zhanwei Liang, Tao Peng, Xueshima Jiao, Yang Zhao, Jie Xie, You Jiang, Bo Meng, Xiang Fang, Xiaoping Yu and Xinhua Dai
Latex Microsphere-Based Bicolor Immunochromatography for Qualitative Detection of Neutralizing Antibody against SARS-CoV-2
Reprinted from: *Biosensors* **2022**, *12*, 103, doi:10.3390/bios12020103 55

Elda A. Flores-Contreras, Reyna Berenice González-González, Iram P. Rodríguez-Sánchez, Juan F. Yee-de León, Hafiz M. N. Iqbal and Everardo González-González
Microfluidics-Based Biosensing Platforms: Emerging Frontiers in Point-of-Care Testing SARS-CoV-2 and Seroprevalence
Reprinted from: *Biosensors* **2022**, *12*, 179, doi:10.3390/bios12030179 65

Wilson A. Ameku, David W. Provance, Carlos M. Morel and Salvatore G. De-Simone
Rapid Detection of Anti-SARS-CoV-2 Antibodies with a Screen-Printed Electrode Modified with a Spike Glycoprotein Epitope
Reprinted from: *Biosensors* **2022**, *12*, 272, doi:10.3390/bios12050272 85

Sabine Szunerits, Hiba Saada, Quentin Pagneux and Rabah Boukherroub
Plasmonic Approaches for the Detection of SARS-CoV-2 Viral Particles
Reprinted from: *Biosensors* **2022**, *12*, 548, doi:10.3390/bios12070548 95

Geert Besselink, Anke Schütz-Trilling, Janneke Veerbeek, Michelle Verbruggen, Adriaan van der Meer, Rens Schonenberg, Henk Dam, Kevin Evers, Ernst Lindhout, Anja Garritsen, Aart van Amerongen, Wout Knoben and Luc Scheres
Asymmetric Mach–Zehnder Interferometric Biosensing for Quantitative and Sensitive Multiplex Detection of Anti-SARS-CoV-2 Antibodies in Human Plasma
Reprinted from: *Biosensors* **2022**, *12*, 553, doi:10.3390/bios12080553 109

Chia-Hsuan Cheng, Yu-Chi Peng, Shu-Min Lin, Hiromi Yatsuda, Szu-Heng Liu, Shih-Jen Liu, Chen-Yen Kuo and Robert Y. L. Wang
Measurements of Anti-SARS-CoV-2 Antibody Levels after Vaccination Using a SH-SAW Biosensor
Reprinted from: *Biosensors* 2022, 12, 599, doi:10.3390/bios12080599 127

Kritika Srinivasan Rajsri, Michael P. McRae, Glennon W. Simmons, Nicolaos J. Christodoulides, Hanover Matz, Helen Dooley, Akiko Koide, Shohei Koide and John T. McDevitt
A Rapid and Sensitive Microfluidics-Based Tool for Seroprevalence Immunity Assessment of COVID-19 and Vaccination-Induced Humoral Antibody Response at the Point of Care
Reprinted from: *Biosensors* 2022, 12, 621, doi:10.3390/bios12080621 137

Nayeli Shantal Castrejón-Jiménez, Blanca Estela García-Pérez, Nydia Edith Reyes-Rodríguez, Vicente Vega-Sánchez, Víctor Manuel Martínez-Juárez and Juan Carlos Hernández-González
Challenges in the Detection of SARS-CoV-2: Evolution of the Lateral Flow Immunoassay as a Valuable Tool for Viral Diagnosis
Reprinted from: *Biosensors* 2022, 12, 728, doi:10.3390/bios12090728 153

Jose Alberto Arano-Martinez, Claudia Lizbeth Martínez-González, Ma Isabel Salazar and Carlos Torres-Torres
A Framework for Biosensors Assisted by Multiphoton Effects and Machine Learning
Reprinted from: *Biosensors* 2022, 12, 710, doi:10.3390/bios12090710 171

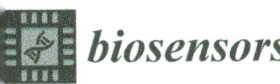

Editorial

Fundamentals of SARS-CoV-2 Biosensors

Carlos Torres-Torres [1,*] and Blanca Estela García-Pérez [2]

[1] Sección de Estudios de Posgrado e Investigación, Escuela Superior de Ingeniería Mecánica y Eléctrica Unidad Zacatenco, Instituto Politécnico Nacional, Mexico City 07738, Mexico
[2] Departamento de Microbiología, Escuela Nacional de Ciencias Biológicas, Instituto Politécnico Nacional, Mexico City 11340, Mexico
* Correspondence: ctorrest@ipn.mx

Citation: Torres-Torres, C.; García-Pérez, B.E. Fundamentals of SARS-CoV-2 Biosensors. *Biosensors* **2022**, *12*, 880. https://doi.org/10.3390/bios12100880

Received: 10 October 2022
Accepted: 10 October 2022
Published: 17 October 2022

Publisher's Note: MDPI stays neutral with regard to jurisdictional claims in published maps and institutional affiliations.

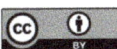

Copyright: © 2022 by the authors. Licensee MDPI, Basel, Switzerland. This article is an open access article distributed under the terms and conditions of the Creative Commons Attribution (CC BY) license (https://creativecommons.org/licenses/by/4.0/).

A beautiful topic in its essence and content is represented by the powerful assistance of sensing methods and techniques for automatically revealing biological agents and biological functions in this era. This Special Issue entitled "Fundamentals of SARS-CoV-2 Biosensors" has been mainly devoted to simultaneously integrate essential and cutting-edge discoveries in the role of coronavirus detection and identification of molecules of immune response as the antibodies neutralizing. This collection of papers is presented as a step towards the development of new alternatives related to current challenges in biosensors emerging for one of the major pandemics of this millennium up to date.

Wei Yin Lim, Boon Leong Lan and Narayanan Ramakrishnan have presented a review on three particular types of biosensors employed for detecting SARS-CoV-2 based on surface plasmon resonance effects, electrochemical measurements and field-effect transistors. Sensing principles and confrontation of the advantages and limitations of these sensors were analyzed. The use of biorecognition elements and plasmonic nanomaterials are proposed in order to improve the sensitivity of the biosensors [1].

Kseniya V. Serebrennikova et al. presented a lateral flow immunoassay (LFIA) including the plasmonic advantages of gold nanoparticles and nanostructures with immobilized antibodies and 4-mercaptobenzoic acid as surface-enhanced Raman scattering (SERS) nanotag. A systematic study of the compositions of SERS nanotags was carried out promoting the acceleration of the typical response time exhibited by LFIA by the incorporation of SERS effects in membrane immuno-analytical systems [2].

Tao Peng et al. showed an investigation about LFIA conducted by both colloidal gold nanoparticles and copper deposition-induced signal amplification. The LFIA coupled with the copper and gold nanostructures yield the enhancement of efficiency and sensitivity in the biosensing processes [3].

Zhanwei Liang et al. developed a point-of-care bicolor LFIA for detecting neutralizing (Nab) antibody against SARS-CoV-2 without sample pretreatment. It is indicated the importance of the principle of NAb-mediated blockage on the interaction between the receptor binding domain of the spike protein and the angiotensin-converting enzyme 2. Red and blue latex microspheres were employed to carry out the measurement and control lines in order to reduce the error bar usually given by monitoring and interpretation of single-colored line data [4].

Elda A. Flores-Contreras et al. reported an analysis about comparative microfluidic platforms employed for SARS-CoV-2 testing. The systems studied were classified according to three different molecules to be detected, which were nucleic acid, antigens, and anti-SARS-CoV-2 antibodies. This manuscript includes a critical report about commercially available alternatives based on microfluidic processes [5].

Wilson A. Ameku et al. designed an electrochemical biosensor for detecting serological immunoglobulin G (IgG) antibodies in sera against spike proteins. How the capture of SARS-CoV-2-specific IgGs generates the formation of an immunocomplex is highlighted. Rapid trace signatures from square-wave voltammetry and the generation of hydroquinone are claimed. Absence of cross-reaction between SARS-CoV-2 and Chagas disease, Chikungunya, Leishmaniosis, Dengue, or new variants of SARS-CoV-2 is guaranteed by this method [6].

Sabine Szunerits, Hiba Saada, Quentin Pagneux and Rabah Boukherroub underlined the powerful potential of portable surface plasmon resonance systems for viral diagnostic and monitoring. A clear review focused on modern biosensing based on surface plasmon resonance phenomena to convert the receptor-binding event of SARS-CoV-2 viral particles into measurable signals was developed. Advantages and details about the key roles of plasmonics for virus particle detection as well as viral protein sensing were analyzed [7].

Geert Besselink et al. proposed a photonic integrated circuit based on an asymmetric Mach–Zehnder interferometer for SARS-CoV-2 biosensing. Attractive advantages of photonics featuring tunable and high analytical sensitivity, signal multiplexing technology, small size, portability, and the potential for high-volume manufacturing were described. Spike proteins, receptor-binding domain, and nucleocapsid proteins as target antigens were experimentally tested in this work [8].

Chia-Hsuan Cheng et al. mentioned the crucial role to detect the amount of anti-SARS-CoV-2 S protein antibodies prior to vaccination. This is regarding the fact that vaccines, apart from inducing antibody production, could cause and adverse effects such as myocarditis, blood clots, muscle pain and fatigue, among others. A shear-horizontal surface acoustic wave biosensor coated with SARS-CoV-2 spike protein is presented in this research to quantify the amount of anti-SARS-CoV-2 S protein antibodies from finger blood. It is reported that mRNA vaccines, such as Moderna or BNT, can originate stronger effects derived by higher concentrations of total anti-SARS-CoV-2 S protein antibodies compared with adenovirus vaccines [9].

Kritika Srinivasan Rajsri et al. described their findings on a rapid quantitative point-of-care serological assay for quantifying anti-SARS-CoV-2 antibodies. the potential use of this proposed system for the timing of booster shots and measuring the level of cross-reactive antibodies is pointed out. A lab-on-a-chip ecosystem is presented as a strategy to easily quantitate the humoral protection against COVID-19. The design proposed includes characteristics for the diagnostic timeline of the disease, seroconversion, and vaccination response spanning multiple doses of immunization in just one test [10].

Nayeli Shantal Castrejón-Jiménez et al. summarized the progress and dynamic evolution of advantages and limitations concerning LFIA techniques for SARS-CoV-2 biosensors. Advanced tools for clinical diagnostics discriminating numerous analytes, including viruses and antibodies were explained. Central pillars for building a realistic tackling of current challenges in diagnostic biosensors were analyzed [11].

Jose Alberto Arano-Martinez et al. elucidated a perspective to explore the future of nonlinear optical processes and machine learning methods to improve the performance of non-invasive biosensors. A straightforward demonstration in the effectiveness of multiphonic interactions assisted by machine learning, neural networks and artificial intelligence in nonlinear systems for SARS-CoV-2 sensing is described. The impact of nonlinearities governed with computer tools and soft computing is emphasized in biosensors suitable for the identification of complex low-dimensional agents, viruses, or biological functions in cells [12].

Original research, critical perspectives and panoramic discussions for envisioning new opportunities in the direction of the progress for SARS-CoV-2 biosensors are analyzed in each of the papers published in this Special Issue.

Author Contributions: Writing—original draft, C.T.-T. and B.E.G.-P.; Writing—review and editing, C.T.-T. and B.E.G.-P. Conceptualization C.T.-T. and B.E.G.-P. All authors contributed equally to the proposal and writing of this manuscript. All authors have read and agreed to the published version of the manuscript.

Funding: This research was funded by Instituto Politécnico Nacional (SIP-2021-2022) and Consejo Nacional de Ciencia y Tecnología (CONACyT).

Acknowledgments: It has been an honor to participate as Guest Editors for this Special Issue in the prestigious Biosensors Journal from MDPI. The Guest Editors appreciate the kind opportunity and support given by the Editorial Board to us in this task. We want to highlight the outstanding work carried out by the staff of the Editorial Office and by the reviewers involved in this Special Issue. We specially thank the brilliant and professional assistance of Vena Luo for her actions in the promotion, selection and organization of activities for publishing this Special Issue. We acknowledge the important work of all authors who submitted their manuscripts. The Guest editors are overjoyed that all these papers have presented immediate applications in the topic of SARS-CoV-2 biosensors, and this Special Issue can become a base for future research.

Conflicts of Interest: The authors declare no conflict of interest.

References

1. Lim, W.Y.; Lan, B.L.; Ramakrishnan, N. Emerging Biosensors to Detect Severe Acute Respiratory Syndrome Coronavirus 2 (SARS-CoV-2): A Review. *Biosensors* **2021**, *11*, 434. [CrossRef]
2. Serebrennikova, K.V.; Byzova, N.A.; Zherdev, A.V.; Khlebtsov, N.G.; Khlebtso, B.N.; Biketo, S.F.; Dzantiev, B.B. Lateral Flow Immunoassay of SARS-CoV-2 Antigen with SERS-Based Registration: Development and Comparison with Traditional Immunoassays. *Biosensors* **2021**, *11*, 510. [CrossRef] [PubMed]
3. Peng, T.; Jiao, X.; Liang, Z.; Zhao, H.; Zhao, Y.; Xie, J.; Jiang, Y.; Yu, X.; Fang, X.; Dai, X. Lateral Flow Immunoassay Coupled with Copper Enhancement for Rapid and Sensitive SARS-CoV-2 Nucleocapsid Protein Detection. *Biosensors* **2022**, *12*, 13. [CrossRef] [PubMed]
4. Liang, Z.; Peng, T.; Jiao, X.; Zhao, Y.; Xie, J.; Jiang, Y.; Meng, B.; Fang, X.; Yu, X.; Dai, X. Latex Microsphere-Based Bicolor Immunochromatography for Qualitative Detection of Neutralizing Antibody against SARS-CoV-2. *Biosensors* **2022**, *12*, 103. [CrossRef] [PubMed]
5. Flores-Contreras, E.A.; González-González, R.B.; Rodríguez-Sánchez, I.P.; Yee-de León, J.F.; Iqbal, H.M.N.; González-González, E. Microfluidics-Based Biosensing Platforms: Emerging Frontiers in Point-of-Care Testing SARS-CoV-2 and Seroprevalence. *Biosensors* **2022**, *12*, 179. [CrossRef] [PubMed]
6. Ameku, W.A.; Provance, D.W.; Morel, C.M.; De-Simone, S.G. Rapid Detection of Anti-SARS-CoV-2 Antibodies with a Screen-Printed Electrode Modified with a Spike Glycoprotein Epitope. *Biosensors* **2022**, *12*, 272. [CrossRef]
7. Szunerits, S.; Saada, H.; Pagneux, Q.; Boukherroub, R. Plasmonic Approaches for the Detection of SARS-CoV-2 Viral Particles. *Biosensors* **2022**, *12*, 548. [CrossRef]
8. Besselink, G.; Schütz-Trilling, A.; Veerbeek, J.; Verbruggen, M.; van der Meer, A.; Schonenberg, R.; Dam, H.; Evers, K.; Lindhout, E.; Garritsen, A.; et al. Asymmetric Mach–Zehnder Interferometric Biosensing for Quantitative and Sensitive Multiplex Detection of Anti-SARS-CoV-2 Antibodies in Human Plasma. *Biosensors* **2022**, *12*, 553. [CrossRef]
9. Cheng, C.-H.; Peng, Y.-C.; Lin, S.-M.; Yatsuda, H.; Liu, S.-H.; Liu, S.-J.; Kuo, C.-Y.; Wang, R.Y.L. Measurements of Anti-SARS-CoV-2 Antibody Levels after Vaccination Using a SH-SAW Biosensor. *Biosensors* **2022**, *12*, 599. [CrossRef] [PubMed]
10. Rajsri, K.S.; McRae, M.P.; Simmons, G.W.; Christodoulides, N.J.; Matz, H.; Dooley, H.; Koide, A.; Koide, S.; McDevitt, J.T. A Rapid and Sensitive Microfluidics-Based Tool for Seroprevalence Immunity Assessment of COVID-19 and Vaccination-Induced Humoral Antibody Response at the Point of Care. *Biosensors* **2022**, *12*, 621. [CrossRef]
11. Castrejón-Jiménez, N.S.; García-Pérez, B.E.; Reyes-Rodríguez, N.E.; Vega-Sánchez, V.; Martínez-Juárez, V.M.; Hernández-González, J.C. Challenges in the Detection of SARS-CoV-2: Evolution of the Lateral Flow Immunoassay as a Valuable Tool for Viral Diagnosis. *Biosensors* **2022**, *12*, 728. [CrossRef] [PubMed]
12. Arano-Martinez, J.A.; Martínez-González, C.L.; Salazar, M.A.; Torres-Torres, C. A Framework for Biosensors Assisted by Multiphoton Effects and Machine Learning. *Biosensors* **2022**, *12*, 710. [CrossRef] [PubMed]

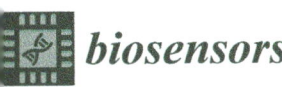

Review

Emerging Biosensors to Detect Severe Acute Respiratory Syndrome Coronavirus 2 (SARS-CoV-2): A Review

Wei Yin Lim, Boon Leong Lan and Narayanan Ramakrishnan *

Electrical and Computer Systems Engineering, School of Engineering and Advanced Engineering Platform, Monash University Malaysia, Bandar Sunway 47500, Selangor, Malaysia; WeiYin.Lim@monash.edu (W.Y.L.); lan.boon.leong@monash.edu (B.L.L.)
* Correspondence: ramakrishnan@monash.edu

Abstract: Coronavirus disease (COVID-19) is a global health crisis caused by the severe acute respiratory syndrome coronavirus 2 (SARS-CoV-2). Real-time reverse transcriptase-polymerase chain reaction (RT-PCR) is the gold standard test for diagnosing COVID-19. Although it is highly accurate, this lab test requires highly-trained personnel and the turn-around time is long. Rapid and inexpensive immuno-diagnostic tests (antigen or antibody test) are available, but these point of care (POC) tests are not as accurate as the RT-PCR test. Biosensors are promising alternatives to these rapid POC tests. Here we review three types of recently developed biosensors for SARS-CoV-2 detection: surface plasmon resonance (SPR)-based, electrochemical and field-effect transistor (FET)-based biosensors. We explain the sensing principles and discuss the advantages and limitations of these sensors. The accuracies of these sensors need to be improved before they could be translated into POC devices for commercial use. We suggest potential biorecognition elements with highly selective target-analyte binding that could be explored to increase the true negative detection rate. To increase the true positive detection rate, we suggest two-dimensional materials and nanomaterials that could be used to modify the sensor surface to increase the sensitivity of the sensor.

Keywords: biosensor; COVID-19 diagnosis; SARS-CoV-2; surface plasmon resonance; field-effect transistor; electrochemical; a point-of-care device

Citation: Lim, W.Y.; Lan, B.L.; Ramakrishnan, N. Emerging Biosensors to Detect Severe Acute Respiratory Syndrome Coronavirus 2 (SARS-CoV-2): A Review. *Biosensors* **2021**, *11*, 434. https://doi.org/10.3390/bios11110434

Received: 6 September 2021
Accepted: 14 October 2021
Published: 2 November 2021

Publisher's Note: MDPI stays neutral with regard to jurisdictional claims in published maps and institutional affiliations.

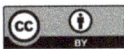

Copyright: © 2021 by the authors. Licensee MDPI, Basel, Switzerland. This article is an open access article distributed under the terms and conditions of the Creative Commons Attribution (CC BY) license (https:// creativecommons.org/licenses/by/ 4.0/).

1. Introduction

COVID-19 is an infectious disease caused by the severe acute respiratory syndrome coronavirus 2 (SARS-CoV-2). COVID-19 was first reported in Wuhan, China in December 2019 and spread rapidly across the world [1,2]. On 11 March 2020, the World Health Organization (WHO) declared the global spread of the novel coronavirus a pandemic and alerted the world to prepare for widespread community transmission [3]. Unfortunately, the transmission rate of SARS-CoV-2 is greater than the coronavirus for the severe acute respiratory syndrome (SARS) and the Middle East respiratory syndrome (MERS) in 2002 and 2012, respectively. COVID-19 was the leading cause of death in 2020 owing to the highly contagious and pathogenic coronavirus SARS-CoV-2. Although various vaccines have been developed and administered in various countries, the pandemic is still ongoing due to the emergence of multiple SARS-CoV-2 variants, particularly the Delta variant, which is much more transmissible. Up to 31 July 2021, there have been more than 197,252,280 confirmed COVID-19 cases globally, with 4,210,452 associated deaths [4].

The SARS-CoV-2 virus rapidly multiplies in the body tissues and triggers the immune system. The symptoms of COVID-19 may appear 2–14 days after exposure to the virus, ranging from mild fever to severe symptoms requiring hospitalization, such as difficulty breathing or shortness of breath [5]. To date, several biomarkers can be used for the detection of SARS-CoV-2: viral nucleic acid (single-stranded ribonucleic acid, RNA), viral protein antigen (spike (S) or nucleocapsid (N)) and antibodies (IgM, IgG or IgA) [6,7]. In general, diagnostic tests for COVID-19 fall into two main categories: viral tests that detect viral nucleic acid and protein antigens, and serological tests that detect anti-SARS-CoV-2 immunoglobulins [8]. The viral nucleic acid and antigen detection tests are used to assess the early stages of active infection, while the antibody tests provide evidence of the previous infection (recovery phase) [9].

Real-time reverse transcription-polymerase chain reaction (RT-PCR) targeting the SARS-CoV-2 RNA is the reference standard diagnostic test for COVID-19. The method is based on the reverse transcription of the viral RNA into complementary DNA (cDNA), followed by isothermally amplifying the specific regions of cDNA and detection by quantitative RT-PCR [10,11]. Although the RT-PCR test has high true positive and true negative detection rates, it is laborious, which leads to a long turn-around time from sample collection to test results. The lengthy RNA isolation steps (which takes approximately 2–4 h) requires highly trained manpower. RT-PCR testing becomes challenging if there are reagent shortages and a large number of samples. PCR tests are therefore not suitable for remote or resource-limited settings. Moreover, false negatives may arise if the sample is collected before the onset of symptoms or due to inadvertent contamination of reagent or specimen [12–14].

To address these limitations, rapid diagnostic tests based on antigen or antibody detection in respiratory samples (e.g., sputum, saliva, throat swab) or blood can provide timely detection at or near the point of care (POC) without the need for sophisticated laboratory facilities. These rapid tests have numerous benefits over the laboratory test, including rapidity of results (within 30 min), lower cost, easy to operate and suitable for large-scale screening outside the laboratory without the need for specialist operators [15–17]. Rapid antigen test is useful for early detection of active infection with a high viral load of SARS-CoV-2. The viral antigen usually appears within a few days after the onset of symptoms before the production of antibodies. A rapid antibody test is more suitable during the convalescent phase of the disease. The prevalence of antibodies in the human blood serum of individuals suspected of being infected with SARS-CoV-2 may take several days or weeks to develop after exposure to the virus. Immunoglobulin M (IgM) will be produced after three to six days of infection and immunoglobulin G (IgG) will be detectable after eight days of infection [18,19]. The Board Decision on Additional Support for Country Responses to COVID-19 has approved 47 and 48 types of rapid SARS-CoV-2 antibody and antigen diagnostic tests, respectively, for home use [20]. However, although these rapid POC tests have high true negative rates, the true positive rates are lower than the RT-PCR test [15,21,22]. The WHO acceptable minimum true positive and true negative rates are 80% and 97%, respectively [23].

Biosensors, which satisfy the WHO's ASSURED criteria: Affordable, Sensitive, Specific, User-friendly, Rapid and Robust, Equipment-free, and Deliverable to end-users [24–26], are potential alternatives to the rapid POC antigen and antibody tests. A biosensor is an analytical device consisting of a biological element (e.g., nucleic acids, enzymes, antibodies, whole cells, or receptors) combined with a transducer for the detection of an analyte. The biological element binds the analyte of interest to the biosensor, and the transducer measures the interaction between the analyte and recognition element and converts the output to a measurable signal proportional to the analyte concentration [27–30]. With the integration of a suitable microfluidic platform and necessary mechanical enclosure, a biosensor can be translated into a POC system, where the sample collection and testing can be performed in the same device [31].

A variety of biosensors have been developed for real-time diagnostic of COVID-19, including surface plasmon resonance (SPR)-based biosensors, electrochemical biosensors and field-effect transistor (FET)-based biosensors. These biosensors have been successfully tested in proof-of-concept studies. However, none of the sensors have been translated into a POC device for commercial use yet. In this paper, we review the most recently developed SPR-based, electrochemical, and FET-based biosensors for SARS-CoV-2 detection. We explain how these sensors work, and discuss their advantages and limitations. Finally, we propose strategies to enhance the sensing performance of these biosensors to meet the WHO minimum requirement for true positive and negative detection rates.

2. Latest Developed Biosensors for COVID-19

Compared to time staking laboratory tests, a biosensor with fast response and high accuracy in the form of a point-of-care device would be an excellent aid for the early diagnosis of SARS-CoV-2 infection. As shown in Figure 1A, generally a biosensor comprises of biosensing elements such as nucleic acids, enzymes, or antibodies that can interact with the target analyte in the form of biological or chemical sample, a transducer that can convert the changes in the biosensing element to an electrical signal, and an amplifier and necessary electronic system to process the electrical signal to digitise the output [27,32]. The COVID-19 outbreak has spurred the development of various types of biosensors with different biosensing platforms that can be used for the diagnosis of COVID-19.

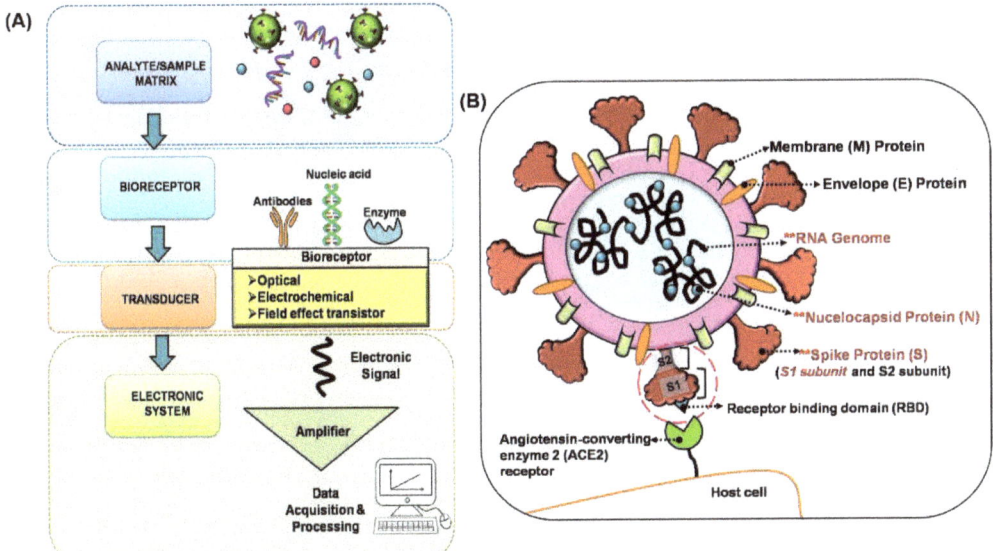

Figure 1. (**A**) Schematic diagram of a biosensor. (**B**) Structure and function of SARS-CoV-2 virus. The main four viral surface proteins are Spike (S), Envelope (E), Membrane (M) and nucleocapsid (N). S protein contains the receptor-binding domain (RBD) that recognises the host cell receptor, i.e., the human angiotensin-converting enzyme 2 (ACE2). E protein contributes to the assembly and morphogenesis of virions. M protein, which is embedded in a lipid bilayer, is responsible for the release of nutrients at the transmembrane and form the viral envelope. N protein binds to the RNA genome to form the nucleocapsid. **Preferred target analyte used for current COVID-19 biosensor development.

SARS-CoV-2 contains four structural proteins, spike (S), membrane (M), envelope (E) and nucleocapsid (N) proteins, as shown in Figure 1B. The S protein is composed of two subunits S1 and S2, which are responsible for the attachment, fusion and entry of the virus. The S1 subunit contains a receptor-binding domain (RBD) that recognises host cell receptors and human angiotensin-converting enzyme 2 (ACE2). The S2 subunit facilitates membrane fusion for virus entry. N proteins bind to the viral RNA genome to form the nucleocapsid. M proteins release nutrients at the transmembrane and form the viral envelope. E proteins are small polypeptides that are responsible for the assembly and release of the virus. The SARS-CoV-2 viral RNA genome consists of open reading frames (ORFs) genes, which encode a total of 16 non–structural proteins (e.g., ORF1ab gene), and at least four structural proteins (e.g., S gene, E gene, M gene, N gene) [33,34]. For SARS-CoV-2 detection, three types of diagnostic tests—on nasopharyngeal swab, throat swab, blood and saliva samples—have been widely used based on (i) virus detection—hybridisation between sequence complementary (capture probe) to the target RNA genome, (ii) antigen protein detection—interaction of monoclonal antigen-specific antibody and virus antigen protein and (iii) antibody detection—interaction of recombinant antigen and target neutralising antibody. As described in the following sections, the current development of biosensors employs these approaches to target SARS-CoV-2 RNA genome (ORF1ab gene, RNA-dependent RNA polymerase (RdRP) gene, S gene, N gene) [35–38], specific antigen protein (S protein (S1 subunit/RBD), N protein) [39–42] and neutralising antibody (IgM, IgG) [35,43].

2.1. Methodology Used in Review Process

We followed the Preferred Reporting Items for Systematic Review and Meta-Analysis (PRISMA) guidelines for the review process. We searched the Web of Science and LENS. ORG databases using these keywords: COVID-19, SARS-CoV-2 and Biosensor, for articles dated from 1 January 2020 to 17 May 2021. A total of 439 articles were retrieved from this comprehensive search. Removal of duplicate and non-journal articles reduced the total to 297 articles. Subsequent screening excluded 143 review articles. Further exclusion of articles not related to three well-established biosensors: surface plasmon resonance, electrochemical and field-effect transistor-based sensors, reduced the total to 15 articles. We require at least experimental proof of concept of SARS-CoV-2 detection for the SPR-based, electrochemical and FET-based biosensors; therefore, we did not further exclude articles that did not report the validation of the sensors in the lab, i.e., report true positive and negative detection rates.

In the following sections, we explain how the three biosensors work and discuss their advantages and limitations. Table 1 presents the summary of these latest biosensors.

2.2. Surface Plasmon Resonance (SPR)/Localised Surface Plasmon Resonance (LSPR) Biosensor

Surface plasmon resonance (SPR) is a well-known sensing technology used for characterising kinetics of ligand–receptor interactions and these types of sensors offer unique real-time and label-free measurement capabilities with high detection sensitivity [44–46]. Figure 2A shows a typical SPR biosensor configuration where biorecognition elements, such as antibodies, are immobilised on the surface of a thin gold film. Surface plasmons are charge density oscillations that propagate along the metal-dielectric (sensing-medium) interface. They are excited by light (monochromatic) that is incident on the metal through a prism (in the prism coupling method) at a particular incident angle, called the resonance angle. Because some energy of the incident light is absorbed by the surface plasmons, the intensity of the reflected light is reduced at the resonance angle. When a sample in liquid form is allowed to flow across the sensor surface, the target analytes in the sample are captured by the immobilised biorecognition elements resulting in a change in the refractive index (RI) of the sensing medium, which shifts the resonance angle, as depicted in Figure 2B. This shift is proportional to the change in analyte mass on the gold film. In SPR imaging (SPRi), the reflected light is imaged using a charge-coupled device (CCD) [47,48]. In another type of SPR configuration known as localised SPR (LSPR), where the thin gold film is replaced by metallic nanoparticles, light incident on the nanoparticles excites coherent oscillations of the electron cloud around each particle, which is called a localised surface plasmon (LSP). Resonance occurs when the frequency of the light matches the LSP oscillation frequency. The analyte detection method is similar to conventional SPR [49,50].

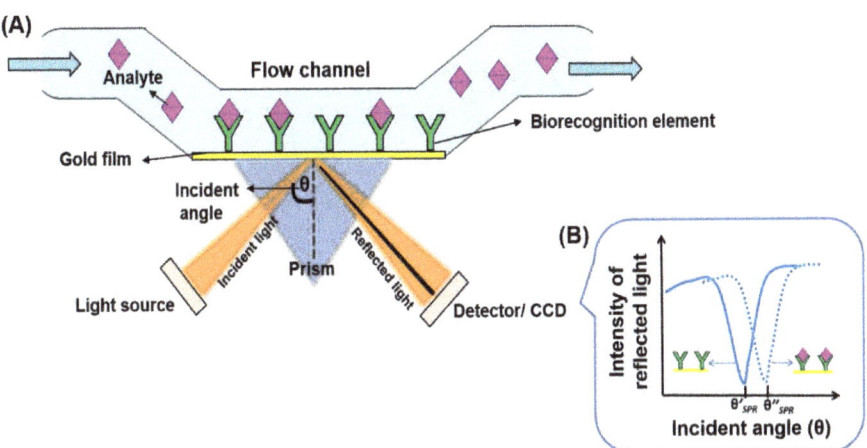

Figure 2. (**A**) Typical Surface Plasmon Resonance (SPR) configuration, (**B**) Resonance angle after antibody immobilisation on sensor surface (θ'_{SPR}) and after analytes bind with immobilised antibodies (θ''_{SPR}). The resonance angle shift is $\theta''_{SPR} - \theta'_{SPR}$.

2.2.1. SPR/LSPR Biosensor for COVID-19

SPR and LSPR technologies have been explored for detecting the SARS-CoV-2 virus. Recent reports on these types of sensors show promising sensitivity with fast and reliable detection. In one of the recent works, a two-dimensional heterostructure, $PtSe_2$/Graphene, was attached to the gold film of the SPR sensor—the sensor configuration is shown in Figure 3A. The sensing region comprises three different ligand-analyte modes: (i) the monoclonal antibodies (mAbs) as ligand and the SARS-CoV-2 virus spike RBD as analyte, (ii) the virus spike RBD as ligand and the virus anti-spike protein (IgM, IgG) as the analyte and (iii) the specific RNA probe as ligand and the virus single-stranded RNA as analyte [35]. The sensor employed BK_7 type prism glass, which generates stronger surface plasmon waves at the metal-dielectric interface. The hetero-structure ($PtSe_2$/Graphene) provided an increased surface area for better adsorption of the target analyte, and hence enhanced sensitivity of the sensor. Graphene's high conductivity, large surface area and chemical stability improved interaction between the target analyte and the ligand [51]. It was observed that the sensitivity tend to increase by $(1 + 0.55) \times L$ times for an increase of L number of graphene layers [35]. Using multiple graphene layers is promising in detecting different analytes such as virus spike RBD, antibodies (IgG or IgM) and viral RNA with a detection sensitivity of 183.33° RIU^{-1}, 153.85° RIU^{-1} and 140.35° RIU^{-1} in SPR angle, respectively.

SPRi-based biosensors for detecting SARS-CoV-2 have also been developed. These sensors follow the principles of SPR and have been utilised to study binding kinetics between biomolecular species in the past [52–54]. SPRi assay was used for quantitative measurement of IgG, IgM and IgA antibodies binding to the RBD spike protein in serum sample [43]. RBD is an ideal target for blocking and neutralisation therapies. This is because viral infection occurs when the S protein on SARS-CoV-2 recognises and binds to the ACE2 receptor on the human host cell through its RBD [55]. Hence, this assay is ideally suited for monitoring the concentration of anti-RBD antibodies of both COVID-19 patients and healthy people who are vaccinated against SARS-CoV-2.

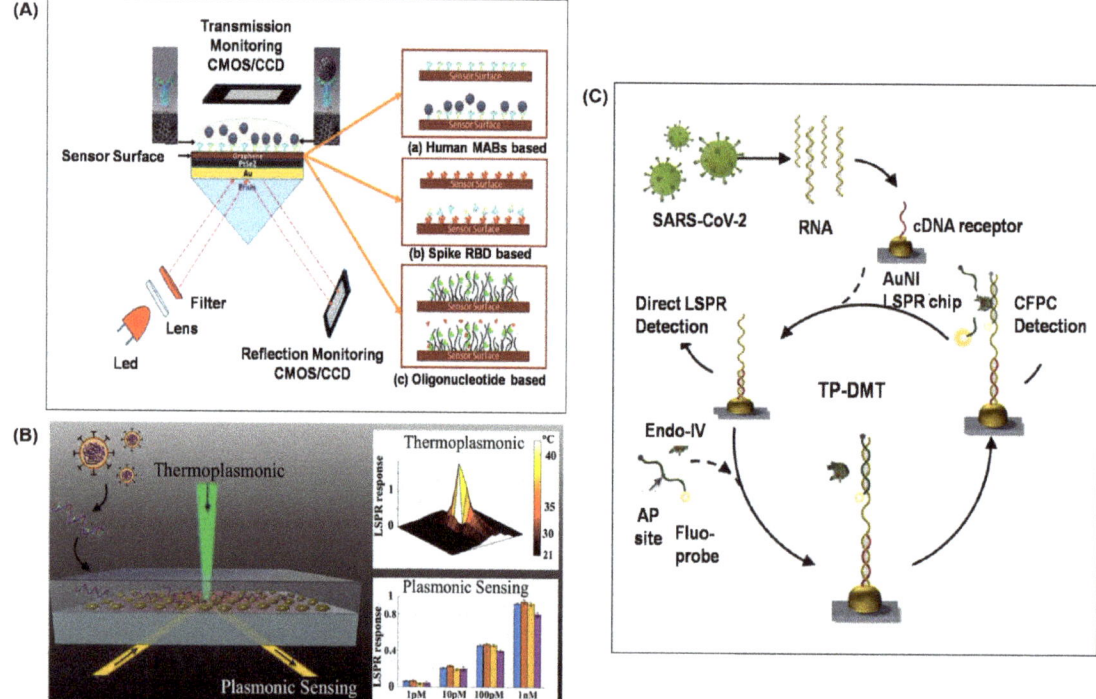

Figure 3. SPR and LSPR biosensor for SARS-CoV-2 detection. (**A**) Graphene-based multiple-layer coated (Bk$_7$/Au/PtSe$_2$/Graphene) SPR biosensor. Reprinted with permission from [35]. (**B**) Dual-functional PPT enhanced LSPR biosensing system. Reprinted with permission from [37]. Copyright 2020, American Chemical Society. (**C**) Thermoplasmonic-assisted dual-mode transducing (TP-DMT) biosensing system. Reprinted with permission from [38]. Copyright 2021, American Chemical Society.

Qiu and co-workers [37,38] demonstrated photothermal-assisted plasmonic sensing (PTAPS) for SARS-CoV-2 detection. Their biosensing device, as shown in Figure 3B, utilises LSPR for the detection of unamplified SARS-CoV-2 [37]. Two-dimensional gold nano-islands (AuNI) played the roles of nanoabsorber, nanoheater and nanotransducer. In this dual-functional system, AuNI functionalised with cDNA receptors were used to detect SARS-CoV-2 RNA through nucleic acid hybridisation. The entire AuNI sensing surface functionalised with a sufficient amount of thiol-cDNA receptor increased sensitivity and inhibit non-specific binding. Non-radiative decay of the resonantly-excited LSPs produces heat that is localised near the AuNI [56]. This plasmonic photothermal (PPT) effect aids the in-situ hybridisation of the RdRp-COVID sequence and its cDNA for SARS-CoV-2 detection. With the use of localised PPT heating, false positive is minimised as the imperfectly matched sequences have difficulty remaining attached to the probe. This LSPR sensor has a detection limit of 0.22 ± 0.08 pM but is highly specific in discriminating the SARS-CoV-2 sequence from similar RdRp-SARS sequence.

Qiu et al. [38] extended the previous PTAPS method by introducing a novel concept of thermoplasmonic-assisted dual-mode transducing (TP-DMT), as shown in Figure 3C. This dual-mode system combines (1) an amplification-free direct viral RNA detection and (2) an amplification-based cyclic fluorescence probe cleavage (CFPC) detection to provide self-validating biosensing readout for quantifying the SARS-CoV-2 sequences within 30 min. The first LSPR signal was based on the hybridisation between the target viral sequences and the functionalised thiol-DNA receptors. The amount of captured sequence is directly proportional to the virus concentration in the sample, and the limit of detection (LOD) was as low as 0.1 ± 0.04 pM. In the CFPC detection, endonuclease IV (site-specific nuclease) was utilised to cleave the apurinic/apyrimidinic (AP)-site modified fluorescent probe from the target viral sequence under local PPT heating. The released fluorescent probe was used to quantify the concentration of the virus, which improved the LOD to 0.275 ± 0.051 femtomolar (fM). This dual-mode sensing method employed two interdependent yet different tests on the AuNI chip, and provides two sensitive readouts of viral sequence to yield remarkably low limits of detection in pM and fM, respectively. When the final readout of the direct viral hybridisation detection exhibited a weak response, the CFPC method was used for verification and it could even detect a trace amount of virus in the sample.

2.2.2. Advantages and Limitations

The SPR-based biosensors we have reviewed for SARS-CoV-2 detection have good sensitivity and reusability. However, they lack selectivity and the refractive index of the biosensors are also affected by temperature, non-specific or specific adsorption on the sensor surface, and changes in buffer concentrations [57]. Hence, the sensor surface needs to be modified with a ligand (e.g., antibody, DNA probe) to selectively capture the target analyte.

On the other hand, SPR-based biosensors allow the integration of nanostructures or nanoparticles to enhance the detection sensitivity [58,59]. The extent of improvement depends strongly on the shape of the nanostructure and the type of metal used [49,59,60]. As mentioned in the previous section, two-dimensional heterostructure [35] and AuNIs [37,38] attached to the gold film in the sensor exhibited maximum sensitivity of $200°$ RIU^{-1} and detection of sample analytes at an ultra-low concentration in the range of pM and fM, respectively. SPR-based sensors allow the tailoring of the sensing medium to improve sensor performance and sensitivity by using multi-layers for the medium or altering the medium thickness [61,62].

However, plasmonic virus detection from clinical specimens is still limited due to surface fouling of the receptor surface and interference of non-specific bindings. Surface fouling limits the application of plasmonic biosensors by blocking recognition element immobilisation and specific binding [63]. It can be prevented by selecting the appropriate sample dilution ratio or the design of ultra-low fouling surfaces with anti-fouling strategies using polymer-based surface chemistry or zwitterionic technology [64,65].

Biosensors with good reusability are highly desirable because it lowers the cost per test. The solvent environment is a key parameter that determines the binding of antibody-antigen. The reversible non-covalent interaction between antibody and antigen can be disrupted by high salt concentration, extreme pH and detergents [66]. Hence, chemical regeneration is the most widely used approach to regenerate the sensor by chemically altering the solvent environment with a regeneration solution (e.g., acid/base, detergent, glycine or urea). SPR sensor could be chemically regenerated for SARS-CoV-2 detection [67].

2.3. Electrochemical Biosensor

Electrochemical biosensors are known for their small size, cost-effectiveness, ease of use and fast response. These types of sensors are extensively used in the development of point of care devices for diagnosing viral infections [68,69]. Among the electrochemical techniques, screen-printed electrode (SPE) technology has aided the development of portable sensors considerably as it provides miniaturised but robust and user-friendly electrodes at low production costs [70,71]. Figure 4 shows a typical configuration of an SPE-based electrochemical sensor employing a three-electrode system: a reference electrode, a counter electrode and a working electrode transduction element for biochemical reaction. The working electrode surface of SPE can be easily modified to immobilise specific biorecognition elements, such as an antibody to target the analyte. The antibody-antigen interaction on the electrode surface is transduced into a measurable electrical quantity.

Alternatively, the catalytic reaction of a signal probe (e.g., enzyme), which labels the detection antibody, forms an electroactive product that releases electrons, which are transduced as a measurable electrochemical signal. The electrochemical measurement can be one of the following: (1) potentiometric-based, (2) amperometric-based, (3) conductometric or impedimetric-based [72,73] to determine the concentration of analyte in a sample. The SPE-based sensor can be integrated with a portable instrument (e.g., potentiostat) or reader (e.g., computer or a smartphone) [74] for digital processing.

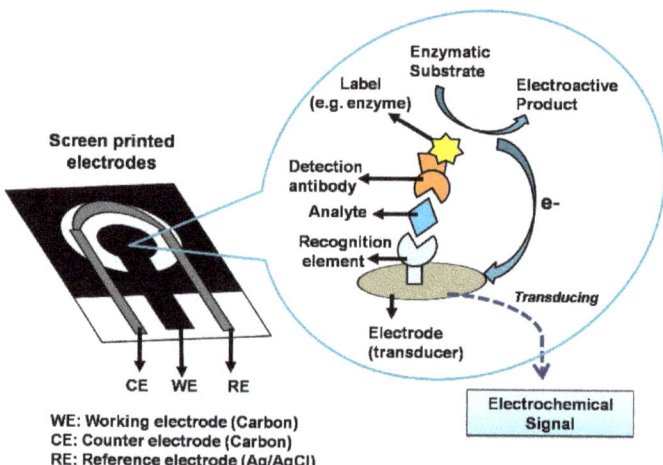

Figure 4. Screen-printed-electrode based electrochemical biosensor. Typical interactions on the working electrode among the biorecognition element, target analyte and detection antibody labelled with an enzyme. As shown, the enzyme oxidises an enzymatic substrate to produce an electroactive product that releases electrons, which are transduced as a measurable electrochemical signal.

Compared to conventional electrode materials (e.g., glassy carbon or carbon paste electrodes), SPEs have the advantage of cost, disposability, size and do not require electrode polishing prior to electrochemical detection. Because of its compact size, SPE only requires a small reagent volume for assay, as low as a few μL. This makes the SPE-based electrochemical biosensor a potential tool for on-site measurement in remote regions with limited resources. Moreover, the electroanalytical performance and sensitivity of the sensor can be enhanced by modifying the SPE working electrode surface with nanomaterials such as gold nanoparticles, graphene and carbon nanotubes to increase the electroactive area of the electrode for further immobilisation of biomolecules such as antibodies, protein or nucleic acid [75–77]. Graphene are two-dimensional carbon nanomaterials, in which the carbon atoms are positioned in a hexagonal honeycomb lattice [78], whereas carbon nanotubes are an allotropic form of carbon that can be rolled up into cylindrical tubes (e.g., single-walled or multi-walled) [79]. They possess characteristic properties of large surface area and excellent electrical conductivity. Hence, they are used as an electro modifier to promote electron transfer between a target analyte and electrode and thereby achieve high detection sensitivity [80,81].

2.3.1. Electrochemical Biosensor for COVID-19

Rural communities bear a higher burden from the COVID-19 outbreak due to limited healthcare resources. The RT-PCR diagnostic method is costly and complicated in procedures, which makes it unsuitable for the low-resource area. Disposable electrochemical biosensors based on SPEs are promising alternatives for rapid, affordable, direct detection of SARS-CoV-2 at the point of care.

Figure 5A shows a recent graphene-based SPE sensor, which is functionalised with a monoclonal anti-spike antibody for detecting SARS-CoV-2 spike antigen. The sensor detected spike protein in a saliva sample, by using square wave voltammetry (SWV) to measure the change of the ferri/ferrocyanide signal, in about 45 min. The ferri/ferrocyanide couple was used as a redox probe and the electrochemical detection was achieved by measuring the peak current of the ferro/ferricyanide redox after the biomolecular binding event on the sensing surface. The peak current is reduced because the target analyte prevented the redox probe from contacting the conductive surface [82]. The LOD of this sensor for spike protein was 20 µg mL^{-1}. However, its sensitivity is lower compared to laboratory ELISA tests, which can detect as low as 3 ng mL^{-1} [39].

In another approach, magnetic beads (MBs)-based immunoassay is coupled with electrochemical detection for viral RNA and antigen detection with high sensitivity. MBs have the potential to reduce the incubation time from hours to minutes and is easily separated from a complex matrix under the action of an external magnetic field; therefore non-specific adsorption is almost negligible [83,84]. Fabiani et al. presented an electrochemical biosensor by combining MBs-based immunoassay and SPE, modified with carbon black, with a portable potentiostat as a reader for SARS-CoV-2 detection in saliva (Figure 5B) [40]. In the MBs-based immunoassay, target protein (S or N protein) in the untreated saliva sample was selectivity captured by the respective monoclonal antibody–bound MB and sandwiched by the respective polyclonal antibody. A secondary antibody attached to the polyclonal antibody is labelled with an alkaline phosphate enzyme. In the electrochemical detection, the labelled beads were drop cast on the working electrode of SPE with 1-naphthyl phosphate to induce the formation of enzymatic by-product 1-napthol. The enzymatic reaction (enzymatic by-product) was electrochemically measured via differential pulse voltammetry (DPV) using a portable potentiostat. The sensor was tested using 24 clinical samples (positive and negative); the true positive rate was 100% and the true negative rate was 88.2% for detecting the S protein. The sensor required 30 min for reaction and exhibited the lowest detection limit of 19 ng mL^{-1} for S proteins and 8 ng mL^{-1} for N proteins, respectively. However, repeated incubation and washing steps are required to perform the MBs-based immunoassay prior to the electrochemical detection.

Chaibun et al. developed an ultrasensitive electrochemical biosensor (as shown in Figure 5C) based on multiplex isothermal rolling circle amplification (RCA) for rapid detection of viral N and S genes of SARS-CoV-2 [36]. The sensor works on a one-step strategy comprised of mixing capture probe-conjugated magnetic bead particle (CP-MBs), silica reporter probe (silica nanoparticles coated redox dye), and the target (viral N and S genes) in a single hybridisation step, followed by a single washing step. The sandwich hybridisation of RCA amplicons with probes that are functionalised with redox-active labels (e.g., methylene blue for N gene and acridine orange for S gene) was detected by DPV. The redox-active reaction could detect as low as 1 copy µL^{-1} of viral N or S genes in less than 2 hours. Moreover, the use of magnetic capture and separation of targets from non-targets reduces the chance of residual contamination and pipetting error, thereby reducing the risk of erroneous results and improving the assay precision [85]. The potentiostat is a key component for reading electrochemical signals, but the traditionally large and expensive bench-top versions limit its use in resource-limited environments. Hence, a portable potentiostat was developed and used, in conjunction with a computer, for electrochemical measurement at the point of use.

The smartphone is the most widely used portable device in the world. It is equipped with powerful connectivity features and researchers have explored the use of smartphones as a wireless diagnostic tool [74,86]. A portable potentiostat with wireless connectivity to a smartphone would facilitate electrochemical analysis at the point-of-use, where access to a computer or wired connection to a device is difficult or impossible [87]. A smartphone-based supersandwich-type electrochemical biosensor was demonstrated as shown in Figure 5D for SARS-CoV-2 RNA detection without nucleic acid amplification and reverse-transcription [88]. The assay employed for sensing utilised two different kinds of primer A and B. The former contains Au@Fe$_3$O$_4$ nanocomposites, the capture probe (CP) and 1 mM hexane-1-thiol (HT). The latter contains Au@p-sulfocalix[8]arene(SCX8)-toluidineblue(TB)-graphene(RGO) nanocomposites, the labelled probe (LP) and the auxiliary probe (AP). Primer A and then B are mixed with the target for 1 h and 2 h, respectively. Subsequently, the sandwich structure formed was dropped on the SPE for electrochemical measurement of TB signal by a smartphone in less than 10 s. TB is a basic thiazine metachromatic dye with a high affinity for nucleic acids, thereby staining tissues with a high DNA and RNA content [89]. This method requires a long incubation time of about 3 h for the formation of sandwich structure and more than 12 h for the preparation of primer A and B. For detection of SARS-CoV-2 in clinical specimens, the true positive rate was 85.5% and 46.2% for confirmed and recovered patients, respectively. The sensor does not require RNA amplification and it only requires two copies of SARS-CoV-2 for an assay, which is advantageous compared to the existing PCR-based RNA assay. The detection limit of the tested samples was found to be 200 copies mL^{-1}.

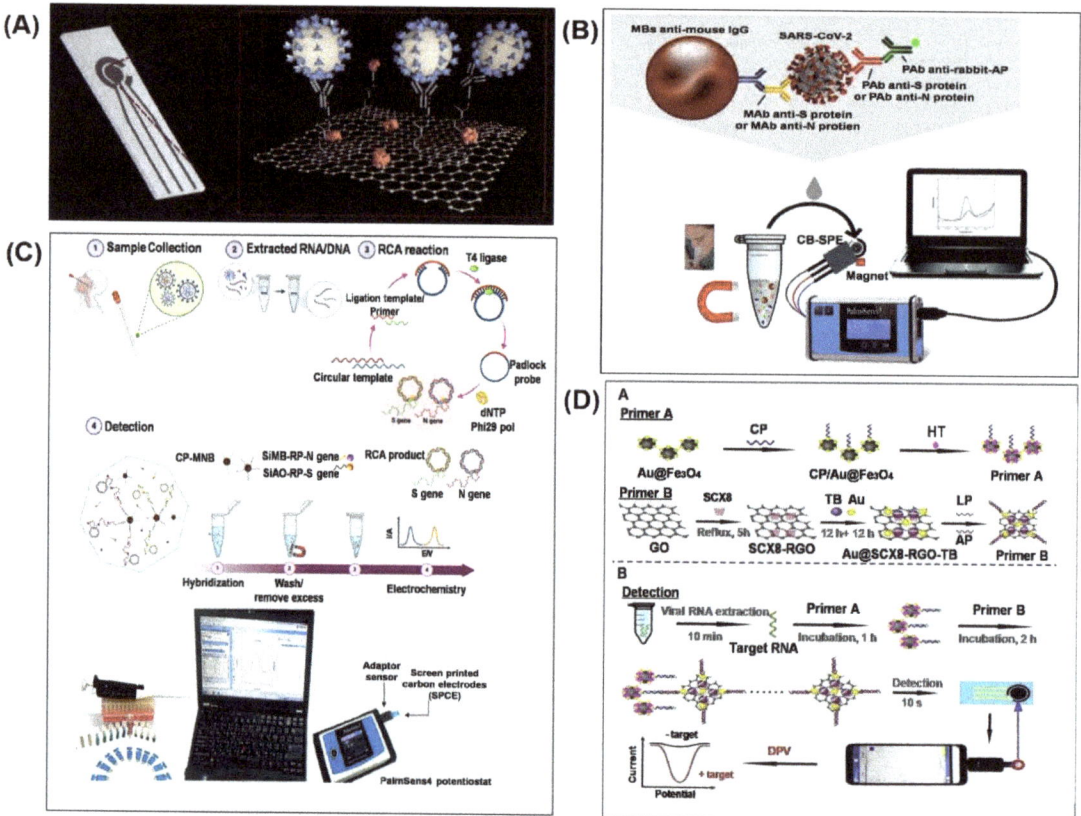

Figure 5. Electrochemical biosensor for SARS-CoV-2 detection. (**A**) Graphene-based electrochemical biosensor. Reprinted with permission from [39]. (**B**) MBs-based electrochemical biosensor. Reprinted with permission from [40]. Copyright 2020, Elsevier B.V. (**C**) Electrochemical biosensor with RCA of the N and S genes. Reprinted with permission from Lertanantawong, B (2021). Copyright 2021 Springer. (**D**) Smartphone-based supersandwich-type electrochemical biosensor. Reprinted with permission from [88]. Copyright 2021, Elsevier B.V.

A few other recently reported works utilised modified screen-printed electrodes with nanostructured materials, as depicted in Figure 6A, to enhance the detection of SARS-CoV-2 spike protein and glycoprotein. In [90], an electrochemical biosensor was fabricated using disposable carbon-based SPE, where the electrode surface was modified with Cu_2O nanocubes. IgG anti-SARS-CoV-2 was attached to staphylococcal protein A (Prot A) that was loaded on the surface (Figure 6B). The larger surface area of the nanocubes provided more active sites to bind IgG and hence allowed more SARS-CoV-2 to be detected. The biosensor exhibited a LOD of 0.04 fg mL^{-1}, and it was 100% successful in detecting true positive and negative samples, based on 16 clinical samples. In [91], the carbon electrode surface was modified with carbon nanofibers (CNF), followed by immobilisation of N protein and antibody for N protein, as depicted in Figure 6C. The CNF not only increased the surface area for more active sites for binding but also allowed a direct collection of nasal samples. The LOD of the sensor was 0.8 pg mL^{-1} for SARS-CoV-2 N protein antigen. In [92], the SPE surface was modified with graphene oxide and gold nanostars, and S spike glycoproteins were used to detect SARS-CoV-2 (Figure 6D). Based on 100 clinical samples, the LOD was 1.68×10^{-22} µg mL^{-1} and the true positive and negative rate was 95% and 60%, respectively.

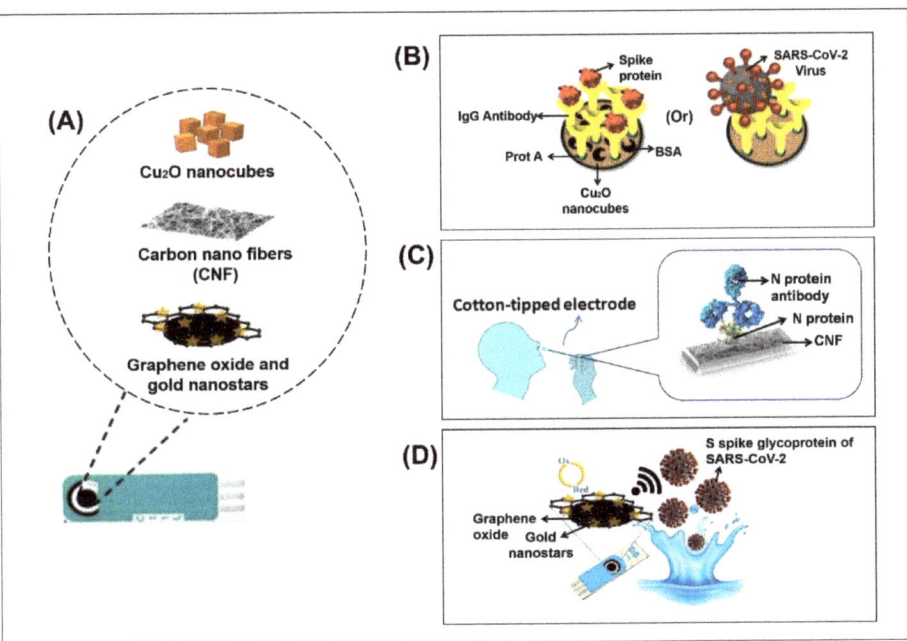

Figure 6. (**A**) Surface modification of screen printed electrodes with nanostructured materials (**B**) Electrochemical immunosensor with Cu_2O nanocube coating for the detection of SARS-CoV-2 spike proteins. Bovine Serum Albumin (BSA) is used as a blocking agent. Reprinted with permission from Roushani, M (2021). Copyright 2021 Springer. (**C**) Cotton-tipped electrochemical immunosensor for the detection of virus nucleocapsid (N) protein. Reprinted with permission [91]. Copyright 2021, American Chemical Society. (**D**) Electrochemical diagnostic kit for the detection of SARS-CoV-2 S spike glycoproteins. Glycoproteins can be traced through the oxidation signals of gold nanostars, which are deposited on the surface of the modified electrode. Reprinted with permission [92]. Copyright 2021, Elsevier B.V.

2.3.2. Advantages and Limitations

The reviewed electrochemical sensors based on SPEs for SARS-CoV-2 detection show excellent portability, with true positive rates ranging between 46.2% and 100%. Typically, commercially available SPEs were used as they are easy to use and disposable. The most commonly used material for the assembly of the working electrode of SPE is carbon, gold and platinum ink. SPEs modified with a range of nanoparticles or nanomaterials are also commercially available. The modification of the sensing surface with a large active surface area (e.g., gold nanoparticles, graphene, carbon nanotubes) increases the number of immobilised biorecognition elements and thus the number of available analyte binding sites, which increases the detection sensitivity of the biosensor. Compared to conventional glassy carbon or carbon paste electrodes, SPEs do not require electrode polishing and electrochemical pre-treatment by electro-deposition. Furthermore, potentiostats are already available in miniaturised formats, which enable on-the-spot or point-of-care applications.

At present, saliva tests offer a promising alternative to nasopharyngeal swabs for COVID-19 diagnosis, since collecting saliva is non-invasive and easy to self-administer [93,94]. However, differences in the sample collection methods—such as cough out (without sputum), split (exclude bubbles) or drooling—can affect the salivary composition and sensitivity to SARS-CoV-2. Consequently, the matrix effect may result in an inaccurate measurement for viscous saliva without any pre-treatment (e.g., dilution with phosphate buffer). However, high dilution of saliva samples with low viral content may lead to a false-negative result. Recently, spike protein detection in saliva samples using an electrochemical biosensor was proposed in [39,40]. It was suggested in [40] that using fresh saliva sampled after drinking a glass of water obviates the need for sample pre-treatment.

2.4. Field Effect Transistor (FET) Biosensor

As shown in Figure 7A, a typical FET-based biosensor consists of a semiconductor substrate with three terminals: (1) the source, (2) the drain and (3) reference or gate in contact with an electrolyte. The source and drain terminals are attached to the semiconducting substrate and a thin oxide layer (insulator) is deposited between these two terminals. Generally, biorecognition elements such as antibodies are immobilised on the oxide layer (sensor surface) to complete the biosensor construction. When a bias voltage is applied across the gate, an electric field is generated and charge carriers flow in the semiconductor channel from the source electrode to the drain electrode. The direction of current depends on the type of channel, either p-type or n-type [95]. The target molecules (e.g., protein, nucleic acid) usually carry charges and they will affect the current when they are bound to the recognition elements immobilised on the sensor surface. The current can thus be monitored as a function of time to detect the target molecules. For the p-type channel, negatively charged target molecules captured by the biorecognition elements accumulate positive charge carriers (holes) in the channel, which increases the current as depicted in Figure 7(Bi). Conversely, if positively charged target molecules bind with the biorecognition elements, the holes are depleted and the current is decreased as depicted in Figure 7(Bii). Different types of nanomaterials can be deposited on the sensor surface, such as silicon nanowires [96,97], carbon nanotubes [98–100] and graphene [42,101–103], for detecting a variety of biological analytes such as proteins, nucleic acids, ions and small molecules, respectively.

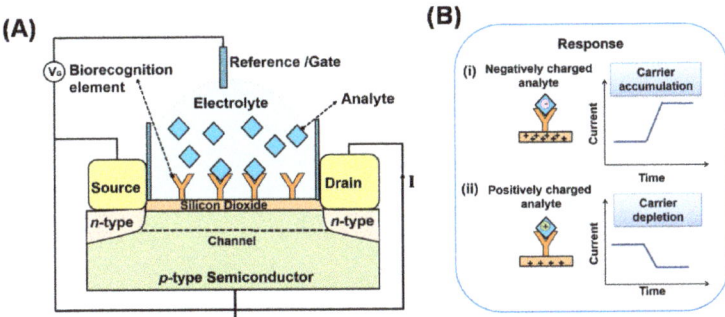

Figure 7. (**A**) Field-effect transistor (FET)-based biosensor with a *p*-type semiconductor channel. (**B**) (**i**) Negatively charged target molecules captured by the biorecognition elements accumulate positive charge carriers (holes) in the channel, which increases the current from the source to the drain electrode. (**ii**) If positively charged target molecules bind with the biorecognition elements, the holes are depleted and the current decreases.

2.4.1. FET Biosensor for COVID-19

Attachment of carbon-based two-dimensional materials and nanotubes (CNTs) on the surface of FET biosensors have been explored to enhance the detection of the target analyte. CNTs and graphene-based FETs have shown high sensitivity in detecting small concentrations of target analyte [104,105].

Recently, a FET biosensor was developed by depositing SARS-CoV-2 spike protein and anti-nucleocapsid protein antibodies functionalised single-walled carbon nanotube (SWCNT) on the sensor surface to detect complimentary SARS-CoV-2 antigens (Figure 8A) [99]. Based on 28 positive samples, the SWCNT-based FET biosensor exhibited a true positive rate of 82.1% and 53.6% for detecting spike protein and nucleocapsid protein, respectively. Based on 10 negative samples, the true negative rate was 70% for both proteins. Overall, the SWCNT-based FET sensor exhibited excellent sensitivity with a LOD of 0.55 fg mL^{-1} and 0.016 fg mL^{-1} in detecting spike protein and nucleocapsid protein, respectively [99]. The sensor has the potential to be used as a rapid SARS-CoV-2 antigen test using clinical nasopharyngeal samples, without pre-processing, in less than 5 min.

In another approach, SARS-CoV-2 spike protein antibodies were functionalised on graphene sheets, which were then deposited on the sensor surface. This graphene-based FET biosensor is depicted in Figure 8B. The sensor was able to detect the SARS-CoV-2 spike antigen protein down to fg mL^{-1} in phosphate-buffered saline samples or clinical transport medium and with a LOD of 2.42×10^2 copies mL^{-1} in clinical samples, at a response rate between 0 and 400 s [42].

However, for viral detection of SARS-CoV-2, the RNA probe is required to detect the presence of complementary nucleic acid sequences (target sequences). To fulfil this need, recently a liquid gated CNT network FET was fabricated on a flexible Kapton film [100], as shown in Figure 8C. The sensor was able to selectively detect a portion of the SARS-CoV-2 RNA through hybridisation. Here, the reverse sequence of the RNA-dependent RNA polymerase gene of SARS-CoV-2 was immobilised onto the CNT sidewalls. The RNA hybridisation was used as the primary signal generator and the liquid gated CNT network FET was used as the signal transducer. The biosensor showed a selective sensing response to the target sequence with a LOD of 10 fM.

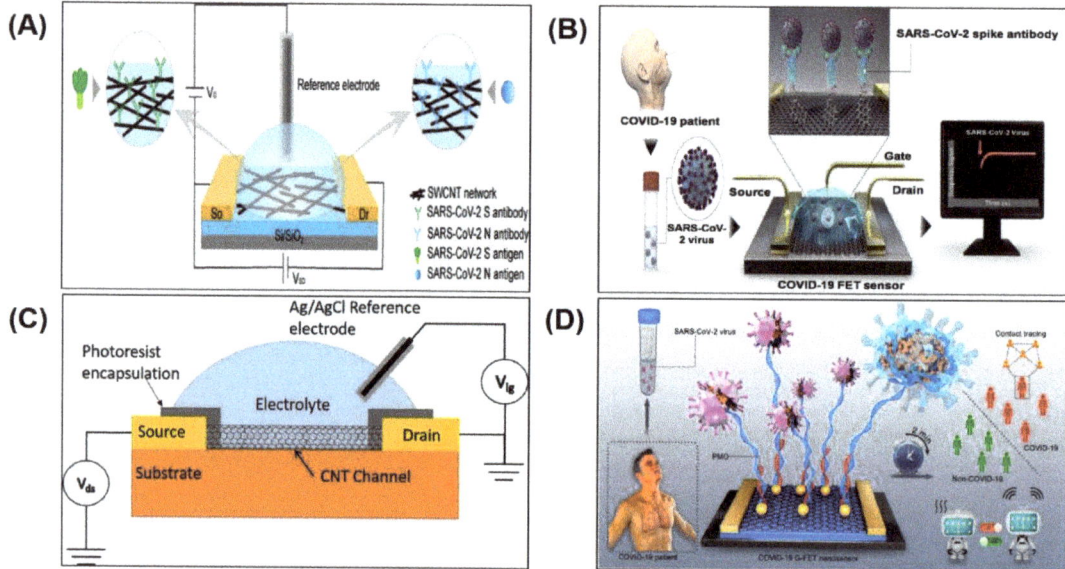

Figure 8. Field-effect transistor biosensor for COVID-19 detection. (**A**) SWCNT-based FET biosensor. Reprinted with permission from [42]. Copyright 2020, American Chemical Society. (**B**) Graphene-based FET biosensor. Reprinted with permission from [99]. Copyright 2021, American Chemical Society. (**C**) CNT-based FET fabricated on a flexible Kapton substrate. Reprinted with permission from [100]. Copyright 2021, Elsevier Ltd. (**D**) PMO-functionalised Graphene-FET biosensor. Reprinted with permission from [106]. Copyright 2021, Elsevier B.V.

In another remarkable FET biosensor, gold nanoparticles (AuNP) decorated graphene sheets and phosphorodiamidate morpholino oligos (PMO) probes were employed on the sensor surface for ultrasensitive and rapid SARS-CoV-2 detection (Figure 8D) [106]. The PMO probe is usually 25 bases in length, and they bind to complementary sequences of RNA or single-stranded DNA according to standard nucleic acid base-pairing [107]. The PMO enabled direct detection of SARS-CoV-2 RNA through the hybridisation between the PMO probe and SARS-CoV-2 RdRp without the need for further PCR amplification. For clinical readiness, an FET biosensor needs to have good reusability [108]. For SARS-CoV-2 RdRp detection, this sensor can be chemically regenerated for reuse by denaturing the PMO-RNA duplex with 8.3 M urea solution for 5 min. The high surface-area-to-volume ratio of AuNP, high conductivity of graphene, and high density of neutral PMO immobilisation provided more responsive testing than using charged oligonucleotide capture probe (e.g., single-stranded DNA probe) [106] for RNA detection. The sensor accuracy was analysed with a receiver operating characteristic (ROC) curve and it achieved an AUC of 0.995.

2.4.2. Advantages and Limitations

Overall, the FET-based sensor provides fast detection and low LOD and does not require additional procedures for labelling during sample preparation. It is low cost, small in size and simple to operate. Nevertheless, the device sensitivity could be further improved, especially at a high concentration of sample analyte as the total number of antibodies anchored on the surface is limited by the small sensor size [109]. Non-specific interaction and screening effect could also diminish response and sensitivity [110]. To prevent non-specific binding, a blocking reagent (e.g., BSA or polyethylene glycol) is required to block the un-reacted active sites, or a covalent coupling (e.g., amide bond) is required to attach the antibody to the sensor [111,112].

The Debye length problem remains an entrenched obstacle [113,114]. A layer of ions in the electrolyte above the sensor surface effectively 'shields' or 'screens' the analytes from the charge carriers in the semiconductor channel. The thickness of this layer is called the Debye length [111]. As shown in Figure 9A, the Debye length under physiological conditions (in 10 mM phosphate buffer saline (PBS) solution) is close to 0.7 nm [115], which is smaller than the size of antibody receptor molecules immobilised on the sensor surface, which are generally 10–15 nm in size [114]. It is difficult to detect analyte-binding that are beyond the Debye length in the physiological environment. There have been attempts to address this problem by using short antibody fragments (e.g., nanobody receptor) or aptamer (Figure 9B), which enable the analyte to bind closer to the sensor surface and achieve a detection limit down to the sub-picomolar range without the loss of selectivity [116].

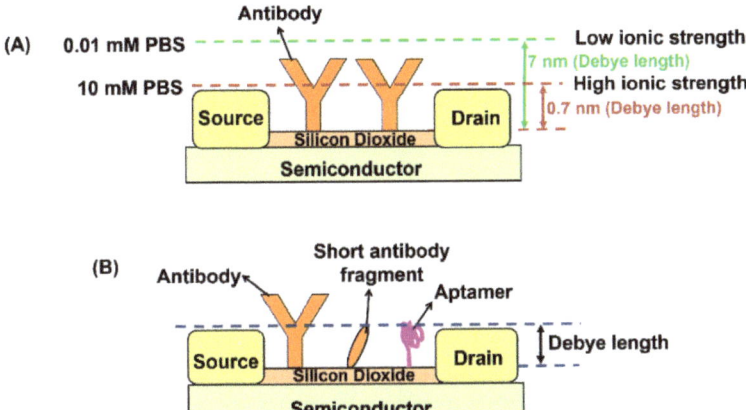

Figure 9. (**A**) The Debye length increases with the reduction of buffer ionic strength. (**B**) Short antibody fragments or aptamers could be used to bring the analyte-binding closer to the sensor surface and within the Debye length.

The Debye length is proportional to the reciprocal of the ionic strength. To increase the Debye length, the electrolyte ionic strength can be lowered by diluting the sample, but this, in turn, dilutes the analyte concentration and may cause a change in protein structure, resulting in the loss of protein activity and binding affinity as well. For example, in [41], the 10 mM PBS buffer was diluted to 0.01 mM, which increased the Debye length from 0.7 nm to 7 nm, comparable to the size of the positive-charged spike protein S1 subunit antibody (7–10 nm). However, dilution makes it difficult to detect low-abundance analytes [117,118].

Table 1. Comparison of the latest developed biosensor: (a) SPR and LSPR, (b) Electrochemical and (c) FET for SARS-CoV-2 detection. In each row, (i), (ii), (iii) represent types of target analyte; 1, 2, 3 represent types of testing sample; [a] represents True Positive Rate (%) and [b] represents True Negative Rate (%).

(a)

Type of Biosensor	Sensing Area & Recognition Element	Target Analyte	Testing Sample	Assay Time	Sensitivity — Limit of Detection (LOD)	Detection Sensitivity (in SPR Angle)	[a] True Positive Rate (%) [b] True Negative Rate (%)	Sample Confirmation Method	Number of Clinical Samples	Ref.
SPR	Graphene-based multiple-layer (BK$_7$/Au/PtSe$_2$/Graphene) modified with specific ligands	(i) Spike RBD (ii) Anti-spike protein (IgG or IgM) (iii) Virus single-stranded RNA	Nasopharyngeal swabs and blood	—	—	(i) 183.3° RIU^{-1} (ii) 153.85° RIU^{-1} (iii) 140.35° RIU^{-1}	—	Not available	Not available	[35]
	Surface Plasmon Resonance imaging (SPRi)	IgG, IgM and IgA	Serum	—	—	—	—	RT-qPCR	384 sera	[43]
LSPR	Gold nanoislands (AuNIs) functionalised with complementary DNA receptor	SARS-CoV-2 sequences	Multigene mixture (RdRp, ORF1ab, and E gene)	—	0.22 ± 0.08 pM	—	—	Not available	Not available	[37]
		SARS-CoV-2 sequences	Nasopharyngeal swabs	30 min	0.1 ± 0.04 pM (Direct viral sequence detection) 0.275 ± 0.051 fM (CFPC detection)	—	—	RT-PCR	8 samples (5 positive and 3 negative samples)	[38]

(b)

Type of Biosensor	Sensing Area & Recognition Element	Target Analyte	Testing Sample	Assay Time	Sensitivity — Limit of Detection (LOD)	[a] True Positive Rate (%) [b] True Negative Rate (%)	Sample Confirmation Method	Number of Clinical Samples	Ref.
Electrochemical	Graphene-based SPE functionalised with a monoclonal anti-spike antibody	Spike protein	Saliva	45 min	20 µg mL^{-1}	—	Not available	Not available	[39]
	Antibodies for S or N proteins immobilised on magnetic beads (MBs)	(i) Spike protein (ii) Nucleocapsid protein	Untreated saliva	30 min	(i) 19 ng mL^{-1} (ii) 8 ng mL^{-1}	[a](i) 100% [b](i) 88.2%	RT-PCR	24 samples (7 positive and 17 negative samples)	[40]
	Sandwich hybridisation of RCA amplicons with probes functionalised with redox-active labels	(i) S gene (ii) N gene	Nasopharyngeal swabs	<2 h	1 copy µL^{-1}	[a](i) 100% [b](i) 100% [a](ii) 100% [b](ii) 100%	qRT-PCR	106 sample (41 positive and 65 negative samples)	[36]
	p-sulfocalix[8]arene functionalised graphene (SCX8-RGO)	SARS-CoV-2 RNA	Throat swabs	<10 s	200 copies mL^{-1}	[a] 85.5% (confirmed patient); 46.2% (recovered patient)	RT-qPCR	88 RNA extracted from 25 SARS-CoV-2-confirmed patients and 8 recovered patients	[88]

Table 1. Cont.

Type of Biosensor	Sensing Area & Recognition Element	Target Analyte	Testing Sample	Assay Time	Sensitivity Limit of Detection (LOD)	[a] True Positive Rate (%) [b] True Negative Rate (%)	Sample Confirmation Method	Number of Clinical Samples	Ref.
	Cu$_2$O nanocubes based SPE immobilised with IgG anti-SARS-CoV-2 spike antibody	Spike protein	1 Nasopharyngeal swabs 2 Saliva	<20 min	0.04 fg mL^{-1}	a (1) 100% b (1) 100% a (2) 100% b (2) 100%	PCR	16 samples (8 positive and 8 negative samples)	[90]
	Carbon nanofiber-based SPE functionalised with nucleocapsid antigen	Nucleocapsid protein	Nasopharyngeal swabs	20 min	0.8 pg mL^{-1}	—	RT-PCR	3 samples (2 positive and 1 negative samples)	[91]
	Graphene oxide-based SPE with 8-hydroxyquinoline and gold nanostars	Viral spike glycoproteins	Nasopharyngeal swabs	1 min	1.68×10^{-22} μg mL^{-1}	a 95% b 60%	RT-PCR	100 samples (60 positive and 40 negative samples)	[92]

Type of Biosensor	Sensing Area & Recognition Element	Target Analyte	Testing Sample	Assay Time	Sensitivity Limit of Detection (LOD)	[a] True Positive Rate (%) [b] True Negative Rate (%)	Sample Confirmation Method	Number of Clinical Samples	Ref.
(c) FET	Single-walled carbon nanotube (SWCNT) functionalised with anti-SARS-CoV-2 spike protein antibody and anti-nucleocapsid protein antibody	(i) Spike protein and (ii) Nucleocapsid protein	Nasopharyngeal swabs	<5 min	(i) 0.55 fg mL^{-1} (ii) 0.016 fg mL^{-1}	a (i) 82.14% a (ii) 53.57% b (i)(ii) 70%	PCR	38 samples (28 positive samples and 10 negative samples)	[99]
	Graphene channel functionalised with SARS-CoV-2 antibody	SARS-CoV-2 RNA	Nasopharyngeal swabs	>1 min	2.42×10^2 copies mL^{-1}	—	RT-PCR	3 SARS-CoV-2-confirmed patients	[42]
	Carbon nanotube channel immobilised with the reverse sequence of the RNA-dependent RNA polymerase gene of SARS-CoV-2	SARS-CoV-2 RNA	Buffer	—	10 fM	—	Not available	Not available	[100]
	Phosphorodiamidate morpholino oligos (PMO) probe immobilised on the AuNP surface	SARS-CoV-2 RNA	1 Buffer, 2 Throat swab 3 Serum	2 min	1 0.37 fM 2 2.29 fM 3 3.99 fM	—	RT-PCR	30 throat swab samples from 20 SARS-CoV-2-confirmed patients and 10 excluded individuals.	[106]

3. Strategies to Enhance the Biosensor Performance

The accuracy of the reviewed biosensors in detecting negative samples are short of the WHO minimum of 97%. This can be improved by choosing biorecognition elements that are highly selective in binding with the target analytes and hence cross-reactivity with unrelated molecules can be avoided to reduce false positives. Moreover, the true positive rate (ranging from 46.2% to 100%) of the biosensors do not all meet the WHO minimum of 80%. This can be improved by increasing the surface area of the sensor site using surface modification techniques to enhance the sensor sensitivity to a low concentration of bioanalytes. These enhancement strategies for COVID-19 biosensor performance are elaborated in the following sections.

3.1. Potential Biorecognition Elements

In general, the detection technique used in biosensors can be classified as labelled or label-free. Labelled biosensors commonly rely on specific labels, such as enzymes (e.g., horseradish peroxidase (HRP), alkaline phosphatase (ALP)), fluorescent molecules or electroactive compounds, to detect analytes. The label helps in signal amplification and increase sensing selectivity, but at the same time, it increases the overall sensor cost and response time. On the other hand, label-free biosensors rely on biorecognition elements to directly detect different types of analyte targets ranging from proteins to DNA and viruses. There is a wide range of biorecognition elements—such as enzyme, antibody, nucleic acid, aptamers, molecularly imprinted polymers—with unique characteristics for the interaction with a specific target of interest [119,120].

In COVID-19 biosensors, antibodies and nucleic acid probes are the most common biorecognition elements used for recognising SARS-CoV-2 biomarkers (e.g., viral proteins, human immunoglobulins or viral RNA) through the formation of antigen-antibody immunocomplex and single-stranded-DNA/oligonucleotide complementary strands complexes, respectively.

In general, monoclonal antibodies are preferred for assay involving binding of a specific antigen. These antibodies are specific to a single epitope of a target molecule, but a slight change in conformation may lead to a dramatically reduced binding capacity [121,122]. However, an alternative approach known as antibody phage display can be employed, where the monoclonal antibodies can be engineered to improve binding affinity with specific viral markers [123,124]. The conventional method of producing monoclonal antibodies requires expensive experimentation with animals and labour-intensive procedures. Besides high cost, the antibodies have a limited lifespan and are susceptible to high temperature [125,126].

Alternatively, high affinity and specificity aptamers have emerged as a substitute to monoclonal antibodies as biorecognition elements in biosensing. Aptamers are artificial single-stranded RNA or DNA oligonucleotides that can be chemically synthesised by an in vitro selection process called Systematic Evolution of Ligands by Exponential Enrichment (SELEX) [127]. Similar to antibodies, aptamers can bind specifically to the target based on structural recognition [127]. Furthermore, aptamers offer many advantages over antibodies, including smaller size, long shelf-life, stable to changes in pH, temperature, and ionic strength [128]. Compared to antibodies, aptamers have a much lower molecular weight (6–30 KDa, 2 nm) than antibodies (150–180 kDa, 15 nm), which allows them to bind with a wide range of potential targets such as ions, small molecules, viruses, and proteins [129–132]. Aptamers also have high thermal stability (up to 95 °C), and they are suitable for repeated use as they can be regenerated easily after denaturation [133]. In particular, when used as a biorecognition element in FET biosensors, the smaller size and compact structure of the aptamers allow the binding event to take place within the Debye length, thus overcoming the Debye length limitation. The bound targets are located closer to the sensor surface, and therefore stronger electrical signal is transduced from the binding event [134].

Phosphorodiamidatemorpholino oligomers (PMO) are uncharged analogues of nucleic acids. Compared to natural nucleic acid probes, the PMO probe offers better stability and higher binding strength owing to its neutral character [135]. RNA and DNA probes are negatively charged in physiological conditions due to their phosphate groups on the nucleic acid backbone. Therefore, electrostatic repulsion exists between the highly negative charged probe and target sequence, which decreases the hybridisation efficiency. Hence, RNA and DNA probes require high ionic strength conditions to shield their intermolecular repulsive force for hybridisations [136]. However, PMO probes have no net charge and they are insensitive to the ionic strength of the buffer, so they can retain their excellent binding affinity to target nucleic acid under the condition of low or high ionic strength [137].

3.2. Potential Nanomaterials for Sensor Surface Modification

With the rapid development of nanotechnology in the past few years, various nanomaterials, such as gold nanoparticles, graphene and carbon nanotubes, have been widely used in the design of biosensors as transduction substrates to enhance sensing performance. Nanomaterials characteristics, such as nano-scale size, larger surface area and higher conductivity, aid in signal amplification [138]. Besides that, the inherent large surface areas of nanomaterials can enhance the loading effect caused by the bioreceptor [139], thereby improving the sensitivity and stability of the biosensor.

In SPR-based sensors, metal nanoparticles (e.g., gold nanoparticles) have been commonly incorporated on the sensor surface [140,141]. As nanoparticles possess unique physical, electronic and chemical properties, large surface area and high free surface energy, biomolecules (e.g., antibody) are strongly adsorbed onto the surface. This improved the SPR detection limit from the nM range to the pM range [142]. The sensitivity improvement by nanomaterials also depends on the type of structures such as nanoshells, nanospheres, nanorods and nanowires. Compared to other shapes, high aspect ratio nanorods (NRs) offer a higher sensitivity to refractive index changes [143,144]. When NRs are used in a sandwich assay format, concentrations in the fM range can be detected [145,146]. In another strategy, dual nanomaterials (e.g., NRs and quasi-spherical nanoparticles (qsNPs)) have yielded attomolar range (aM) detection, which is about a 10-fold enhancement in sensitivity compared to sensor employing a single type of nanoparticles [141].

In addition, two-dimensional materials such as graphene are widely used in SPR, FET and electrochemical based biosensors. The high surface area to volume ratio and carbon-based ring structures of graphene enhances the adsorption of biorecognition elements onto the sensor surface [147,148]. Adding graphene-based materials on the gold film of SPR sensors allow detection down to fg/mL of mass change [149]. Graphene and reduced graphene oxide possess excellent electronic properties, which allow them to be used as sensor surface material in FET [150] and electrochemical sensors [151]. Due to the excellent electronic and adsorption properties of these materials, the LOD of the FET biosensor reported in [147] is 1 fM and 10 fM for the detection of the Japanese encephalitis and avian influenza virus, respectively. However, graphene yields a small current on-off ratio in FETs, which limits its sensitivity [136]. A large on-off ratio is required to reduce static leakage current for the sensor. To achieve this, two-dimensional semiconducting transition metal dichalcogenides (TMDCs) (e.g., molybdenum disulfide (MoS_2) nanoflakes, tungsten disulfide (WS_2) nanosheets) and black phosphorus (BP) can be explored. TMDCs have a larger bandgap than graphene and excellent characteristics such as large surface area and high electron transfer [152,153]. BP has adjustable band gap value and high carrier mobility [154,155].

4. Conclusions

The recently developed SPR-based, electrochemical and FET-based biosensors for SARS-CoV-2 detection we have reviewed are promising alternatives to currently available point of care (POC) tests. However, in addition to the limitations we have highlighted, none of the sensors met the WHO minimum requirement for true positive and true negative detection rates. Some of the sensors met the former requirement, but none met the latter requirement. The detection accuracies (particularly the true negative/false positive rate) need to be significantly improved before the sensors could be translated into POC devices for commercial use. The biorecognition elements and sensor surface modification materials we have suggested could be explored to improve the true negative and true positive rate, respectively.

Author Contributions: W.Y.L.—conceptualisation, writing—original draft; N.R.—conceptualisation, review and editing, supervision and funding acquisition; B.L.L.—conceptualisation, review and editing and funding acquisition. All authors have read and agreed to the published version of the manuscript.

Funding: This work was supported by Monash University Malaysia Grants: STG-000047 and PLT-000012.

Institutional Review Board Statement: Not applicable.

Informed Consent Statement: Not applicable.

Data Availability Statement: Not applicable.

Conflicts of Interest: The authors declare no conflict of interest.

References

1. Wu, J.T.; Leung, K.; Leung, G.M. Nowcasting and forecasting the potential domestic and international spread of the 2019-nCoV outbreak originating in Wuhan, China: A modelling study. *Lancet* **2020**, *395*, 689–697. [CrossRef]
2. Huang, C.; Wang, Y.; Li, X.; Ren, L.; Zhao, J.; Hu, Y.; Zhang, L.; Fan, G.; Xu, J.; Gu, X.; et al. Clinical features of patients infected with 2019 novel coronavirus in Wuhan, China. *Lancet* **2020**, *395*, 497–506. [CrossRef]
3. WHO Director-General's Opening Remarks at the Media Briefing on COVID-19-2020. Available online: https://www.who.int/director-general/speeches/detail/who-director-general-s-opening-remarks-at-the-media-briefing-on-covid-19---11-march-2020 (accessed on 19 May 2021).
4. World Health Organization Coronavirus (COVID-19) Dashboard. Available online: https://covid19.who.int/ (accessed on 31 July 2021).
5. Fu, L.; Wang, B.; Yuan, T.; Chen, X.; Ao, Y.; Fitzpatrick, T.; Li, P.; Zhou, Y.; Lin, Y.-F.; Duan, Q.; et al. Clinical characteristics of coronavirus disease 2019 (COVID-19) in China: A systematic review and meta-analysis. *J. Infect.* **2020**, *80*, 656–665. [CrossRef]
6. Zhang, L.; Guo, H. Biomarkers of COVID-19 and technologies to combat SARS-CoV-2. *Adv. Biomark. Sci. Technol.* **2020**, *2*, 1–23. [CrossRef] [PubMed]
7. Asif, M.; Ajmal, M.; Ashraf, G.; Muhammad, N.; Aziz, A.; Iftikhar, T.; Wang, J.; Liu, H. The role of biosensors in COVID-19 outbreak. *Curr. Opin. Electrochem.* **2020**, *23*, 174–184. [CrossRef]
8. Bastos, M.L.; Tavaziva, G.; Abidi, S.K.; Campbell, J.R.; Haraoui, L.-P.; Johnston, J.C.; Lan, Z.; Law, S.; MacLean, E.; Trajman, A.; et al. Diagnostic accuracy of serological tests for covid-19: Systematic review and meta-analysis. *BMJ* **2020**, *370*, m2516. [CrossRef]
9. Rasmi, Y.; Li, X.; Khan, J.; Ozer, T.; Choi, J.R. Emerging point-of-care biosensors for rapid diagnosis of COVID-19: Current progress, challenges, and future prospects. *Anal. Bioanal. Chem.* **2021**, *413*, 4137–4159. [CrossRef] [PubMed]
10. Corman, V.M.; Landt, O.; Kaiser, M.; Molenkamp, R.; Meijer, A.; Chu, D.K.; Bleicker, T.; Brünink, S.; Schneider, J.; Schmidt, M.L.; et al. Detection of 2019 novel coronavirus (2019-nCoV) by real-time RT-PCR. *Eurosurveillance* **2020**, *25*, 2000045. [CrossRef]
11. Udugama, B.; Kadhiresan, P.; Kozlowski, H.N.; Malekjahani, A.; Osborne, M.; Li, V.Y.; Chen, H.; Mubareka, S.; Gubbay, J.B.; Chan, W.C. Diagnosing COVID-19: The disease and tools for detection. *ACS Nano* **2020**, *14*, 3822–3835. [CrossRef]
12. Sethuraman, N.; Jeremiah, S.S.; Ryo, A. Interpreting diagnostic tests for SARS-CoV-2. *JAMA* **2020**, *323*, 2249–2251. [CrossRef] [PubMed]
13. Tahamtan, A.; Ardebili, A. Real-time RT-PCR in COVID-19 detection: Issues affecting the results. *Expert Rev. Mol. Diagn.* **2020**, *20*, 453–454. [CrossRef]
14. Chen, Z.; Li, Y.; Wu, B.; Hou, Y.; Bao, J.; Deng, X. A patient with COVID-19 presenting a false-negative reverse transcriptase polymerase chain reaction result. *Korean J. Radiol.* **2020**, *21*, 623. [CrossRef]
15. Boum, Y.; Fai, K.N.; Nikolay, B.; Mboringong, A.B.; Bebell, L.M.; Ndifon, M.; Abbah, A.; Essaka, R.; Eteki, L.; Luquero, F.; et al. Performance and operational feasibility of antigen and antibody rapid diagnostic tests for COVID-19 in symptomatic and asymptomatic patients in Cameroon: A clinical, prospective, diagnostic accuracy study. *Lancet Infect. Dis.* **2021**, *21*, 1089–1096. [CrossRef]
16. Berger, A.; Nsoga, M.T.N.; Perez-Rodriguez, F.J.; Aad, Y.A.; Sattonnet-Roche, P.; Gayet-Ageron, A.; Jaksic, C.; Torriani, G.; Boehm, E.; Kronig, I.; et al. Diagnostic accuracy of two commercial SARS-CoV-2 Antigen-detecting rapid tests at the point of care in community-based testing centers. *PLoS ONE* **2021**, *16*, e0248921. [CrossRef]

17. Corman, V.M.; Haage, V.C.; Bleicker, T.; Schmidt, M.L.; Mühlemann, B.; Zuchowski, M.; Jo, W.K.; Tscheak, P.; Möncke-Buchner, E.; Müller, M.A.; et al. Comparison of seven commercial SARS-CoV-2 rapid point-of-care antigen tests: A single-centre laboratory evaluation study. *Lancet Microbe* **2021**, *2*, e311–e319. [CrossRef]
18. Gowri, A.; Kumar, A.; Anand, S. Recent advances in nanomaterials based biosensors for point of care (PoC) diagnosis of covid-19-A minireview. *TrAC Trends Anal. Chem.* **2021**, *137*, 116205. [CrossRef]
19. Gao, H.-X.; Li, Y.-N.; Xu, Z.-G.; Wang, Y.-L.; Wang, H.-B.; Cao, J.-F.; Yuan, D.-Q.; Li, L.; Xu, Y.; Zhang, Z.; et al. Detection of serum immunoglobulin M and immunoglobulin G antibodies in 2019 novel coronavirus infected patients from different stages. *Chin. Med. J.* **2020**, *133*, 1479. [CrossRef]
20. The Global Fund. List of SARS-CoV-2 Diagnostic Test Kits and Equipments Eligible for Procurement According to Board Decision on Additional Support for Country Responses to COVID-19 (GF/B42/EDP11). Available online: https://www.theglobalfund.org/media/9629/covid19_diagnosticproducts_list_en.pdf (accessed on 4 August 2021).
21. Mak, G.C.; Cheng, P.K.; Lau, S.S.; Wong, K.K.; Lau, C.; Lam, E.T.; Chan, R.C.; Tsang, D.N. Evaluation of rapid antigen test for detection of SARS-CoV-2 virus. *J. Clin. Virol.* **2020**, *129*, 104500. [CrossRef]
22. Scohy, A.; Anantharajah, A.; Bodéus, M.; Kabamba-Mukadi, B.; Verroken, A.; Rodriguez-Villalobos, H. Low performance of rapid antigen detection test as frontline testing for COVID-19 diagnosis. *J. Clin. Virol.* **2020**, *129*, 104455. [CrossRef]
23. Antigen-Detection in the Diagnosis of SARS-CoV-2 Infection Using Rapid Immunoassays. Available online: https://www.who.int/publications/i/item/antigen-detection-in-the-diagnosis-of-sars-cov-2infection-using-rapid-immunoassays (accessed on 19 May 2021).
24. Omidfar, K.; Ahmadi, A.; Syedmoradi, L.; Khoshfetrat, S.M.; Larijani, B. Point-of-care biosensors in medicine: A brief overview of our achievements in this field based on the conducted research in EMRI (endocrinology and metabolism research Institute of Tehran University of medical sciences) over the past fourteen years. *J. Diabetes Metab. Disord.* **2020**, 1–5. [CrossRef]
25. Mabey, D.; Peeling, R.W.; Ustianowski, A.; Perkins, M.D. Diagnostics for the developing world. *Nat. Rev. Microbiol.* **2004**, *2*, 231–240. [CrossRef]
26. Land, K.J.; Boeras, D.I.; Chen, X.-S.; Ramsay, A.R.; Peeling, R.W. REASSURED diagnostics to inform disease control strategies, strengthen health systems and improve patient outcomes. *Nat. Microbiol.* **2019**, *4*, 46–54. [CrossRef]
27. Bhalla, N.; Jolly, P.; Formisano, N.; Estrela, P. Introduction to biosensors. *Essays Biochem.* **2016**, *60*, 1–8.
28. Metkar, S.K.; Girigoswami, K. Diagnostic biosensors in medicine—A review. *Biocatal. Agric. Biotechnol.* **2019**, *17*, 271–283. [CrossRef]
29. Yoo, S.M.; Lee, S.Y. Optical biosensors for the detection of pathogenic microorganisms. *Trends Biotechnol.* **2016**, *34*, 7–25. [CrossRef]
30. Bastos, A.R.; Vicente, C.; Oliveira-Silva, R.; Silva, N.J.; Tacão, M.; da Costa, J.P.; Lima, M.; André, P.S.; Ferreira, R.A. Integrated optical Mach-Zehnder interferometer based on organic-inorganic hybrids for photonics-on-a-chip biosensing applications. *Sensors* **2018**, *18*, 840. [CrossRef]
31. Chen, Y.-T.; Lee, Y.-C.; Lai, Y.-H.; Lim, J.-C.; Huang, N.-T.; Lin, C.-T.; Huang, J.-J. Review of integrated optical biosensors for point-of-care applications. *Biosensors* **2020**, *10*, 209. [CrossRef]
32. Yi, Z.; Sayago, J. Transistors as an Emerging Platform for Portable Amplified Biodetection in Preventive Personalized Point-of-Care Testing. In *Different Types of Field-Effect Transistors: Theory and Applications*; Pejovic, M.M., Pejovic, M.M., Eds.; InTechOpen: London, UK, 2017; Volume 165, pp. 165–181.
33. Rastogi, M.; Pandey, N.; Shukla, A.; Singh, S.K. SARS coronavirus 2: From genome to infectome. *Respir. Res.* **2020**, *21*, 318. [CrossRef]
34. Helmy, Y.A.; Fawzy, M.; Elaswad, A.; Sobieh, A.; Kenney, S.P.; Shehata, A.A. The COVID-19 pandemic: A comprehensive review of taxonomy, genetics, epidemiology, diagnosis, treatment, and control. *J. Clin. Med.* **2020**, *9*, 1225. [CrossRef]
35. Akib, T.B.A.; Mou, S.F.; Rahman, M.; Rana, M.; Islam, M.; Mehedi, I.M.; Mahmud, M.; Kouzani, A.Z. Design and Numerical Analysis of a Graphene-Coated SPR Biosensor for Rapid Detection of the Novel Coronavirus. *Sensors* **2021**, *21*, 3491. [CrossRef]
36. Chaibun, T.; Puenpa, J.; Ngamdee, T.; Boonapatcharoen, N.; Athamanolap, P.; O'Mullane, A.P.; Vongpunsawad, S.; Poovorawan, Y.; Lee, S.Y.; Lertanantawong, B. Rapid electrochemical detection of coronavirus SARS-CoV-2. *Nat. Commun.* **2021**, *12*, 802. [CrossRef] [PubMed]
37. Qiu, G.; Gai, Z.; Tao, Y.; Schmitt, J.; Kullak-Ublick, G.A.; Wang, J. Dual-functional plasmonic photothermal biosensors for highly accurate severe acute respiratory syndrome coronavirus 2 detection. *ACS Nano* **2020**, *14*, 5268–5277. [CrossRef] [PubMed]
38. Qiu, G.; Gai, Z.; Saleh, L.; Tang, J.; Gui, T.; Kullak-Ublick, G.A.; Wang, J. Thermoplasmonic-Assisted Cyclic Cleavage Amplification for Self-Validating Plasmonic Detection of SARS-CoV-2. *ACS Nano* **2021**, *15*, 7536–7546. [CrossRef] [PubMed]
39. Mojsoska, B.; Larsen, S.; Olsen, D.A.; Madsen, J.S.; Brandslund, I.; Alatraktchi, F.A. Rapid SARS-CoV-2 Detection Using Electrochemical Immunosensor. *Sensors* **2021**, *21*, 390. [CrossRef] [PubMed]
40. Fabiani, L.; Saroglia, M.; Galatà, G.; De Santis, R.; Fillo, S.; Luca, V.; Faggioni, G.; D'Amore, N.; Regalbuto, E.; Salvatori, P.; et al. Magnetic beads combined with carbon black-based screen-printed electrodes for COVID-19: A reliable and miniaturized electrochemical immunosensor for SARS-CoV-2 detection in saliva. *Biosens. Bioelectron.* **2021**, *171*, 112686. [CrossRef]
41. Zhang, X.; Qi, Q.; Jing, Q.; Ao, S.; Zhang, Z.; Ding, M.; Wu, M.; Liu, K.; Wang, W.; Ling, Y.; et al. Electrical probing of COVID-19 spike protein receptor binding domain via a graphene field-effect transistor. *arXiv* **2020**, arXiv:2003.12529.

42. Seo, G.; Lee, G.; Kim, M.J.; Baek, S.-H.; Choi, M.; Ku, K.B.; Lee, C.-S.; Jun, S.; Park, D.; Kim, H.G.; et al. Rapid detection of COVID-19 causative virus (SARS-CoV-2) in human nasopharyngeal swab specimens using field-effect transistor-based biosensor. *ACS Nano* **2020**, *14*, 5135–5142. [CrossRef] [PubMed]
43. Schasfoort, R.B.; van Weperen, J.; van Amsterdam, M.; Parisot, J.; Hendriks, J.; Koerselman, M.; Karperien, M.; Mentink, A.; Bennink, M.; Krabbe, H.; et al. Presence and strength of binding of IgM, IgG and IgA antibodies against SARS-CoV-2 during CoViD-19 infection. *Biosens. Bioelectron.* **2021**, *183*, 113165. [CrossRef]
44. Sarcina, L.; Mangiatordi, G.F.; Torricelli, F.; Bollella, P.; Gounani, Z.; Österbacka, R.; Macchia, E.; Torsi, L. Surface Plasmon Resonance Assay for Label-Free and Selective Detection of HIV-1 p24 Protein. *Biosensors* **2021**, *11*, 180. [CrossRef] [PubMed]
45. Chang, C.-C. Recent Advancements in Aptamer-Based Surface Plasmon Resonance Biosensing Strategies. *Biosensors* **2021**, *11*, 233. [CrossRef]
46. Sun, D.; Wu, Y.; Chang, S.-J.; Chen, C.-J.; Liu, J.-T. Investigation of the recognition interaction between glycated hemoglobin and its aptamer by using surface plasmon resonance. *Talanta* **2021**, *222*, 121466. [CrossRef]
47. Scarano, S.; Mascini, M.; Turner, A.P.; Minunni, M. Surface plasmon resonance imaging for affinity-based biosensors. *Biosens. Bioelectron.* **2010**, *25*, 957–966. [CrossRef]
48. Spoto, G.; Minunni, M. Surface plasmon resonance imaging: What next? *J. Phys. Chem. Lett.* **2012**, *3*, 2682–2691. [CrossRef] [PubMed]
49. Cao, J.; Galbraith, E.K.; Sun, T.; Grattan, K.T.V. Comparison of surface plasmon resonance and localized surface plasmon resonance-based optical fibre sensors. In Proceedings of the Sensors & Their Applications XVIAt, Cork, Ireland, 12–14 September 2011; p. 012050.
50. Jatschka, J.; Dathe, A.; Csáki, A.; Fritzsche, W.; Stranik, O. Propagating and localized surface plasmon resonance sensing—A critical comparison based on measurements and theory. *Sens. Bio-Sens. Res.* **2016**, *7*, 62–70. [CrossRef]
51. Mohan, V.B.; Lau, K.-T.; Hui, D.; Bhattacharyya, D. Graphene-based materials and their composites: A review on production, applications and product limitations. *Compos. B Eng.* **2018**, *142*, 200–220. [CrossRef]
52. Shen, M.; Joshi, A.A.; Vannam, R.; Dixit, C.K.; Hamilton, R.G.; Kumar, C.V.; Rusling, J.F.; Peczuh, M.W. Epitope-Resolved Detection of Peanut-Specific IgE Antibodies by Surface Plasmon Resonance Imaging. *ChemBioChem* **2018**, *19*, 199–202. [CrossRef] [PubMed]
53. Smith, E.A.; Corn, R.M. Surface plasmon resonance imaging as a tool to monitor biomolecular interactions in an array based format. *Appl. Spectrosc.* **2003**, *57*, 320A–332A. [CrossRef]
54. Garcia, B.H., II; Goodman, R.M. Use of surface plasmon resonance imaging to study viral RNA: Protein interactions. *J. Virol. Methods* **2008**, *147*, 18–25. [CrossRef]
55. Tai, W.; He, L.; Zhang, X.; Pu, J.; Voronin, D.; Jiang, S.; Zhou, Y.; Du, L. Characterization of the receptor-binding domain (RBD) of 2019 novel coronavirus: Implication for development of RBD protein as a viral attachment inhibitor and vaccine. *Cell. Mol. Immunol.* **2020**, *17*, 613–620. [CrossRef]
56. Kim, M.; Lee, J.H.; Nam, J.M. Plasmonic photothermal nanoparticles for biomedical applications. *Adv. Sci.* **2019**, *6*, 1900471. [CrossRef]
57. Schasfoort, R.B. Introduction to surface plasmon resonance. In *Handbook of Surface Plasmon Resonance*, 2nd ed.; Schasfoort, R.B., Ed.; Royal Society of Chemistry: London, UK, 2017; pp. 1–26.
58. Iravani, S. Nano-and biosensors for the detection of SARS-CoV-2: Challenges and opportunities. *Mater. Adv.* **2020**, *1*, 3092–3103. [CrossRef]
59. Mauriz, E. Recent progress in plasmonic biosensing schemes for virus detection. *Sensors* **2020**, *20*, 4745. [CrossRef] [PubMed]
60. Xu, X.; Ying, Y.; Li, Y. Gold nanorods based LSPR biosensor for label-free detection of alpha-fetoprotein. *Procedia Eng.* **2011**, *25*, 67–70. [CrossRef]
61. Moznuzzaman, M.; Islam, M.R.; Khan, I. Effect of layer thickness variation on sensitivity: An SPR based sensor for formalin detection. *Sens. Bio-Sens. Res.* **2021**, *32*, 100419. [CrossRef]
62. Xia, G.; Zhou, C.; Jin, S.; Huang, C.; Xing, J.; Liu, Z. Sensitivity enhancement of two-dimensional materials based on genetic optimization in surface plasmon resonance. *Sensors* **2019**, *19*, 1198. [CrossRef] [PubMed]
63. Unser, S.; Bruzas, I.; He, J.; Sagle, L. Localized surface plasmon resonance biosensing: Current challenges and approaches. *Sensors* **2015**, *15*, 15684–15716. [CrossRef] [PubMed]
64. Mauriz, E. Low-Fouling Substrates for Plasmonic Sensing of Circulating Biomarkers in Biological Fluids. *Biosensors* **2020**, *10*, 63. [CrossRef]
65. Liu, B.; Liu, X.; Shi, S.; Huang, R.; Su, R.; Qi, W.; He, Z. Design and mechanisms of antifouling materials for surface plasmon resonance sensors. *Acta Biomater.* **2016**, *40*, 100–118. [CrossRef] [PubMed]
66. Janeway, C.A., Jr.; Travers, P.; Walport, M.; Shlomchik, M.J. The interaction of the antibody molecule with specific antigen. In *Immunobiology: The Immune System in Health and Disease*, 5th ed.; Garland Science: New York, NY, USA, 2001; pp. 71–76.
67. Djaileb, A.C.; Benjamin, C.; Jodaylami, M.H.; Thibault, V.; Coutu, J.; Stevenson, K.; Forest, S.; Live, L.S.; Boudreau, D.; Pelletier, J.N.; et al. A rapid and quantitative serum test for SARS-CoV-2 antibodies with portable surface plasmon resonance sensing. *ChemRxiv* **2020**. [CrossRef]
68. Zhao, Z.; Huang, C.; Huang, Z.; Lin, F.; He, Q.; Tao, D.; Jaffrezic-Renault, N.; Guo, Z. Advancements in electrochemical biosensing for respiratory virus detection: A review. *TrAC Trends Anal. Chem.* **2021**, *139*, 116253. [CrossRef]

69. Balkourani, G.; Brouzgou, A.; Archonti, M.; Papandrianos, N.; Song, S.; Tsiakaras, P. Emerging materials for the electrochemical detection of COVID-19. *J. Electroanal. Chem.* **2021**, *893*, 115289. [CrossRef]
70. Da Silva, E.T.; Souto, D.E.; Barragan, J.T.; Giarola, J.d.F.; de Moraes, A.C.; Kubota, L.T. Electrochemical biosensors in point-of-care devices: Recent advances and future trends. *ChemElectroChem* **2017**, *4*, 778–794. [CrossRef]
71. Taleat, Z.; Khoshroo, A.; Mazloum-Ardakani, M. Screen-printed electrodes for biosensing: A review (2008–2013). *Microchim. Acta* **2014**, *181*, 865–891. [CrossRef]
72. Thévenot, D.R.; Toth, K.; Durst, R.A.; Wilson, G.S. Electrochemical biosensors: Recommended definitions and classification. *Biosens. Bioelectron.* **2001**, *16*, 121–131. [CrossRef]
73. Grieshaber, D.; MacKenzie, R.; Vörös, J.; Reimhult, E. Electrochemical biosensors-sensor principles and architectures. *Sensors* **2008**, *8*, 1400–1458. [CrossRef] [PubMed]
74. Sun, A.; Wambach, T.; Venkatesh, A.; Hall, D.A. A low-cost smartphone-based electrochemical biosensor for point-of-care diagnostics. In Proceedings of the IEEE Biomedical Circuits and Systems Conference (BioCAS) Proceedings, Lausanne, Switzerland, 22–24 October 2014; pp. 312–315.
75. Torres-Rivero, K.; Florido, A.; Bastos-Arrieta, J. Recent Trends in the Improvement of the Electrochemical Response of Screen-Printed Electrodes by Their Modification with Shaped Metal Nanoparticles. *Sensors* **2021**, *21*, 2596. [CrossRef]
76. Nelis, J.L.; Migliorelli, D.; Jafari, S.; Generelli, S.; Lou-Franco, J.; Salvador, J.P.; Marco, M.P.; Cao, C.; Elliott, C.T.; Campbell, K. The benefits of carbon black, gold and magnetic nanomaterials for point-of-harvest electrochemical quantification of domoic acid. *Microchim. Acta* **2020**, *187*, 164. [CrossRef]
77. Silva, T.A.; Moraes, F.C.; Janegitz, B.C.; Fatibello-Filho, O. Electrochemical biosensors based on nanostructured carbon black: A review. *J. Nanomater.* **2017**, *2017*, 4571614. [CrossRef]
78. Sur, U.K. Graphene: A Rising Star on the Horizon of Materials Science. *Int. J. Electrochem.* **2012**, *2012*, 237689. [CrossRef]
79. Eatemadi, A.; Daraee, H.; Karimkhanloo, H.; Kouhi, M.; Zarghami, N.; Akbarzadeh, A.; Abasi, M.; Hanifehpour, Y.; Joo, S.W. Carbon nanotubes: Properties, synthesis, purification, and medical applications. *Nanoscale Res. Lett.* **2014**, *9*, 393. [CrossRef]
80. Duekhuntod, W.; Karuwan, C.; Tuantranont, A.; Nacapricha, D.; Teerasong, S. A Screen Printed Graphene Based Electrochemical Sensor for Single Drop Analysis of Hydroquinone in Cosmetic Products. *Int. J. Electrochem. Sci.* **2019**, *14*, 7631–7642. [CrossRef]
81. Gupta, S.; Murthy, C.; Prabha, C.R. Recent advances in carbon nanotube based electrochemical biosensors. *Int. J. Biol. Macromol.* **2018**, *108*, 687–703. [CrossRef]
82. Layqah, L.A.; Eissa, S. An electrochemical immunosensor for the corona virus associated with the Middle East respiratory syndrome using an array of gold nanoparticle-modified carbon electrodes. *Microchim. Acta* **2019**, *186*, 224. [CrossRef] [PubMed]
83. Schmalenberg, M.; Beaudoin, C.; Bulst, L.; Steubl, D.; Luppa, P.B. Magnetic bead fluorescent immunoassay for the rapid detection of the novel inflammation marker YKL40 at the point-of-care. *J. Immunol. Methods* **2015**, *427*, 36–41. [CrossRef] [PubMed]
84. Sista, R.S.; Eckhardt, A.E.; Srinivasan, V.; Pollack, M.G.; Palanki, S.; Pamula, V.K. Heterogeneous immunoassays using magnetic beads on a digital microfluidic platform. *Lab Chip* **2008**, *8*, 2188–2196. [CrossRef]
85. Molinero-Fernández, Á.; Moreno-Guzmán, M.; López, M.Á.; Escarpa, A. Magnetic Bead-Based Electrochemical Immunoassays On-Drop and On-Chip for Procalcitonin Determination: Disposable Tools for Clinical Sepsis Diagnosis. *Biosensors* **2020**, *10*, 66. [CrossRef]
86. Zhang, D.; Liu, Q. Biosensors and bioelectronics on smartphone for portable biochemical detection. *Biosens. Bioelectron.* **2016**, *75*, 273–284. [CrossRef]
87. Ainla, A.; Mousavi, M.P.; Tsaloglou, M.-N.; Redston, J.; Bell, J.G.; Fernández-Abedul, M.T.; Whitesides, G.M. Open-source potentiostat for wireless electrochemical detection with smartphones. *Anal. Chem.* **2018**, *90*, 6240–6246. [CrossRef]
88. Zhao, H.; Liu, F.; Xie, W.; Zhou, T.-C.; OuYang, J.; Jin, L.; Li, H.; Zhao, C.-Y.; Zhang, L.; Wei, J. Ultrasensitive supersandwich-type electrochemical sensor for SARS-CoV-2 from the infected COVID-19 patients using a smartphone. *Sens. Actuators B* **2021**, *327*, 128899. [CrossRef]
89. Sridharan, G.; Shankar, A.A. Toluidine blue: A review of its chemistry and clinical utility. *J. Oral Maxillofac. Pathol.* **2012**, *16*, 251. [CrossRef]
90. Rahmati, Z.; Roushani, M.; Hosseini, H.; Choobin, H. Electrochemical immunosensor with Cu_2O nanocube coating for detection of SARS-CoV-2 spike protein. *Microchim. Acta* **2021**, *188*, 105. [CrossRef]
91. Eissa, S.; Zourob, M. Development of a low-cost cotton-tipped electrochemical immunosensor for the detection of SARS-CoV-2. *Anal. Chem.* **2020**, *93*, 1826–1833. [CrossRef] [PubMed]
92. Hashemi, S.A.; Behbahan, N.G.G.; Bahrani, S.; Mousavi, S.M.; Gholami, A.; Ramakrishna, S.; Firoozsani, M.; Moghadami, M.; Lankarani, K.B.; Omidifar, N. Ultra-sensitive viral glycoprotein detection NanoSystem toward accurate tracing SARS-CoV-2 in biological/non-biological media. *Biosens. Bioelectron.* **2021**, *171*, 112731. [CrossRef]
93. Wyllie, A.L.; Fournier, J.; Casanovas-Massana, A.; Campbell, M.; Tokuyama, M.; Vijayakumar, P.; Geng, B.; Muenker, M.C.; Moore, A.J.; Vogels, C.B.; et al. Saliva is more sensitive for SARS-CoV-2 detection in COVID-19 patients than nasopharyngeal swabs. *MedRxiv* **2020**. [CrossRef]
94. Hill, C.; Thuret, J.-Y. The sensitivity and costs of testing for SARS-CoV-2 infection with saliva versus nasopharyngeal swabs. *Ann. Intern. Med.* **2021**, *174*, 582. [CrossRef] [PubMed]
95. Lee, C.-S.; Kim, S.K.; Kim, M. Ion-sensitive field-effect transistor for biological sensing. *Sensors* **2009**, *9*, 7111–7131. [CrossRef]

96. Chua, J.H.; Chee, R.-E.; Agarwal, A.; Wong, S.M.; Zhang, G.-J. Label-free electrical detection of cardiac biomarker with complementary metal-oxide semiconductor-compatible silicon nanowire sensor arrays. *Anal. Chem.* **2009**, *81*, 6266–6271. [CrossRef]
97. Zhang, G.-J.; Zhang, L.; Huang, M.J.; Luo, Z.H.H.; Tay, G.K.I.; Lim, E.-J.A.; Kang, T.G.; Chen, Y. Silicon nanowire biosensor for highly sensitive and rapid detection of Dengue virus. *Sens. Actuators B* **2010**, *146*, 138–144. [CrossRef]
98. Allen, B.L.; Kichambare, P.D.; Star, A. Carbon nanotube field-effect-transistor-based biosensors. *Adv. Mater.* **2007**, *19*, 1439–1451. [CrossRef]
99. Shao, W.; Shurin, M.R.; Wheeler, S.E.; He, X.; Star, A. Rapid Detection of SARS-CoV-2 Antigens Using High-Purity Semiconducting Single-Walled Carbon Nanotube-Based Field-Effect Transistors. *ACS Appl. Mater. Interfaces* **2021**, *13*, 10321–10327. [CrossRef]
100. Thanihaichelvan, M.; Surendran, S.; Kumanan, T.; Sutharsini, U.; Ravirajan, P.; Valluvan, R.; Tharsika, T. Selective and electronic detection of COVID-19 (Coronavirus) using carbon nanotube field effect transistor-based biosensor: A proof-of-concept study. *Mater. Today Proc.* **2021**, in press. [CrossRef]
101. Chen, Y.; Ren, R.; Pu, H.; Guo, X.; Chang, J.; Zhou, G.; Mao, S.; Kron, M.; Chen, J. Field-effect transistor biosensor for rapid detection of Ebola antigen. *Sci. Rep.* **2017**, *7*, 10974. [CrossRef]
102. Tu, J.; Gan, Y.; Liang, T.; Hu, Q.; Wang, Q.; Ren, T.; Sun, Q.; Wan, H.; Wang, P. Graphene FET array biosensor based on ssDNA aptamer for ultrasensitive Hg^{2+} detection in environmental pollutants. *Front. Chem.* **2018**, *6*, 333. [CrossRef] [PubMed]
103. Zhu, Y.; Hao, Y.; Adogla, E.A.; Yan, J.; Li, D.; Xu, K.; Wang, Q.; Hone, J.; Lin, Q. A graphene-based affinity nanosensor for detection of low-charge and low-molecular-weight molecules. *Nanoscale* **2016**, *8*, 5815–5819. [CrossRef] [PubMed]
104. Yao, X.; Zhang, Y.; Jin, W.; Hu, Y.; Cui, Y. Carbon Nanotube Field-Effect Transistor-Based Chemical and Biological Sensors. *Sensors* **2021**, *21*, 995. [CrossRef]
105. Min, S.J.; Kim, J.W.; Kim, J.H.; Choi, J.H.; Park, C.W.; Min, N.K. Effect of Varying the Semiconducting/Metallic Tube Ratio on the Performance of Mixed Single-Walled Carbon Nanotube Network Gas Sensors. *J. Nanomater.* **2017**, *2017*, 8761064. [CrossRef]
106. Li, J.; Wu, D.; Yu, Y.; Li, T.; Li, K.; Xiao, M.-M.; Li, Y.; Zhang, Z.-Y.; Zhang, G.-J. Rapid and unamplified identification of COVID-19 with morpholino-modified graphene field-effect transistor nanosensor. *Biosens. Bioelectron.* **2021**, *183*, 113206. [CrossRef]
107. Mei, J.; Li, Y.-T.; Zhang, H.; Xiao, M.-M.; Ning, Y.; Zhang, Z.-Y.; Zhang, G.-J. Molybdenum disulfide field-effect transistor biosensor for ultrasensitive detection of DNA by employing morpholino as probe. *Biosens. Bioelectron.* **2018**, *110*, 71–77. [CrossRef] [PubMed]
108. Wadhera, T.; Kakkar, D.; Wadhwa, G.; Raj, B. Recent advances and progress in development of the field effect transistor biosensor: A review. *J. Electron. Mater.* **2019**, *48*, 7635–7646. [CrossRef]
109. Vu, C.A.; Chen, W.Y. Field-effect transistor biosensors for biomedical applications: Recent advances and future prospects. *Sensors* **2019**, *19*, 4214. [CrossRef]
110. Poghossian, A.; Jablonski, M.; Molinnus, D.; Wege, C.; Schöning, M.J. Field-effect sensors for virus detection: From Ebola to SARS-CoV-2 and plant viral enhancers. *Front. Plant Sci.* **2020**, *11*, 598103. [CrossRef]
111. Sung, D.; Koo, J. A review of BioFET's basic principles and materials for biomedical applications. *Biomed. Eng. Lett.* **2021**, *11*, 85–96. [CrossRef]
112. Star, A.; Gabriel, J.-C.P.; Bradley, K.; Grüner, G. Electronic detection of specific protein binding using nanotube FET devices. *Nano Lett.* **2003**, *3*, 459–463. [CrossRef]
113. Syu, Y.-C.; Hsu, W.-E.; Lin, C.-T. Field-effect transistor biosensing: Devices and clinical applications. *ECS J. Solid State Sci. Technol.* **2018**, *7*, Q3196. [CrossRef]
114. Alabsi, S.S.; Ahmed, A.Y.; Dennis, J.O.; Khir, M.M.; Algamili, A. A Review of Carbon Nanotubes Field Effect-Based Biosensors. *IEEE Access* **2020**, *8*, 69509–69521. [CrossRef]
115. Chu, C.-H.; Sarangadharan, I.; Regmi, A.; Chen, Y.-W.; Hsu, C.-P.; Chang, W.-H.; Lee, G.-Y.; Chyi, J.-I.; Chen, C.-C.; Shiesh, S.-C.; et al. Beyond the Debye length in high ionic strength solution: Direct protein detection with field-effect transistors (FETs) in human serum. *Sci. Rep.* **2017**, *7*, 5256. [CrossRef]
116. Filipiak, M.S.; Rother, M.; Andoy, N.M.; Knudsen, A.C.; Grimm, S.B.; Bachran, C.; Swee, L.K.; Zaumseil, J.; Tarasov, A. Label-free immunodetection in high ionic strength solutions using carbon nanotube transistors with nanobody receptors. In Proceedings of the Eurosensors 2017, Paris, France, 3–6 September 2017; p. 491.
117. Kesler, V.; Murmann, B.; Soh, H.T. Going beyond the Debye Length: Overcoming Charge Screening Limitations in Next-Generation Bioelectronic Sensors. *ACS Nano* **2020**, *14*, 16194–16201. [CrossRef]
118. Sun, J.; Liu, Y. Matrix effect study and immunoassay detection using electrolyte-gated graphene biosensor. *Micromachines* **2018**, *9*, 142. [CrossRef]
119. Morales, M.A.; Halpern, J.M. Guide to selecting a biorecognition element for biosensors. *Bioconjug. Chem.* **2018**, *29*, 3231–3239. [CrossRef]
120. Alhalaili, B.; Popescu, I.N.; Kamoun, O.; Alzubi, F.; Alawadhia, S.; Vidu, R. Nanobiosensors for the Detection of Novel Coronavirus 2019-nCoV and Other Pandemic/Epidemic Respiratory Viruses: A Review. *Sensors* **2020**, *20*, 6591. [CrossRef]
121. Lipman, N.S.; Jackson, L.R.; Trudel, L.J.; Weis-Garcia, F. Monoclonal versus polyclonal antibodies: Distinguishing characteristics, applications, and information resources. *ILAR J.* **2005**, *46*, 258–268. [CrossRef]
122. Sadeghalvad, M.; Rezaei, N. Introduction on Monoclonal Antibodies. In *Monoclonal Antibodies*; Rezaei, N., Ed.; IntechOpen: London, UK, 2021; pp. 1–21.
123. Limsakul, P.; Charupanit, K.; Moonla, C.; Jeerapan, I. Advances in emergent biological recognition elements and bioelectronics for diagnosing COVID-19. *Emergent Mater.* **2021**, *4*, 231–247. [CrossRef]

124. Alfaleh, M.A.; Alsaab, H.O.; Mahmoud, A.B.; Alkayyal, A.A.; Jones, M.L.; Mahler, S.M.; Hashem, A.M. Phage display derived monoclonal antibodies: From bench to bedside. *Front. Immunol.* **2020**, *11*, 1986. [CrossRef]
125. Lim, S.A.; Ahmed, M.U. Introduction to food biosensors. In *Food Biosensors*; Minhaz Uddin Ahmed, M.Z., Tamiya, E., Eds.; Food Chemistry, Function and Analysis; The Royal Society of Chemistry: Cambridge, UK, 2016; pp. 1–21.
126. Cesewski, E.; Johnson, B.N. Electrochemical biosensors for pathogen detection. *Biosens. Bioelectron.* **2020**, *159*, 112214. [CrossRef]
127. Zhang, Y.; Lai, B.S.; Juhas, M. Recent advances in aptamer discovery and applications. *Molecules* **2019**, *24*, 941. [CrossRef]
128. Purohit, B.; Vernekar, P.R.; Shetti, N.P.; Chandra, P. Biosensor nanoengineering: Design, operation, and implementation for biomolecular analysis. *Sens. Int.* **2020**, *1*, 100040. [CrossRef]
129. Yang, D.; Liu, X.; Zhou, Y.; Luo, L.; Zhang, J.; Huang, A.; Mao, Q.; Chen, X.; Tang, L. Aptamer-based biosensors for detection of lead (ii) ion: A review. *Anal. Methods* **2017**, *9*, 1976–1990. [CrossRef]
130. Ruscito, A.; DeRosa, M.C. Small-molecule binding aptamers: Selection strategies, characterization, and applications. *Front. Chem.* **2016**, *4*, 14. [CrossRef]
131. Zou, X.; Wu, J.; Gu, J.; Shen, L.; Mao, L. Application of aptamers in virus detection and antiviral therapy. *Front. Microbiol.* **2019**, *10*, 1462. [CrossRef]
132. Xiong, H.; Yan, J.; Cai, S.; He, Q.; Peng, D.; Liu, Z.; Liu, Y. Cancer protein biomarker discovery based on nucleic acid aptamers. *Int. J. Biol. Macromol.* **2019**, *132*, 190–202. [CrossRef]
133. Zhou, J.; Rossi, J. Aptamers as targeted therapeutics: Current potential and challenges. *Nat. Rev. Drug Discov.* **2017**, *16*, 181–202. [CrossRef]
134. Lee, J.-O.; So, H.-M.; Jeon, E.-K.; Chang, H.; Won, K.; Kim, Y.H. Aptamers as molecular recognition elements for electrical nanobiosensors. *Anal. Bioanal. Chem.* **2008**, *390*, 1023–1032. [CrossRef]
135. Bagi, A.; Soelberg, S.D.; Furlong, C.E.; Baussant, T. Implementing Morpholino-Based Nucleic Acid Sensing on a Portable Surface Plasmon Resonance Instrument for Future Application in Environmental Monitoring. *Sensors* **2018**, *18*, 3259. [CrossRef]
136. Zhang, A.; Lieber, C.M. Nano-bioelectronics. *Chem. Rev.* **2016**, *116*, 215–257. [CrossRef]
137. Xiong, Y.; McQuistan, T.J.; Stanek, J.W.; Summerton, J.E.; Mata, J.E.; Squier, T.C. Detection of unique Ebola virus oligonucleotides using fluorescently-labeled phosphorodiamidate morpholino oligonucleotide probe pairs. *Anal. Biochem.* **2018**, *557*, 84–90. [CrossRef]
138. Malhotra, B.D.; Ali, M.A. Nanomaterials in Biosensors: Fundamentals and Applications. In *Nanomaterials for Biosensors*; Malhotra, B.D., Ali, M.A., Eds.; William Andrew Publishing: Norwich, UK; New York, NY, USA, 2018; pp. 1–74.
139. Holzinger, M.; Le Goff, A.; Cosnier, S. Nanomaterials for biosensing applications: A review. *Front. Chem.* **2014**, *2*, 63. [CrossRef]
140. Mei, Z.; Wang, Y.; Tang, L. Gold nanorod array biochip for label-free, multiplexed biological detection. *Methods Mol. Biol.* **2017**, *1571*, 129–141.
141. Baek, S.H.; Wark, A.W.; Lee, H.J. Dual nanoparticle amplified surface plasmon resonance detection of thrombin at subattomolar concentrations. *Anal. Chem.* **2014**, *86*, 9824–9829. [CrossRef]
142. Antiochia, R.; Bollella, P.; Favero, G.; Mazzei, F. Nanotechnology-based surface plasmon resonance affinity biosensors for in vitro diagnostics. *Int. J. Anal. Chem.* **2016**, *2016*, 2981931. [CrossRef]
143. Hong, Y.; Huh, Y.-M.; Yoon, D.S.; Yang, J. Nanobiosensors based on localized surface plasmon resonance for biomarker detection. *J. Nanomater.* **2012**, *2012*, 759830. [CrossRef]
144. Shrivastav, A.M.; Cvelbar, U.; Abdulhalim, I. A comprehensive review on plasmonic-based biosensors used in viral diagnostics. *Commun. Biol.* **2021**, *4*, 70. [CrossRef]
145. Law, W.-C.; Yong, K.-T.; Baev, A.; Prasad, P.N. Sensitivity improved surface plasmon resonance biosensor for cancer biomarker detection based on plasmonic enhancement. *ACS Nano* **2011**, *5*, 4858–4864. [CrossRef]
146. Choi, J.-W.; Kang, D.-Y.; Jang, Y.-H.; Kim, H.-H.; Min, J.; Oh, B.-K. Ultra-sensitive surface plasmon resonance based immunosensor for prostate-specific antigen using gold nanoparticle–antibody complex. *Colloids Surf. A* **2008**, *313*, 655–659. [CrossRef]
147. Roberts, A.; Chauhan, N.; Islam, S.; Mahari, S.; Ghawri, B.; Gandham, R.K.; Majumdar, S.; Ghosh, A.; Gandhi, S. Graphene functionalized field-effect transistors for ultrasensitive detection of Japanese encephalitis and Avian influenza virus. *Sci. Rep.* **2020**, *10*, 14546. [CrossRef]
148. Song, B.; Li, D.; Qi, W.; Elstner, M.; Fan, C.; Fang, H. Graphene on Au (111): A highly conductive material with excellent adsorption properties for high-resolution bio/nanodetection and identification. *ChemPhysChem* **2010**, *11*, 585–589. [CrossRef] [PubMed]
149. Nurrohman, D.T.; Chiu, N.-F. A review of graphene-based surface plasmon resonance and surface-enhanced raman scattering biosensors: Current status and future prospects. *Nanomaterials* **2021**, *11*, 216. [CrossRef]
150. Xu, S.; Zhan, J.; Man, B.; Jiang, S.; Yue, W.; Gao, S.; Guo, C.; Liu, H.; Li, Z.; Wang, J.; et al. Real-time reliable determination of binding kinetics of DNA hybridization using a multi-channel graphene biosensor. *Nat. Commun.* **2017**, *8*, 14902. [CrossRef]
151. Joshi, S.R.; Sharma, A.; Kim, G.-H.; Jang, J. Low cost synthesis of reduced graphene oxide using biopolymer for influenza virus sensor. *Mater. Sci. Eng.* **2020**, *108*, 110465. [CrossRef] [PubMed]
152. Ryder, C.R.; Wood, J.D.; Wells, S.A.; Hersam, M.C. Chemically tailoring semiconducting two-dimensional transition metal dichalcogenides and black phosphorus. *ACS Nano* **2016**, *10*, 3900–3917. [CrossRef]
153. Wen, W.; Song, Y.; Yan, X.; Zhu, C.; Du, D.; Wang, S.; Asiri, A.M.; Lin, Y. Recent advances in emerging 2D nanomaterials for biosensing and bioimaging applications. *Mater. Today* **2018**, *21*, 164–177. [CrossRef]

154. Cai, Y.; Zhang, J.; Zhou, Y.; Chen, C.; Lin, F.; Wang, L. Refractive index sensor with alternative high performance using black phosphorus in the all-dielectric configuration. *Opt. Express* **2021**, *29*, 23810–23821. [CrossRef] [PubMed]
155. Li, X.; Yu, Z.; Xiong, X.; Li, T.; Gao, T.; Wang, R.; Huang, R.; Wu, Y. High-speed black phosphorus field-effect transistors approaching ballistic limit. *Sci. Adv.* **2019**, *5*, 1–5. [CrossRef] [PubMed]

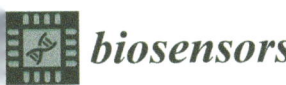

Article

Lateral Flow Immunoassay of SARS-CoV-2 Antigen with SERS-Based Registration: Development and Comparison with Traditional Immunoassays

Kseniya V. Serebrennikova [1], Nadezhda A. Byzova [1], Anatoly V. Zherdev [1], Nikolai G. Khlebtsov [2,3], Boris N. Khlebtsov [2], Sergey F. Biketov [4] and Boris B. Dzantiev [1,*]

1. A.N. Bach Institute of Biochemistry, Research Center of Biotechnology, Russian Academy of Sciences, 119071 Moscow, Russia; ksenijasereb@mail.ru (K.V.S.); nbyzova@inbi.ras.ru (N.A.B.); zherdev@inbi.ras.ru (A.V.Z.)
2. Institute of Biochemistry and Physiology of Plants and Microorganisms, Russian Academy of Sciences, 410049 Saratov, Russia; khlebtsov_n@ibppm.ru (N.G.K.); khlebtsov_b@ibppm.ru (B.N.K.)
3. Faculty of Nano- and Biomedical Technologies, Saratov State University, 410012 Saratov, Russia
4. State Research Center for Applied Microbiology and Biotechnology, 142279 Obolensk, Moscow Region, Russia; biketov@mail.ru
* Correspondence: dzantiev@inbi.ras.ru; Tel.: +7-495-954-31-42

Abstract: The current COVID-19 pandemic has increased the demand for pathogen detection methods that combine low detection limits with rapid results. Despite the significant progress in methods and devices for nucleic acid amplification, immunochemical methods are still preferred for mass testing without specialized laboratories and highly qualified personnel. The most widely used immunoassays are microplate enzyme-linked immunosorbent assay (ELISA) with photometric detection and lateral flow immunoassay (LFIA) with visual results assessment. However, the disadvantage of ELISA is its considerable duration, and that of LFIA is its low sensitivity. In this study, the modified LFIA of a specific antigen of the causative agent of COVID-19, spike receptor-binding domain, was developed and characterized. This modified LFIA includes the use of gold nanoparticles with immobilized antibodies and 4-mercaptobenzoic acid as surface-enhanced Raman scattering (SERS) nanotag and registration of the nanotag binding by SERS spectrometry. To enhance the sensitivity of LFIA-SERS analysis, we determined the optimal compositions of SERS nanotags and membranes used in LFIA. For benchmark comparison, ELISA and conventional colorimetric LFIA were used with the same immune reagents. The proposed method combines a low detection limit of 0.1 ng/mL (at 0.4 ng/mL for ELISA and 1 ng/mL for qualitative LFIA) with a short assay time equal to 20 min (at 3.5 h for ELISA and 15 min for LFIA). The results obtained demonstrate the promise of using the SERS effects in membrane immuno-analytical systems.

Keywords: SARS-CoV-2; immunochromatography; test strips; surface antigen; Raman spectra

1. Introduction

The current COVID-19 pandemic has challenged the global healthcare system [1,2]. The SARS-CoV-2 virus causing this disease has four main structural proteins (spike, envelope, membrane, and nucleocapsid), which contribute to the assembly of the virus and its penetration into target cells (in the case of spike protein) [3,4]. Both spike and nucleocapsid proteins are considered antigens for the serodiagnosis of SARS-CoV-2. The incubation period for COVID-19 after the virus enters the host is estimated to be 5–6 days [5,6]. During this time, the patient is contagious, and the virus is easily transmitted from person to person by airborne droplets or direct contact.

To prevent high mortality and the risk of a severe course of the disease, timely and rapid detection of SARS-CoV-2 as well as the differential diagnoses from other coronavirus infections and influenza or SARS viruses is required [7–10]. The use of polymerase chain reaction or other amplification techniques for this purpose is associated with a long duration, specialized and expensive equipment, and skilled personnel [11,12]. Therefore, accurate point-of-care COVID-19 tests are attracting a lot of attention thanks to their speed, ease of use, and potential for diagnostic implementation. Immunoassay techniques, such as microplate enzyme-linked immunosorbent assay (ELISA) and lateral flow immunoassay (LFIA), provide more simple testing than the amplification techniques. The effectiveness of both methods for rapid mass screening of COVID-19 in routine clinical practice has been confirmed [13,14]. However, the principle of visual colorimetric detection underlining the assessment of LFIA testing results limits the sensitivity and reliability of this method. In contrast, the main disadvantage of ELISA is prolonged (several hours) testing.

To overcome the sensitivity barrier of common LFIA, the integration of surface-enhanced Raman scattering (SERS) nanotags with LFIA based on specific antigen-antibody interactions, resulting in the detection of SERS signals for quantitative interpretation of the results, was proposed [15]. The enhancing possibilities of Raman signals are attributed to the enhanced electromagnetic field near the noble metal surface under conditions of plasmon resonance [16]. According to theoretical calculations, the decrease in the detection limit provided by SERS signal enhancement can reach up to eight orders of magnitude. However, such results are rarely reached, and the typical gain in sensitivity is limited to one to two orders of magnitude [17,18]. The effectiveness of the implementation of SERS nanotags in LFIA tests for the detection of various analytes was evaluated in a review by Khlebtsov et al. [15]. The SERS-based LFIAs were successfully applied for quantitative detection of antibiotics [19], biomarkers [20–23], allergens [24], pathogens [25,26], and so on. To date, only a few researchers have proposed the integration of SERS nanotags with LFIA to improve the efficiency of COVID-19 diagnostics through serological IgM and IgG testing [18,27], whereas in the case of SARS-CoV-2 antigen detection, the SERS technique was not earlier applied.

In this study, we developed a novel SERS-based LFIA for the detection of the SARS-CoV-2 spike receptor-binding domain (RBD). A conjugate of anti-SARS-CoV-2 spike RBD antibodies with 4-mercaptobenzoic acid (MBA)-modified spherical gold nanoparticles (AuNPs) was synthesized and used as a SERS nanotag. Parameters such as the loading of the Raman reporter molecule and concentration of specific antibodies in the SERS nanotag as well as the choice of the analytical membrane for the SERS-based LFIA were optimized. After the conventional sandwich LFIA procedure, the intensity of MBA Raman scattering in the test zone was measured for quantitative assessment of the analyte. The analytical performance of SERS-based LFIA was compared with ELISA and standard AuNP-based LFIA for SARS-CoV-2 spike RBD detection using the same immunoreagents. The effectivity of SERS-based LFIA for COVID-19 diagnosis was confirmed by detecting spike RBD protein in the SARS-CoV-2 lysate. Compared to the previously mentioned LFIAs for anti-SARS-CoV-2 IgM/IgG detection, which are not recommended for use as the only diagnostic tool as well as for controlling the spread of the virus, the proposed test for determining SARS-CoV-2 Spike RBD, on the contrary, will allow for detecting the virus in the first days following infection.

2. Materials and Methods

2.1. Materials, Chemicals, and Apparatuses

Monoclonal anti-RBD antibodies (MAb), clones RBDF5 and RBDB2, and recombinant RBD were provided by HyTest (Moscow, Russia). Inactivated SARS-CoV-2 virions (2019-nCoV/Victoria/1/2020) in the form of infected Vero cells lysate were obtained from the State Research Center of Virology and Biotechnology «Vector» (Novosibirsk Region, Russia). Goat anti-mouse IgG (GAMI) antibodies were obtained from Arista Biologicals (Allentown, PA, USA). Hydrogen tetrachloroaurate(III) ($HAuCl_4$), sodium citrate, sodium azide, bovine serum albumin (BSA), d-biotin-N-hydroxysuccinimide ester, dimethyl sulfoxide (DMSO), streptavidin conjugated with horseradish peroxidase (STR–HRP), 3,3′,5,5′-

tetramethylbenzidine dihydrochloride (TMB), sucrose, Tris, Tween-20, Triton X-100, and 4-mercaptobenzoic acid were purchased from Sigma-Aldrich (St. Louis, MO, USA). All other chemicals were of analytical grade and used without further purification. All solutions were prepared with ultrapure water (Millipore Corporation, Burlington, MA, USA) with the resistivity of 18.2 MΩ.

The nitrocellulose membranes (CNPC-15 µm, CNPF-10 µm, and 90CNPH), conjugate fiberglass pad (PT-R7), sample pad (GFB-R4), and absorbent pad (AP045) were obtained from Mdi Easypack (Advanced Microdevices; Ambala Cantonment, Haryana, India). Absorption spectra were acquired using spectrophotometer UV-2450 (Shimadzu, Kyoto, Japan). Raman spectra were obtained using Peak seeker Pro 785 Raman spectrometer (Agiltron Inc.; Woburn, MA, USA). The 96-well transparent polystyrene microplates for ELISA were purchased from Corning Costar (Tewksbury, MA, USA). The ELISA results were measured using a Zenyth 3100 microplate spectrophotometer (Anthos Labtec Instruments; Wals, Austria). Transmission electron microscopy (TEM) images were obtained with a JEM-100C electron microscope (JEOL, Tokyo, Japan) operating at 80 kV. The nitrocellulose membranes were processed using an IsoFlow dispenser (Imagene Technology; Lebanon, NH, USA). Test strips were cut using an automatic guillotine Index Cutter-1 (A-Point Technologies; Gibbstown, NJ, USA). The intensity of the coloration was recorded using a CanoScan 9000F (Canon; Tochigi, Japan) scanner. The scanned images were digitally processed by TotalLAB software (Cleaver Scientific; Rugby, UK).

2.2. Biotinylation of Antibody RBDF5

Biotinylation of MAb RBDF5 was carried out as described previously [28]. The molar ratio of biotin to MAb was 10:1. A freshly prepared solution of d-biotin-N-hydroxysuccinimide ester with a concentration of 1 mM in DMSO was added to 200 µL of MAb solution with a concentration of 100 µM in 50 mM PBS containing 0.1 M NaCl (pH 7.4). The mixture was incubated for 2 h on a shaker at room temperature. Thereafter, dialysis against PBS was performed to remove the unbound low molecular weight reagents.

2.3. Sandwich ELISA of RBD

An amount of 100 µL of MAb RBDB2 with a concentration of 1 µg/mL in PBS was added to microplate wells. After incubation at 4 °C for 16 h and four washes by PBS containing 0.05% Triton X-100 (PBST), 100 µL of PBST solutions, containing RBD from 0.5 µg/mL to 0.5 ng/mL, were added and left to bind at 37 °C for 1 h. After the second washing step, 100 µL of biotinylated MAb RBDF5 with a concentration of 1 µg/mL was added to the wells. After incubation at 37 °C for 1 h and washing with PBST, 100 µL of STR–HRP (diluted 1:5000 with PBST) was added to the wells. Following a 1 h incubation at 37 °C, the wells were washed four times with PBST and one time with distilled water, and 100 µL of the substrate solution (0.4 mM TMB and 3 mM H_2O_2 in 40 mM sodium citrate buffer, pH 4.0) was added to the wells. After a further 15 min for the color development, 50 µL of 1 M H_2SO_4 were added to stop the reaction. The resulting optical density at 450 nm (OD450) was measured.

2.4. Preparation of AuNP

AuNPs were prepared using the citrate method [29]. An amount of 10 mL of a 0.01% aqueous solution of $HAuCl_4$ was heated to boiling with the subsequent addition of 0.1 mL of sodium citrate under vigorous stirring. After boiling for 25 min to complete the reduction reaction, the colloidal solution was cooled to room temperature. The AuNP solution was kept in a glass bottle at 4 °C for future use.

2.5. Preparation of Antibody RBDF5 Conjugate with AuNP

MAb RBDF5 were conjugated with AuNPs (RBDF5–AuNP) as described by Panferov et al. [30]. Before the conjugation, the MAb were dialyzed against 10 mM Tris buffer, pH 9.0, for 1 h, at 4 °C. The pH of the AuNP solution was adjusted to 9.0 with 0.1 M K_2CO_3, and then the MAb were added with a concentration of 10 µg/mL. After 45 min stirring, BSA was added to the mixture at a final concentration of 0.25% in solution. The resultant mixture was centrifuged at 15,000× g for 15 min to remove unbound antibodies, followed by sediment resuspension in a 10 mM Tris buffer containing 1% BSA, 1% sucrose, and 0.05% NaN_3 (pH 8.5), and storage at 4 °C.

2.6. Preparation of SERS Nanotag

To prepare the MBA-modified AuNPs (Au^{MBA}), 1 mM MBA solution was added to 10 mL AuNPs to a final concentration in a solution of 1–10 µM. The solution was kept under constant stirring for 3 h to ensure self-assembly of the reporter molecule on the surface of the AuNP. Au^{MBA} were characterized by absorption spectra and TEM.

Anti-RBDF5 antibody-labeled Au^{MBA} (SERS nanotag) was prepared by physical adsorption of antibodies onto AuNPs. First, 10 mL of the Au^{MBA} solution was centrifuged, and the precipitate was redispersed in Milli-Q. After that, 1 mL of Au^{MBA} was adjusted to pH 8.5 with K_2CO_3, and 100 µL of MAb (MAb concentration was from 50 to 250 µg/mL) was added. The mixture was left under constant stirring for 3 h. Finally, 50 µL of 10% BSA was added to block nonspecific binding sites on the surface of the AuNPs. The resulting solution was left to incubate overnight. The next day, the SERS nanotag was centrifuged at 6000 rpm for 20 min at 4 °C, and the pellet was resuspended in PBS containing 5% BSA, 0.025% Tween 20, and 0.05% NaN_3. The SERS nanotag solution was stored at 4 °C for future use.

2.7. Manufacturing of Tests Strips for LFIA

The nitrocellulose membranes were processed using an IsoFlow dispenser. To form the control zone (CZ), a GAMI solution with a concentration of 0.5 mg/mL in PBS was used. To form the test zone (TZ), a solution of MAb RBDB2 with a concentration of 1.0 mg/mL in PBS was used. Of each solution, 32 µL was applied per 240 mm of the width of the sheet of the nitrocellulose membranes. For standard LFIA, the conjugate RBDF5–AuNP (OD = 4.0) was sprayed onto the conjugate membrane in 400 µL per 240 mm membrane length. To form test strips for SERS-based LFIA, the SERS nanotag was applied to the conjugate membrane through the same protocol. After dispensing, all membranes were left to dry at room temperature for about 20 h. The obtained sheets with applied reactants were assembled, including the separation and absorption membranes, and were cut into strips 3.5 mm wide.

2.8. LFIA and Data Processing

Standard AuNP-based LFIA and SERS-based LFIA were performed at room temperature, and solutions of spike RBD protein were prepared in PBST with concentrations from 0.01 to 100 ng/mL and added to the microplate wells in a volume of 100 µL. The test strips were immersed in a vertical position with their lower end for 1 min in an aliquot of the sample, after which they were placed on a horizontal surface. The intensity of the TZ coloration was assessed after 10 min and recorded using a scanner, after which the images were digitally processed by TotalLAB software. The LFIA results were presented as the dependence of the colorimetric intensity on the log concentration to produce a sigmoidal curve.

2.9. SERS-Based LFIA and Data Processing

After the conventional procedure of LFIA, SERS spectra of the TZ were recorded with a Peak seeker Pro 785 Raman spectrometer (785 nm, 30 mW, the integration time was 10 s). The measurements were carried out in three independent repetitions (for three different points inside TZ and for two sets of test strips). The peak intensity of the SERS nanotag at 1076 cm^{-1} was used to quantify SESR signal. The background signal was counted as three times the standard deviation of the signal from the analytical membrane and nonspecifically adsorbed nanotags.

2.10. Spike RBD Protein Detection in the Lysate of SARS-CoV-2 Infected Vero Cell

The effectivity and reliability of the developed SERS-based LFIA were assessed by detecting the spike RBD protein in Vero cell lysates that contained infectious SARS-CoV-2 virions [30]. The inactivation of SARS-CoV-2 virus was performed by treatment with β-propiolactone. Since the concentration of epitopes could not be determined, solutions of the viral lysate in PBST to be analyzed were prepared by serial dilutions in the microplate wells, followed by the SERS-based LFIA procedure described in Section 2.5.

3. Results

3.1. Principle of SERS-Based LFIA for Detection of SARS-CoV-2 RBD

The principle of SERS-based LFIA depicted in Figure 1 is similar to the standard sandwich scheme of LFIA, except for the composition of the immunoconjugate (SERS nanotag in this case), which provides a detectable SERS signal for quantitative analysis of SARS-CoV-2 RBD spike protein. When the sample reached the conjugate pad, the RBD interacted with the SERS nanotag to form an immunocomplex, SERS Nanotag–RBD. The immunocomplex continued to move along the analytical membrane and was captured by immobilized anti-RBD MAb in the TZ, forming a colored band corresponding to the sandwich immunocomplex anti-RBD MAb–RBD–SERS Nanotag. The excess of SERS nanotag continued to move to the CZ, where it was captured by GAMI, forming a colored control band. Thus, the presence of the target protein in the sample results in the formation of two colored bands. Accordingly, the intensity of the characteristic peaks in the SERS spectra from the SERS nanotag is directly proportional to the protein content in the sample and can be used to graph a calibration curve for the quantitative determination of the RBD.

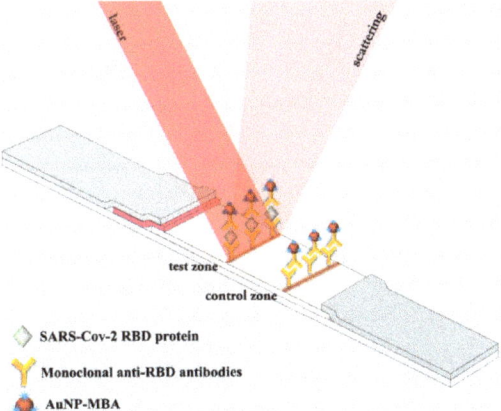

Figure 1. Schematic principle of SERS-based LFIA for RBD protein detection using SERS nanotag.

3.2. Characterization of AuNP and MBA-Modified AuNP

The structure and morphology of AuNP and Au^{MBA} were characterized by TEM and absorption spectroscopy. The TEM image revealed the monodispersed nanoparticles with a diameter distribution in the range of 24.2–40.3 nm. The average diameter of AuNPs was 31.4 ± 3.6 nm with an ellipticity of 1.1 (Figure 2A). In this study, non-covalent conjugation was preferable since this method is gentle and straightforward and allows antibodies to be immobilized on the surface of nanoparticles modified by reporter molecules with minimal conformational changes. Since 4-mercaptobenzoic acid molecules are adsorbed on the surface of AuNPs through the S-atom, and the binding of antibodies to AuNPs is dominated by electrostatic interactions between the negatively charged surface of nanoparticles promoted by carboxylic groups of MBA and antibodies containing a positive charge, it is assumed that the reporter does not significantly affect the adsorption of antibodies [31,32].

For adsorption of MBA on the surface of AuNP through thiol groups, different amounts of MBA were added to 10 mL of the colloidal solution so that its final concentration was from 1 to 10 µM. TEM measurements of AuNPs modified by 1 µM MBA demonstrated a slight increase in the average diameter up to 31.3 ± 2.9 nm with an ellipticity of 1.2 (Figure 2B). The diameter distribution was from 23.8 nm to 40.2 nm.

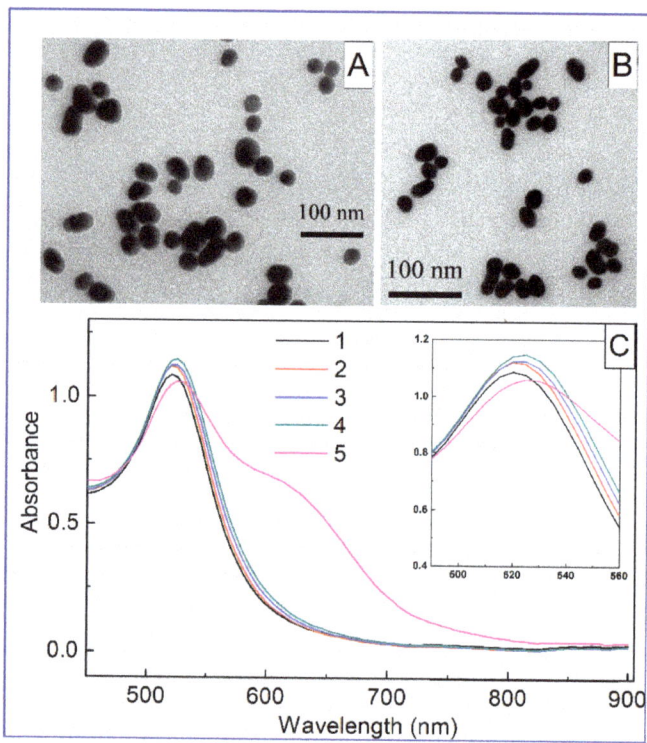

Figure 2. TEM image of bare AuNPs (**A**) and MBA-modified AuNP (**B**). (**C**) Absorbance spectra of bare AuNP (1) and Au^{MBA} at 1 µM (2), 3 µM (3), 5 µM (4), and 10 µM (5) concentrations. The inset shows an enlarged portion of spectra.

Figure 2C displays the spectra of nanoparticles after incubation with MBA. Bare AuNPs demonstrate surface plasmon resonance at 525 nm. AuNP solutions functionalized with 1 µM, 3 µM, and 5 µM MBA demonstrate a gradual shift in the absorption peak (insert in Figure 2C), which is associated with the formation of an MBA shell around the nanoparticles and an increase in the aggregation of nanoparticles. However, the Au^{MBA} functionalized with 10 µM MBA aggregated, as evidenced by the shift of the peak and broadening of the absorption spectrum. Therefore, further experiments continued with AuNPs containing 1 µM, 3 µM, and 5 µM MBA.

3.3. The Optimization of Experimental Conditions of SERS-Based LFIA

To achieve the best performance of SERS-based LFIA, several experimental conditions were investigated. The concentrations of capture antibodies and GAMI applied to the analytical membrane to form TZ and CZ, respectively, were adjusted in a previous study [30]. In this work, the parameters that affect the performance of the SERS-based LFIA were optimized, namely, the MBA and MAb RBDF5 content in SERS nanotag and the choice of the analytical membrane. At the first stage, AuNPs modified with MBA, where the concentration of reporter molecule was 1 µM, 3 µM, and 5 µM, were obtained and 2 µL of the as-prepared Au^{MBA} probes with the AuNPs concentration of 30 nM was pipetted onto the analytical membrane in the form of a spot. Comparison of the Raman intensity of the characteristic band at 1076 cm^{-1} versus the MBA concentration, illustrated in Figure 3A, showed a higher value of Raman signal for the Au^{MBA} containing 3 µM MBA. A slight decrease in the SERS intensity when applying AuNPs modified with 5 µM MBA can be explained by the inverse effect of aggregation of nanoparticles, which leads to an unreproducible SERS signal and photodamage of analyte in the hot spot [33,34]. Further investigation of the dependences of the Raman intensity on the MBA concentration in the SERS nanotag after conjugation with MAb RBDF5, carried out as in the previous experiment, revealed similar results (Figure 3A). Therefore, for the development of the SERS-based LFIA, two SERS nanotags containing 1 µM and 3 µM of MBA were chosen.

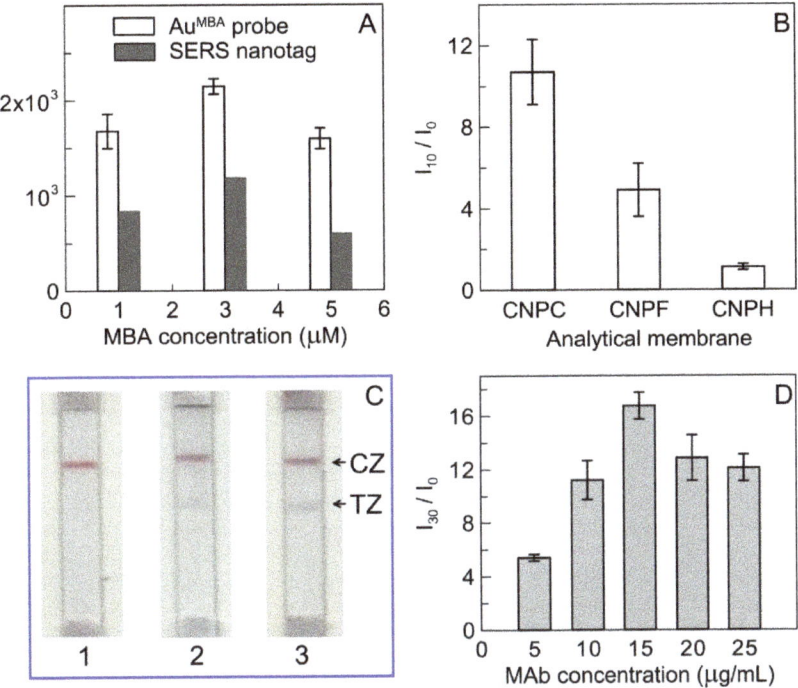

Figure 3. (**A**) Dependence of the Raman intensity on the concentration of MBA in the Au^{MBA} probe and SERS nanotag. (**B**) Optimization of analytical membrane. (**C**) Images of test strips after conventional procedure of LFIA using SERS nanotags with 1 µM (1), 3 µM (2), and 5 µM (3) of MBA. (**D**) Optimization of antibody concentration to prepare SERS nanotags; the positive control contains 10 or 30 ng/mL of RBD. PBS containing 1% v/v Tween 20 is used as a negative control.

The choice of the analytical membrane is an important step in the SERS-based LFIA development because it contributes to the flow rate of the SERS nanotag and to the binding of the SERS nanotag–RBD immunoprobe to the immobilized MAb in the TZ. The effect of three analytical membranes (namely, CNPC, CNPF, and CNPH) was investigated. The pore size and flow rate for the used analytical membranes differ at no more than one and a half times (https://mdimembrane.com/, accessed on 30 October 2021). The membranes differ also in the used additional reactants to vary protein-binding capacity, but the chemical nature of these reactants is a know-how of the manufacturer. It may be noted that the lowest colorimetric signal for membrane CNPH accords to the maximal flow rate that could be insufficient to complete the immunoreaction. The highest colorimetric signal for membrane CNPC was confirmed by the SERS measurements, according to its higher protein binding capacity than CNPF. As shown in Figure 3B, the normalized intensity (I/I_0) of the characteristic band at 1076 cm^{-1} was significantly higher than the bands for CNPF and CNPH. Therefore, CNPC membrane was chosen for further study.

At the next stage, the selected SERS nanotags were immobilized on the conjugate pad, and the standard procedure of colorimetric LFIA was carried out. As shown in the images of the scanned test strips after analysis (Figure 3C), in the case of the SERS nanotag containing 3 µM MBA, a background signal was observed in the absence of the target RBD. Thus, the obtained results showed that the SERS nanotag containing 1 µM MBA is optimal for SERS-based LFIA.

Another important parameter affecting the sensitivity of the SERS-based LFIA is the MAb load in the SERS nanotag. In the preparation of SERS nanotag, different amounts of anti-RBDF5 MAb were added so that the final concentration of MAb in the solution was from 5 to 25 µg/mL. The effect of MAb concentration on normalized SERS intensity (I/I_0) was investigated (Figure 3D). An increase in the normalized SERS intensity was observed with an increase in the concentration of MAb up to 15 µg/mL, whereas a further increase in a load of antibodies in the SERS nanotag was accompanied by a plateau for the dependence of I/I_0 on MAb concentration. Thus, 15 µg/mL of MAb RBDF5 is the optimal concentration for the preparation of the SERS nanotag, which provides the highest signal-to-background ratio.

3.4. SERS-Based LFIA for RBD Detection

To assess the analytical performance of SERS-based LFIA, RBD solutions were prepared in the range from 0.01 to 100 ng/mL by diluting the analyte in PBST. After the completion of the colorimetric LFIA procedure, the color changes provided by the binding of the SERS nanotag in the TZ were observed (Figure 4A). In the colorimetric-based LFIA, a red band was visually observed where the analyte concentration was above 1 ng/mL. The quantitative assessment of colorimetric-based LFIA resulted in a 1.2 ng/mL detection limit and an operating range from 4.2 to 60.4 ng/mL (Figure 4B). The duration of the colorimetric LFIA was 15 min. Figure 4C displays the average SERS spectra acquired in the TZ for different analyte concentrations. According to the sandwich scheme of analysis, with an increase in the RBD concentration, the SERS intensity at 1076 cm^{-1} generated from the SERS nanotag gradually increases. Compared to colorimetric LFIA, characteristic MBA bands are observed in the SERS spectra without the target analyte. This phenomenon may be associated with the nonspecific binding of the SERS nanotag on the analytical membrane. Starting from the analyte concentration of 0.1 ng/mL, the characteristic peak of the SERS nanotag is reliably distinguishable from the background signal. The calibration curve represented by the dependence of the SERS signal intensity on the analyte concentration is shown in Figure 4D. The detection limit of RBD was defined as the minimum concentration at which the signal was three times the standard deviation of the background signal. The limit of RBD detection was calculated to be 0.1 ng/mL, with a working range from 0.1 to 10 ng/mL. Comparison of the results obtained by colorimetric LFIA with SERS-based LFIA for RBD detection demonstrated enhanced sensitivity by one order of magnitude. Based on the molecular weights of RBD, protein S and SARS-CoV-2 virion and S protein content in the virion [35–37], the given LOD value corresponds to 4 pM RBD (or protein S monomer). This concentration can be achieved in the case of complete lysis while maintaining the antigenic properties of SARS-CoV-2 virions at a concentration of 0.06 pM.

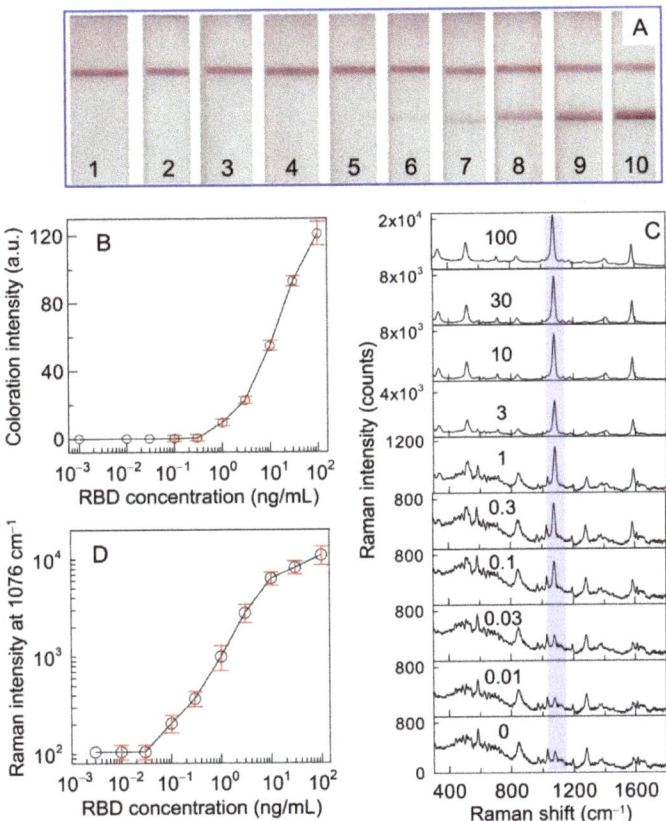

Figure 4. (**A**) Photographic images of LFIA strips after application of RBD at concentrations 0 (1), 0.01 (2). 0.03 (3), 0.1 (4), 0.3 (5), 1 (6), 3 (7), 10 (8), 30 (9), and 100 ng/mL (10). The top and bottom lines correspond to the control and test zones, respectively. (**B**) Calibration curve obtained after conventional LFIA procedure using SERS nanotags. The error bars indicate the STD for three measurements; (**C**) SERS spectra measured in the test line for RBD concentrations from 0.01 to 100 ng/mL. (**D**) Calibration curve of SERS-LFIA for RBD. The bars show the STD of the Raman signal at 1076 cm^{-1}, measured from three independent SERS-based LFIA runs.

The effectiveness of the developed SERS-based LFIA was evaluated in the determination of RBD protein in the SARS-CoV-2 lysate. SARS-CoV-2-inactivated virions were diluted multiple times in PBST and applied to the sample pad. Figure 5 demonstrates photographic images of test strips after completion of colorimetric LFIA procedure (Figure 5A) and compares the calibration curves obtained for colorimetric (Figure 5B) and SERS (Figure 5D) detection, respectively. The background signal consists of two sources: (1) the membrane background and (2) the signal from nonspecifically captured nanoparticles when the buffer is used instead of an analyte solution. In SERS-based LFIA for protein determination in lysate, the second contribution seems to be more intensive compared to that for RBD detection due to enhanced signal from nonspecifically captured particles. As follows from the SERS spectra acquired in the TZ after the analysis of the lysate, the SERS intensity of the band at 1076 cm^{-1} decreased with increasing sample dilution (Figure 5C). The spike protein was detected colorimetrically under conditions when the lysate was diluted 222 times, while SERS-based LFIA allowed for identifying the protein when the lysate was diluted 1250 times.

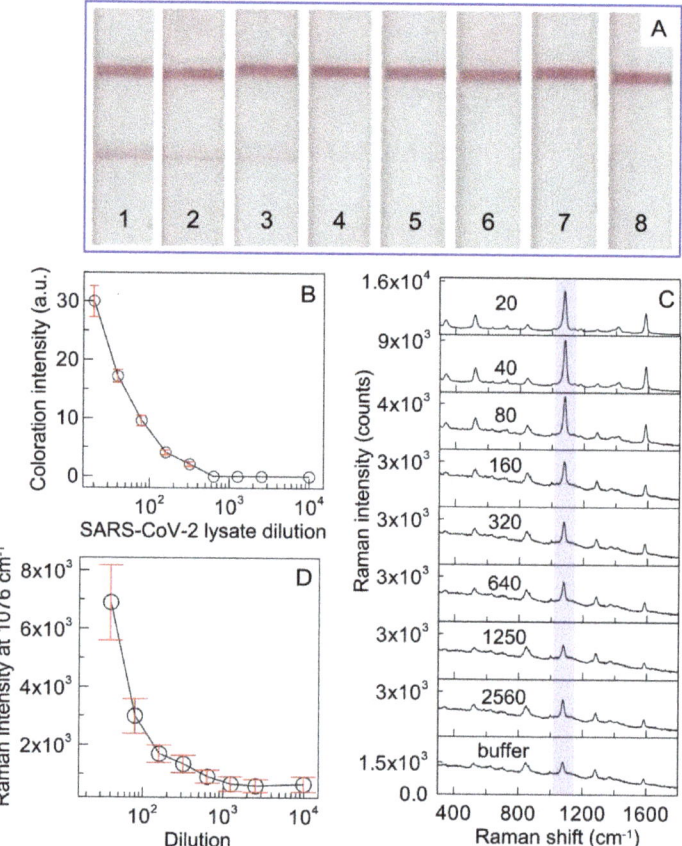

Figure 5. (**A**) Photographic images of LFIA strips after application of the lysate at sequential two-fold dilutions of 20 (1), 40 (2), 80 (3), 160 (4), 320 (5), 640 (6), 1280 (7), and 2560 (8); (**B**) Calibration curve obtained after conventional LFIA procedure using SERS nanotags as immunoprobe for spike RBD detection in SARS-CoV-2 viral lysate. The error bars indicate the STD for three measurements; (**C**) SERS spectra measured in the TZ for different lysate dilutions. The numbers mean the dilution. (**D**) Dependence of the SERS intensity on the lysate dilution. The bars show the STD of the Raman signal at 1076 cm^{-1}, measured at five points in the middle of the test line.

3.5. Comparison of SERS-Based LFIA with ELISA and Standard AuNP-Based LFIA

Of particular interest when integrating an immunoassay with quantitative readout techniques is the comparison of the achieved analytical characteristics with those obtained by standard ELISA and AuNP-based LFIA methods. For the grounded conclusion from the experimental data, three formats of immunoassay were carried out using the same immunoreagents. Moreover, the concentration of capture MAb immobilized on the analytical membrane and detecting MAb in the labeled immunoconjugate was the same for standard LFIA and SERS-based LFIA using SERS nanotag. The calibration curve of ELISA for RBD is shown in Figure 6A. Under optimized conditions, the ELISA demonstrated a working range between 7.8 and 59.9 ng/mL with a detection limit of RBD at 0.4 ng/mL. The time of analysis was 3.5 h. After assembly of standard LFIA test strips with pre-impregnated immunocomponents, analysis of samples containing RBD in the range from 0.01 to 100 ng/mL showed a visual limit of detection at 1 ng/mL. Instrumental assessment of the LFIA results with plotting the dependence of the staining intensity of the TZ on the RBD concentration revealed a working range between 1.3 and 35.4 ng/mL with a detection limit of 0.5 ng/mL (Figure 6B). The standard qualitative AuNP-based LFIA takes 15 min. Comparing the three formats of immunoassay, it should be noted that the proposed SERS-based LFIA format combines the advantages of the considered standard ELISA and LFIA and provides an increase in the sensitivity owing to the implementation of SERS as a readout technique. Clearly, the integration of LFIA with the SERS technique involves using an additional device—a Raman spectrometer. However, today—thanks to the popularity and advantages of this method—the SERS technique is developing toward miniaturization and cost reduction. Recently, the successful development and applications of handheld Raman spectrometers were demonstrated for LFIA of various biomarkers [22,38]. The miniaturization and cost reduction of SERS-based readers makes them a promising and potential tool for developing rapid, highly sensitive, and quantitative on-site LFIA tests. In view of the aforementioned, the current study can be considered as confirmation of the prospects for further technical development of SERS-based LFIA.

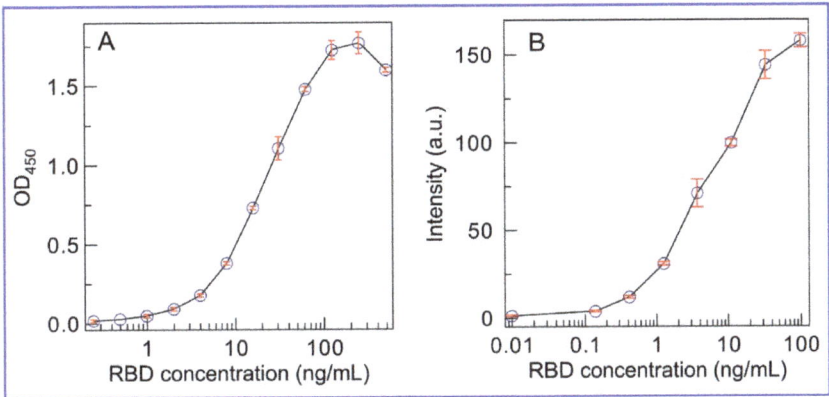

Figure 6. Calibration curves for spike RBD protein using ELISA (**A**) and standard AuNP-based LFIA (**B**). The error bars indicate the STD for three measurements.

4. Discussion

In the context of the ongoing COVID-19 pandemic, the development of new technologies for early detection of the virus and determination of the body's response to the virus, complementing the laborious PCR testing and expanding the range of diagnostic techniques, is a priority area of research worldwide. Rapid lateral flow assay is a valuable tool for diagnosing and monitoring various diseases [39–42]. To date, rapid diagnostics of COVID-19 to determine the antigen and the presence of IgG/IgM antibodies to SARS-CoV-2 to prevent the spread of the virus is carried out using lateral flow tests [43,44]. In parallel, other methods of virus identification are being developed, including electrochemical sensors, colorimetric tests, and SERS sensors [45–47]. The latter has limitations associated with complex procedures for preparing the metal substrate, and in the case of direct SERS detection, with the difficulty of obtaining an intrinsic spectrum of the target analyte.

This study offers an integrated approach of lateral flow assay with a highly sensitive SERS detection, where the concentration of the analyte in one place and its highly specific determination is provided by the immunochemical principles of the analysis. The AuNP modified by MBA and conjugated with anti-RBD MAb were used as a SERS nanotag for quantitative LFIA detection. Compared to the preparation of SERS substrates, ensuring the reproducibility of SERS biosensors, the colloidal gold solution used in this work is easy to synthesize, is homogeneous, and allows for the measurements of AuNPs-based SERS nanotags on portable Raman spectrometers with high laser power and long exposure times. To achieve high analytical characteristics, the concentration of the reporter molecule and MAb in the SERS nanotag as well as the type of analytical membrane were optimized. Summarizing the results obtained, the proposed SERS-based LFIA demonstrates good performance for the detection of spike RBD protein and exhibits the effectiveness for identifying spike RBD protein in the viral lysate.

Comparison of the analytical performance of the developed SERS-based LFIA with those obtained by the membrane-based tests for detection of RBD of surface S-protein of SARS-CoV-2 is shown in Table 1. According to the overviewed membrane-based immunoassay techniques, the proposed SERS-based LFIA demonstrates comparable, and in some cases, superior performance for RBD determination.

Table 1. Comparison of different SERS detection strategies for SARS-CoV-2 spike RBD protein.

Sensor	Limit of Detection	Sample	Ref.
Colloidal gold-based immunochromatographic strip	62.5 ng/mL	Standard solution	[48]
Chemiluminescence paper assay using Co–Fe@hemin-peroxidase nanozyme	0.1 ng/mL	Standard solution	[49]
LFIA using gold-enhanced AuNP	1 pg/mL	Saliva	[30]
Paper-based antigen test	0.07 nM	Standard solution	[50]
LFIA using mesoporous Si encapsulated up-conversion nanoparticles	1.6 ng/mL	Standard solution	[51]
SERS-based LFIA	0.1 ng/mL	Standard solution	This work

5. Conclusions

In this study, the SERS-based LFIA, combining the specificity and rapidity of traditional ELISA and LFIA methods with susceptible SERS readout technique, was developed for SARS-CoV-2 spike RBD protein detection. Comparison of the three immunoassay formats revealed a decrease in the order of magnitude in the antigen detection limit after quantitative measurement of the Raman intensities of the captured SERS nanotag. The SERS-based LFIA allows for the quantitative determination of RBD in 20 min. The developed SERS-based LFIA was validated by spike RBD protein determination in inactivated SARS-CoV-2 virions. In summary, the proposed SERS-based LFIA is an alternative and complementary approach to current laboratory methods providing early, rapid, and on-site diagnosis of COVID-19.

Author Contributions: Conceptualization, K.V.S., N.A.B. and B.B.D.; methodology, N.G.K. and B.B.D.; validation, K.V.S., N.A.B. and S.F.B.; formal analysis, K.V.S. and A.V.Z.; investigation, K.V.S., N.A.B. and B.N.K.; resources, S.F.B. and B.B.D.; data curation, A.V.Z. and B.B.D.; writing—original draft preparation, K.V.S.; writing—review and editing, all authors; visualization, K.V.S., N.A.B., B.N.K.; supervision, B.B.D.; project administration, S.F.B. and B.B.D.; funding acquisition, S.F.B. and B.B.D. All authors have read and agreed to the published version of the manuscript.

Funding: This research was funded by the Ministry of Science and Higher Education of Russia, grant number 075-15-2019-1671, 31 October 2019.

Institutional Review Board Statement: Not applicable.

Informed Consent Statement: Not applicable.

Data Availability Statement: Data are presented in the article. Initial instrumental output data are available upon request from corresponding author.

Conflicts of Interest: The authors declare no conflict of interest.

References

1. Gorbalenya, A.E.; Baker, S.C.; Baric, R.S.; de Groot, R.J.; Drosten, C.; Gulyaeva, A.A.; Haagmans, B.L.; Lauber, C.; Leontovich, A.M.; Neuman, B.W.; et al. The species severe acute respiratory syndrome-related coronavirus: Classifying 2019-nCoV and naming it SARS-CoV-2. *Nat. Microbiol.* **2020**, *5*, 536–544. [CrossRef]
2. Synowiec, A.; Szczepański, A.; Barreto-Duran, E.; Lie, L.K.; Pyrc, K. Severe acute respiratory syndrome coronavirus 2 (SARS-CoV-2): A systemic infection. *Clin. Microbiol. Rev.* **2021**, *34*, e00133-20. [CrossRef] [PubMed]
3. Mariano, G.; Farthing, R.J.; Lale-Farjat, S.L.M.; Bergeron, J.R.C. Structural characterization of SARS-CoV-2: Where we are, and where we need to be. *Front. Mol. Biosci.* **2020**, *7*, 605236. [CrossRef] [PubMed]
4. Chen, W.; Feng, P.; Liu, K.; Wu, M.; Lin, H. Computational identification of small interfering RNA targets in SARS-CoV-2. *Virol. Sin.* **2020**, *35*, 359–361. [CrossRef]

5. Wassie, G.T.; Azene, A.G.; Bantie, G.M.; Dessie, G.; Aragaw, A.M. Incubation period of severe acute respiratory syndrome novel coronavirus 2 that causes coronavirus disease 2019: A systematic review and meta-analysis. *Curr. Ther. Res. Clin. Exp.* **2020**, *93*, 100607. [CrossRef]
6. Zaki, N.; Mohamed, E.A. The estimations of the COVID-19 incubation period: A scoping reviews of the literature. *J. Infect. Public Health* **2021**, *14*, 638–646. [CrossRef] [PubMed]
7. Tsatsakis, A.; Calina, D.; Falzone, L.; Petrakis, D.; Mitrut, R.; Siokas, V.; Pennisi, M.; Lanza, G.; Libra, M.; Doukas, S.G.; et al. SARS-CoV-2 pathophysiology and its clinical implications: An integrative overview of the pharmacotherapeutic management of COVID-19. *Food Chem. Toxicol.* **2020**, *146*, 111769. [CrossRef]
8. Vaira, L.A.; Salzano, G.; Deiana, G.; De Riu, G. Anosmia and ageusia: Common findings in COVID-19 patients. *Laryngoscope* **2020**, *130*, 1787. [CrossRef]
9. Bouadma, L.; Wiedemann, A.; Patrier, J.; Surénaud, M.; Wicky, P.-H.; Foucat, E.; Diehl, J.-L.; Hejblum, B.P.; Sinnah, F.; de Montmollin, E.; et al. Immune alterations in a patient with SARS-CoV-2-related acute respiratory distress syndrome. *J. Clin. Immunol.* **2020**, *40*, 1082–1092. [CrossRef]
10. WHO. *Coronavirus Disease (COVID-19): Situation Report*, 60th ed.; Coronavirus Disease; WHO: Geneva, Switzerland, 2019.
11. Kanji, J.N.; Zelyas, N.; MacDonald, C.; Pabbaraju, K.; Khan, M.N.; Prasad, A.; Hu, J.; Diggle, M.; Berenger, B.M.; Tipples, G. False negative rate of COVID-19 PCR testing: A discordant testing analysis. *Virol. J.* **2021**, *18*, 13. [CrossRef] [PubMed]
12. Lascarrou, J.-B.; Colin, G.; Le Thuaut, A.; Serck, N.; Ohana, M.; Sauneuf, B.; Geri, G.; Mesland, J.-B.; Ribeyre, G.; Hussenet, C.; et al. Predictors of negative first SARS-CoV-2 RT-PCR despite final diagnosis of COVID-19 and association with outcome. *Sci. Rep.* **2021**, *11*, 2388. [CrossRef]
13. Schuler, C.F.; Gherasim, C.; O'Shea, K.; Manthei, D.M.; Chen, J.; Giacherio, D.; Troost, J.P.; Baldwin, J.L.; Baker, J.R. Accurate point-of-care serology tests for COVID-19. *PLoS ONE* **2021**, *16*, e0248729. [CrossRef] [PubMed]
14. Pickering, S.; Batra, R.; Snell, L.B.; Merrick, B.; Nebbia, G.; Douthwaite, S.; Patel, A.; Ik, M.T.K.; Patel, B.; Charalampous, T.; et al. Comparative performance of SARS-CoV-2 lateral flow antigen tests and association with detection of infectious virus in clinical specimens: A single-centre laboratory evaluation study. *Lancet Microbe* **2021**, *2*, e461–e471. [CrossRef]
15. Khlebtsov, B.; Khlebtsov, N. Surface-enhanced Raman scattering-based lateral-flow immunoassay. *Nanomaterials* **2020**, *10*, 2228. [CrossRef]
16. Ding, S.-Y.; You, E.-M.; Tian, Z.-Q.; Moskovits, M. Electromagnetic theories of surface-enhanced Raman spectroscopy. *Chem. Soc. Rev.* **2017**, *46*, 4042–4076. [CrossRef]
17. Khlebtsov, B.N.; Bratashov, D.N.; Byzova, N.A.; Dzantiev, B.B.; Khlebtsov, N.G. SERS-based lateral flow immunoassay of troponin I by using gap-enhanced Raman tags. *Nano Res.* **2019**, *12*, 413–420. [CrossRef]
18. Chen, S.; Meng, L.; Wang, L.; Huang, X.; Ali, S.; Chen, X.; Yu, M.; Yi, M.; Li, L.; Chen, X.; et al. SERS-based lateral flow immunoassay for sensitive and simultaneous detection of anti-SARS-CoV-2 IgM and IgG antibodies by using gap-enhanced Raman nanotags. *Sens. Actuators B Chem.* **2021**, *348*, 130706. [CrossRef]
19. Fan, R.; Tang, S.; Luo, S.; Liu, H.; Zhang, W.; Yang, C.; He, L.; Chen, Y. Duplex surface enhanced Raman scattering-based lateral flow immunosensor for the low-level detection of antibiotic residues in milk. *Molecules* **2020**, *25*, 5249. [CrossRef]
20. Hassanain, W.A.; Spoors, J.; Johnson, C.L.; Faulds, K.; Keegan, N.; Graham, D. Rapid ultra-sensitive diagnosis of *Clostridium difficile* infection using a SERS-based lateral flow assay. *Analyst* **2021**, *146*, 4495–4505. [CrossRef]
21. Ma, Y.; Liu, H.; Chen, Y.; Gu, C.; Wei, G.; Jiang, T. Improved lateral flow strip based on hydrophilic−hydrophobic SERS substrate for ultra−sensitive and quantitative immunoassay. *Appl. Surf. Sci.* **2020**, *529*, 147121. [CrossRef]
22. Li, Y.; Liu, X.; Guo, J.; Zhang, Y.; Guo, J.; Wu, X.; Wang, B.; Ma, X. Simultaneous detection of inflammatory biomarkers by SERS nanotag-based lateral flow assay with portable cloud Raman spectrometer. *Nanomaterials* **2021**, *11*, 1496. [CrossRef] [PubMed]
23. Liu, X.; Yang, X.; Li, K.; Liu, H.; Xiao, R.; Wang, W.; Wang, C.; Wang, S. Fe3O4@Au SERS tags-based lateral flow assay for simultaneous detection of serum amyloid A and C-reactive protein in unprocessed blood sample. *Sens. Actuators B Chem.* **2020**, *320*, 128350. [CrossRef]
24. Xi, J.; Yu, Q. The development of lateral flow immunoassay strip tests based on surface enhanced Raman spectroscopy coupled with gold nanoparticles for the rapid detection of soybean allergen β-conglycinin. *Spectrochim. Acta Part A Mol. Biomol. Spectrosc.* **2020**, *241*, 118640. [CrossRef]
25. Huo, C.; Li, D.; Hu, Z.; Li, G.; Hu, Y.; Sun, H. A novel lateral flow assay for rapid and sensitive nucleic acid detection of *Avibacterium paragallinarum*. *Front. Vet. Sci.* **2021**, *8*, 738558. [CrossRef] [PubMed]
26. Shi, L.; Xu, L.; Xiao, R.; Zhou, Z.; Wang, C.; Wang, S.; Gu, B. Rapid, quantitative, high-sensitive detection of *Escherichia coli* O157:H7 by gold-shell silica-core nanospheres-based surface-enhanced Raman scattering lateral flow immunoassay. *Front. Microbiol.* **2020**, *11*, 596005. [CrossRef] [PubMed]
27. Liu, H.; Dai, E.; Xiao, R.; Zhou, Z.; Zhang, M.; Bai, Z.; Shao, Y.; Qi, K.; Tu, J.; Wang, C.; et al. Development of a SERS-based lateral flow immunoassay for rapid and ultra-sensitive detection of anti-SARS-CoV-2 IgM/IgG in clinical samples. *Sens. Actuators B Chem.* **2021**, *329*, 129196. [CrossRef]
28. Bayer, E.A.; Wilchek, M. Protein biotinylation. *Methods Enzymol.* **1990**, *184*, 138–160. [CrossRef] [PubMed]
29. Wuithschick, M.; Birnbaum, A.; Witte, S.; Sztucki, M.; Vainio, U.; Pinna, N.; Rademann, K.; Emmerling, F.; Kraehnert, R.; Polte, J.R. Turkevich in new robes: Key questions answered for the most common gold nanoparticle synthesis. *ACS Nano* **2015**, *9*, 7052–7071. [CrossRef] [PubMed]

30. Panferov, V.G.; Byzova, N.A.; Biketov, S.F.; Zherdev, A.V.; Dzantiev, B.B. Comparative study of in situ techniques to enlarge gold nanoparticles for highly sensitive lateral flow immunoassay of SARS-CoV-2. *Biosensors* **2021**, *11*, 229. [CrossRef]
31. Ma, W.G.; Fang, Y.; Hao, G.L.; Wang, W.G. Adsorption behaviors of 4-mercaptobenzoic acid on silver and gold films. *Chin. J. Chem. Phys.* **2011**, *23*, 659. [CrossRef]
32. Oliveira, M.J.; de Almeida, P.M.; Nunes, D.; Fortunato, E.; Martins, R.; Pereira, E.; Byrne, H.J.; Águas, H.; Franco, R. Design and simple assembly of gold nanostar bioconjugates for surface-enhanced Raman spectroscopy immunoassays. *Nanomaterials* **2019**, *9*, 1561. [CrossRef]
33. Israelsen, N.D.; Wooley, D.; Hanson, C.; Vargis, E. Rational design of Raman-labeled nanoparticles for a dual-modality, light scattering immunoassay on a polystyrene substrate. *J. Biol. Eng.* **2016**, *10*, 2. [CrossRef] [PubMed]
34. Kleinman, S.; Frontiera, R.; Henry, A.-I.; Dieringer, J.; van Duyne, R. Creating, characterizing, and controlling chemistry with SERS hot spots. *Phys. Chem. Chem. Phys.* **2015**, *15*, 21–36. [CrossRef]
35. Ke, Z.; Oton, J.; Qu, K.; Cortese, M.; Zila, V.; McKeane, L.; Nakane, T.; Zivanov, J.; Neufeldt, C.J.; Cerikan, B.; et al. Structures and distributions of SARS-CoV-2 spike proteins on intact virions. *Nature* **2020**, *588*, 498–502. [CrossRef] [PubMed]
36. Huang, Y.; Yang, C.; Xu, X.F.; Xu, W.; Liu, S.W. Structural and functional properties of SARS-CoV-2 spike protein: Potential antivirus drug development for COVID-19. *Acta Pharmacol. Sin.* **2020**, *41*, 1141–1149. [CrossRef]
37. Sender, R.; Bar-On, Y.M.; Gleizer, S.; Bernsthein, B.; Flamholz, A.; Phillips, R.; Milo, R. The total number and mass of SARS-CoV-2 virions. *Proc. Natl. Acad. Sci. USA* **2021**, *118*, e2024815118. [CrossRef]
38. Xiao, R.; Lu, L.; Rong, Z.; Wang, C.; Peng, Y.; Wang, F.; Sun, M.; Dong, J.; Wang, D.; et al. Portable and multiplexed lateral flow immunoassay reader based on SERS for highly sensitive point-of-care testing. *Biosens. Bioelectron.* **2020**, *168*, 112524. [CrossRef] [PubMed]
39. Di Nardo, F.; Chiarello, M.; Cavalera, S.; Baggiani, C.; Anfossi, L. Ten years of lateral flow immunoassay technique applications: Trends, challenges and future perspectives. *Sensors* **2021**, *21*, 5185. [CrossRef]
40. Byzova, N.A.; Zherdev, A.V.; Vengerov, Y.Y.; Starovoitova, T.A.; Dzantiev, B.B. A triple immunochromatographic test for simultaneous determination of cardiac troponin I, fatty acid binding protein, and C-reactive protein biomarkers. *Microchim. Acta* **2017**, *184*, 463–471. [CrossRef]
41. Serebrennikova, K.V.; Samsonova, J.V.; Osipov, A.P. A semi-quantitative rapid multi-range gradient lateral flow immunoassay for procalcitonin. *Microchim. Acta* **2019**, *186*, 423. [CrossRef]
42. Wang, K.; Qin, W.; Hou, Y.; Xiao, K.; Yan, W. The application of lateral flow immunoassay in point of care testing: A review. *Nano Biomed. Eng.* **2016**, *8*, 172–183. [CrossRef]
43. Bernasconi, L.; Oberle, M.; Gisler, V.; Ottiger, C.; Fankhauser, H.; Schuetz, P.; Fux, C.A.; Hammerer-Lercher, A. Diagnostic performance of a SARS-CoV-2 IgG/IgM lateral flow immunochromatography assay in symptomatic patients presenting to the emergency department. *Clin. Chem. Lab. Med.* **2020**, *58*, e159–e161. [CrossRef] [PubMed]
44. Basgalupp, S.; dos Santos, G.; Bessel, M.; Garcia, L.; de Moura, A.C.; Rocha, A.C.; Brito, E.; de Miranda, G.; Dornelles, T.; Dartora, W.; et al. Diagnostic properties of three SARS-CoV-2 antibody tests. *Diagnostics* **2021**, *11*, 1441. [CrossRef]
45. Vadlamani, B.S.; Uppal, T.; Verma, S.C.; Misra, M. Functionalized TiO2 nanotube-based electrochemical biosensor for rapid detection of SARS-CoV-2. *Sensors* **2020**, *20*, 5871. [CrossRef] [PubMed]
46. Büyüksünetçi, Y.T.; Çitil, B.E.; Tapan, U.; Anık, U. Development and application of a SARS-CoV-2 colorimetric biosensor based on the peroxidase-mimic activity of γ-Fe2O3 nanoparticles. *Microchim. Acta* **2021**, *188*, 335. [CrossRef]
47. Daoudi, K.; Ramachandran, K.; Alawadhi, H.; Boukherroub, R.; Dogheche, E.; Khakani, M.; Gaidi, M. Ultra-sensitive and fast optical detection of the spike protein of the SARS-CoV-2 using AgNPs/SiNWs nanohybrid based sensors. *Surf. Interfaces* **2021**, *27*, 101454. [CrossRef]
48. Li, G.; Wang, A.; Chen, Y.; Sun, Y.; Du, Y.; Wang, X.; Ding, P.; Jia, R.; Wang, Y.; Zhang, G. Development of a colloidal gold-based immunochromatographic strip for rapid detection of severe acute respiratory syndrome coronavirus 2 spike protein. *Front. Immunol.* **2021**, *12*, 635677. [CrossRef] [PubMed]
49. Liu, D.; Ju, C.; Han, C.; Shi, R.; Chen, X.; Duan, D.; Yan, J.; Yan, X. Nanozyme chemiluminescence paper test for rapid and sensitive detection of SARS-CoV-2 antigen. *Biosens. Bioelectron.* **2020**, *173*, 112817. [CrossRef] [PubMed]
50. Hristov, D.; Rijal, H.; Gomez-Marquez, J.; Hamad-Schifferli, K. Developing a paper-based antigen assay to differentiate between coronaviruses and SARS-CoV-2 spike variants. *Anal. Chem.* **2021**, *93*, 7825–7832. [CrossRef] [PubMed]
51. Guo, J.; Chen, S.; Tian, S.; Liu, K.; Ni, J.; Zhao, M.; Kang, Y.; Ma, X.; Guo, J. 5G-enabled ultra-sensitive fluorescence sensor for proactive prognosis of COVID-19. *Biosens. Bioelectron.* **2021**, *181*, 113160. [CrossRef] [PubMed]

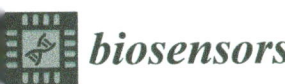

Communication

Lateral Flow Immunoassay Coupled with Copper Enhancement for Rapid and Sensitive SARS-CoV-2 Nucleocapsid Protein Detection

Tao Peng [1], Xueshima Jiao [1,2], Zhanwei Liang [1,2], Hongwei Zhao [3], Yang Zhao [1], Jie Xie [1], You Jiang [1], Xiaoping Yu [2], Xiang Fang [1] and Xinhua Dai [1,*]

1. Technology Innovation Center of Mass Spectrometry for State Market Regulation, Center for Advanced Measurement Science, National Institute of Metrology, Beijing 100029, China; pengtao@nim.ac.cn (T.P.); s20090710020@cjlu.edu.cn (X.J.); s20090710033@cjlu.edu.cn (Z.L.); zhaoy@nim.ac.cn (Y.Z.); xiejie@nim.ac.cn (J.X.); jiangyou@nim.ac.cn (Y.J.); fangxaing@nim.ac.cn (X.F.)
2. College of Life Sciences, China Jiliang University, Hangzhou 310018, China; yxp@cjlu.edu.cn
3. College of Ecology and Environment, Hainan University, Haikou 570228, China; hwzhao@hainanu.edu.cn
* Correspondence: daixh@nim.ac.cn; Tel.: +86-010-6452-4962; Fax: +86-010-6452-4962

Abstract: The coronavirus disease 2019 (COVID-19) pandemic caused by severe acute respiratory coronavirus 2 (SARS-CoV-2) is still raging all over the world. Hence, the rapid and sensitive screening of the suspected population is in high demand. The nucleocapsid protein (NP) of SARS-CoV-2 has been selected as an ideal marker for viral antigen detection. This study describes a lateral flow immunoassay (LFIA) based on colloidal gold nanoparticles for rapid NP antigen detection, in which sensitivity was improved through copper deposition-induced signal amplification. The detection sensitivity of the developed LFIA for NP antigen detection (using certified reference materials) under the optimized parameters was 0.01 µg/mL and was promoted by three orders of magnitude to 10 pg/mL after copper deposition signal amplification. The LFIA coupled with the copper enhancement technique has many merits such as low cost, high efficiency, and high sensitivity. It provides an effective approach to the rapid screening, diagnosis, and monitoring of the suspected population in the COVID-19 outbreak.

Keywords: SARS-CoV-2; nucleocapsid protein; signal amplification; copper deposition

1. Introduction

The coronavirus disease 2019 (COVID-19) pandemic caused by severe acute respiratory coronavirus 2 (SARS-CoV-2) has spread to 216 countries, and the cumulative number of confirmed cases has exceeded 200 million around the world. Some vaccines have been developed and administered, but the cumulative number of confirmed cases continues to increase every day. Thus, rapid screening, early detection, and timely diagnosis are still the main measures to prevent and control SARS-CoV-2 transmission. Rapid antibody detection was used as the supplementary means of nucleic acid detection for COVID-19 diagnosis before 2021 [1–3]. However, antibody detection has become meaningless for the screening of suspected populations since the beginning of vaccination against COVID-19. Nucleic acid detection is considered the gold standard, but its use is limited because of the time-consuming process, relatively high cost, and high professional and equipment requirements [4]. Hence, direct, rapid, point-of-care viral antigen detection methods without pretreatment are highly needed, especially in countries with serious outbreaks.

Coronavirus particles contain four structural proteins, namely, the nucleocapsid protein (NP), envelope protein, membrane protein, and spike protein [5]. Among them, the NP has been considered an ideal target for early diagnosis since the severe acute respiratory syndrome (SARS) outbreak in 2003 because the NP is predominantly and profusely expressed by severe acute respiratory syndrome coronavirus (SARS-CoV) [6]. The NP antigen can be detected up to 1 day before the appearance of clinical symptoms; thus, NP is considered one of the best markers for SARS-CoV detection [7]. SARS-CoV-2 has high genetic similarity to SARS-CoV [8]; therefore, theoretically, the NP antigen of SARS-CoV-2 can also be used as the diagnostic marker for COVID-19.

Mass spectrometry assays [9], electrochemical immunosensor assays [10,11], and lateral flow immunoassays (LFIAs) [12] have been developed for the detection of the SARS-CoV-2 NP antigen. Immunoassays, which are based on the specific reactions between antigen and antibody, may be a good choice for NP antigen detection because of their simple, convenient, and quick process. The LFIA, which combines chromatography technology with conventional immunoassay and nanomaterials, is considered the most attractive point-of-care testing device because it exhibits several advantages, including simple technical requirements, rapid detection capability, portability, affordability, high detection accuracy, and high efficiency [13]. Recently, colloidal gold nanoparticles (GCNPs), latex beads, fluorescent microspheres, and quantum dots have been used as labels to develop LFIAs for the rapid and sensitive screening of the NP antigen. For instance, Kim et al. [14] developed a cellulose nanobead-based LFIA platform using NP-specific single-chain variable fragment-crystallizable fragment fusion antibodies; Nichols' group [12] described a half-strip LFIA with latex beads as the indicator, and Diao et al. [15] developed a fluorescence LFIA to rapidly detect the SARS-CoV-2 NP antigen in the laboratory. In addition, several antigen detection kits based on LFIAs have been approved by the National Medical Products Administration and marked as "Conformité Européenne". However, the sensitivity of antigen detection was unsatisfactory compared with that of the reverse transcription-polymerase chain reaction assay [16,17]. Hence, the promotion of LFIA sensitivity is key for the rapid detection of SARS-CoV-2 NP antigen.

Wang's group have applied a high-performance quantum dot nanobead [18] and magnetic quantum dot with a triple quantum dot shell [19] as novel labels to improve the sensitivity of the LFIA and accurately diagnose SARS-CoV-2; both labels exhibited good performances with sensitivity of 5.0 and 0.5 pg/mL in NP antigen detection, respectively. In addition, a robust Co–Fe@hemin-peroxidase nanozyme was used to amplify the immune reaction signal of a chemiluminescence paper assay with high sensitivity [20]. At present, GCNPs are the most common and popular signal indicators in LFIA because of their extraordinary physicochemical properties, such as good optical vision and high stability. Many strategies, such as silver staining, double labelling, enzyme catalysis, and a biotin-avidin system, have been applied to promote the sensitivity of GCNP-based LFIAs [21]. In addition to these strategies, GCNP-induced copper deposition can also enhance the LFIA signal and has the advantages of low cost, safety, and easy storage. Theoretically, Cu^{2+} is reduced into Cu^+ in the presence of ascorbic acid, and then Cu^+ is converted into Cu, which is deposited with the assistance of GCNPs and remarkably enhances the optical signal intensity of the LFIA. Liu's group has taken advantage of this feature to improve the sensitivity of the colorimetric immunoassay and LFIA, which exhibited good performances in rapid detection [22–24].

In this work, a GCNP-based LFIA coupled with copper deposition-induced signal amplification has been developed for rapid SARS-CoV-2 NP antigen detection. As shown in the scheme in Figure 1A, the developed NP antigen detection system includes a GCNP-based LFIA test strip, copper deposition, a simple homemade device for signal amplification, and a lysis buffer. In theory, the LFIA for NP antigen detection was based on the sandwich mode. Briefly, the test line without a red band indicates that the sample is negative for the antigen; the red band appears in the presence of the NP antigen, and the signal intensity of the test line is positively correlated with the NP antigen concentration. First, the LFIA test strips were immersed in $CuSO_4$ solution. Then, the Cu^{2+} ions were reduced into Cu^+ ions with the addition of L-sodium ascorbate (L-AANa) solution. Finally, with the assistance of the GCNPs captured on the test and control lines, the Cu^+ ions were converted into Cu and deposited on the surface of GCNPs, which remarkably enhanced the visual signal intensity. Consequently, the sensitivity of LFIA for NP antigen detection improved considerably (Figure 1B). The developed direct, rapid point-of-care detection method for the SARS-CoV-2 NP antigen via copper deposition signal amplification was predicted to be a convenient supplementary approach to rapidly and effectively screen the suspected population in the COVID-19 pandemic.

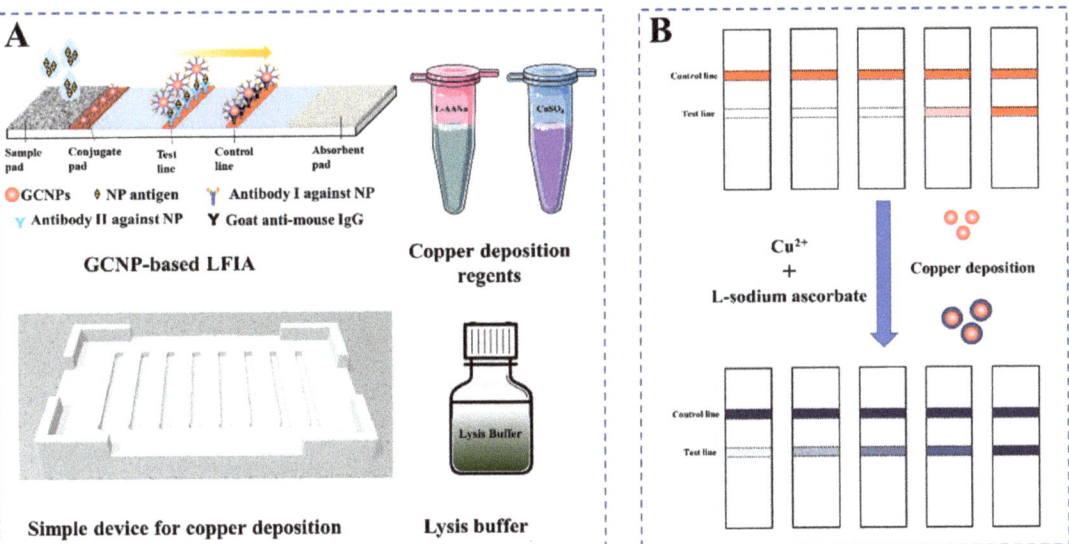

Figure 1. The diagram of GCNP-based LFIA coupled with copper deposition-introduced signal amplification for NP antigen detection. (**A**) Elements of the developed NP antigen detection system. (**B**) Results of antigen detection and signal amplification.

2. Materials and Methods

2.1. Reagents and Apparatus

Mouse monoclonal antibodies I (No. DA027) and II (No. CSB-MA33255A2m) against SARS-CoV-2 NP antigen were purchased from Shanghai Jin'an Biotechnology Co. Ltd. (Shanghai, China) and Wuhan Huamei Biotechnology Co. Ltd. (Wuhan, China), respectively. Goat anti-mouse IgG was purchased from Beijing Yongjia Venture Company (Beijing, China). The NP solution reference material for COVID-19 (Code: GBW(E)091097) was provided by the National Institute of Metrology (Beijing, China). Chloroauric acid ($HAuCl_4 \cdot 3H_2O$) was purchased from Sigma–Aldrich Chemical Corporation (St. Louis, Mo, USA). Copper sulfate pentahydrate ($CuSO_4 \cdot 5H_2O$), L-AANa, trisodium citrate, PEG_{20000}, bovine serum albumin (BSA), and Tween-20 were purchased from Aladdin Reagent Co., Ltd. (Shanghai, China). Sample pad, glass-fiber membrane, PVC pad, and absorbent pad were obtained from Kinbio Tech Co., Ltd. (Shanghai, China). Nitrocellulose (NC) membrane was purchased from Sartorius (Gottingen, Germany). All solvents and other chemicals were of analytical reagent grade.

The XYZ 3D film spraying instrument, CNC cutting machine (CTS300), and microcomputer automatic cutting machine (ZQ2402) were supplied by Kinbio Tech Co., Ltd. (Shanghai, China). Ultrapure water was purified with Milli-Q system from Millipore Corp. (Bedford, MA, USA).

2.2. Preparation of GCNPs

GCNPs were prepared according to the reference [25]. Briefly, 1 mL of $HAuCl_4 \cdot 3H_2O$ solution (1%, w/v) was added to 99 mL of ultrapure water and heated to boil. Then, 1.8 mL of 1% (w/v) sodium citrate solution was added quickly under rapid stirring. After the solution turned clear red, the solution was heated for another 5 min. The GCNP solution was cooled to room temperature naturally and then stored at 4 °C.

2.3. Synthesis of GCNP-Antibody I Detection Probes

The GCNP solution was adjusted to pH 8.0 by adding 0.2 M K_2CO_3 and then stirred with a constant speed mixer. Mouse monoclonal antibody I against NP antigen was diluted with phosphate buffer and added drop by drop under rapid stirring. After 1 h, 1% (w/v) PEG_{20000} solution and 10% (w/v) BSA solution were added successively to block the spare sites on the GCNPs for 20 min. The mixture was centrifuged at 8000 rpm at 4 °C for 30 min to remove the unconjugated free antibodies. The supernatant was discarded, and the precipitate was resuspensed with 1.0 M Tris-HCl containing 0.5% polyvinylpyrrolidone K30, 10% sucrose, 1% BSA, and 0.05% ProClin300. Finally, the GCNP-antibody I detection probe solution was obtained and stored at 4 °C until use.

2.4. Preparation of LFIA Test Strips

The LFIA test strip was composed of a sample pad, a conjugated pad, a NC membrane, an absorbent paper, and an adhesive PVC bottom plate. The prepared GCNP-antibody I detection probe solution was sprayed on the conjugated pad using an XYZ 3D film spraying instrument at a spray rate of 3 μL/cm, and the pad was dried at 37 °C for 2 h with a vacuum dryer. Goat anti-mouse IgG and mouse monoclonal antibody II were dispensed onto the NC membrane as the control and test lines, respectively, and then dried at 37 °C for 16 h. The fabricated LFIA test strip was cut into 3.0 mm-wide strips, stored at room temperature, and kept dry.

2.5. Copper Deposition-Induced Signal Amplification on the LFIA Strip

The NP antigen solution reference material was diluted into a series of standard solutions at concentrations of 1.0, 1.0×10^{-1}, 1.0×10^{-2}, 1.0×10^{-3}, 1.0×10^{-4}, 1.0×10^{-5}, and 1.0×10^{-6} μg/mL, and 10 μL of each solution was mixed with 80 μL of lysis buffer (0.4% SDS, 0.6% TritonX-100, and 0.4% PVP were dissolved in 1.0 M Tris-HCl, pH 8.0) for 3 min. Each liquid was added to the sample pad of the LFIA strips, and the results could be observed by the naked eye after 15 min. Then, the strips were placed into the homemade device with the copper enhancement solution (50 mM L-AANa and 50 Mm $CuSO_4$), and the results were obtained after 3 min.

3. Results and Discussion

3.1. Validation of GCNP-Mediated Copper Deposition

The developed LFIA test strips were used to detect 0–10 μg/mL NP antigen to validate whether the signal was amplified by GCNP-mediated copper deposition. As shown in Figure 2, 0.1 μg/mL of the NP antigen could be distinguished from the negative before signal amplification. $CuSO_4$ and L-AANa solutions with the same volume were added sequentially to the test strips. After 3 min, the red bands turned into black bands, and the LFIA strip for 0.01 μg/mL NP antigen detection also presented a clear band on the test line, which suggests that the detection sensitivity was successfully promoted by GCNP-mediated copper deposition.

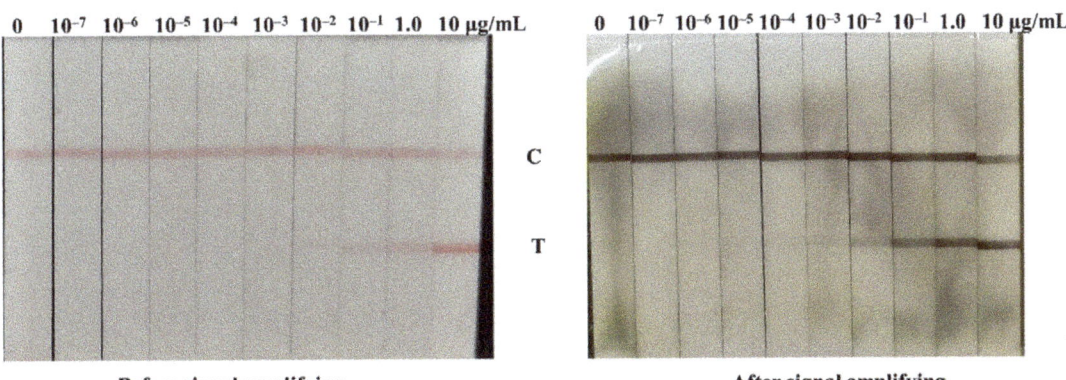

Figure 2. Comparison of the detection sensitivity before and after signal amplifying introduced by copper deposition.

3.2. Optimization of the Parameters

Six anti-NP antibodies were obtained from different companies and primarily evaluated by LFIA. Antibodies I and II from Shanghai Jin'an Biotechnology Co. Ltd. and Wuhan Huamei Biotechnology Co. Ltd. were selected in the present work (Figure S1). First, the pH and antibody amount of the GCNP-antibody I detection probe were optimized. Different volumes (4, 6, 8, and 10 µL) of 0.2 M K_2CO_3 solution were added to 1 mL of GCNP solution in order to adjust the pH of the detection probes. As shown in Figure 3A, the probes on the conjugated pad released completely, and the test line showed a clear red band without nonspecific adsorption when 8 µL of 0.2 M K_2CO_3 solution was added. Under the optimized pH, different amounts of antibody I (5, 10, 20, and 40 µg) was diluted with phosphate buffer, and then added into 1 mL of the GCNP solution. The prepared detection probes were evaluated with 0.1 µg/mL of the NP antigen; the result suggested that 10 µg of antibody I is the optimum amount (Figure 3B). Moreover, the UV-vis spectra of the GCNPs and detection probes (Figure S2) indicate that the characteristic absorption peak red shifted, which demonstrates that the antibody I conjugated with the GCNPs successfully. The amount of goat anti-mouse IgG coated on the control line seemed to have no significant influence on the detection result (Figure 3C); thus, 0.3 mg/mL of goat anti-mouse IgG was selected, in consideration of the cost.

The sensitivity of the strip was affected by the amount of antibody coated on the test line. The mouse monoclonal antibody II against the NP antigen was diluted to 0.2, 0.4, 0.6, and 0.8 mg/mL with PBS buffer (0.01 M, pH = 7.4) and then sprayed on the NC membrane as the test lines. The positive sample with 0.1 µg/mL of the NP antigen was used to select the optimum amount of the antibody II. Based on the result in Figure 4A, 0.6 mg/mL of antibody II was selected. In addition, the liquid flow rate on the NC membrane is related to the width of the LFIA test strips, and a slower flow rate leads to a better immune reaction, which may directly impact the sensitivity of the LFIA. Hence, the fabricated LFIA was cut into 3.0, 3.5, and 4.0 mm widths to investigate the influence of test strip width on the sensitivity of the strip. The results in Figure 4B suggested that the color of the test line on the strip with a 3.0 mm width was the clearest. The results confirmed that the flow rate of liquid on the narrow test strip was the lowest, which increased the reaction time between the target and the detection probes and resulted in the improvement of the signal intensity.

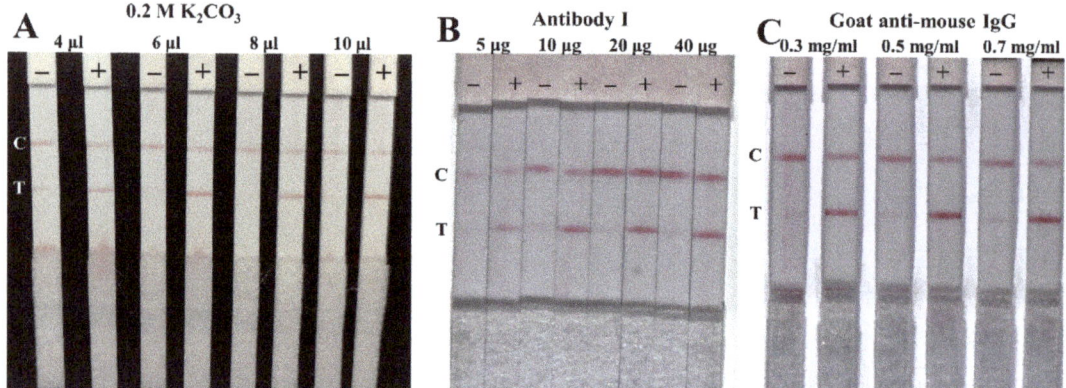

Figure 3. Optimization of the amount of 0.2 M K$_2$CO$_3$ solution used (**A**), antibody I used in the detection probes (**B**), and goat anti-mouse IgG on the control line (**C**). The positive sample was buffer spiked with 0.1 μg/mL of the NP antigen.

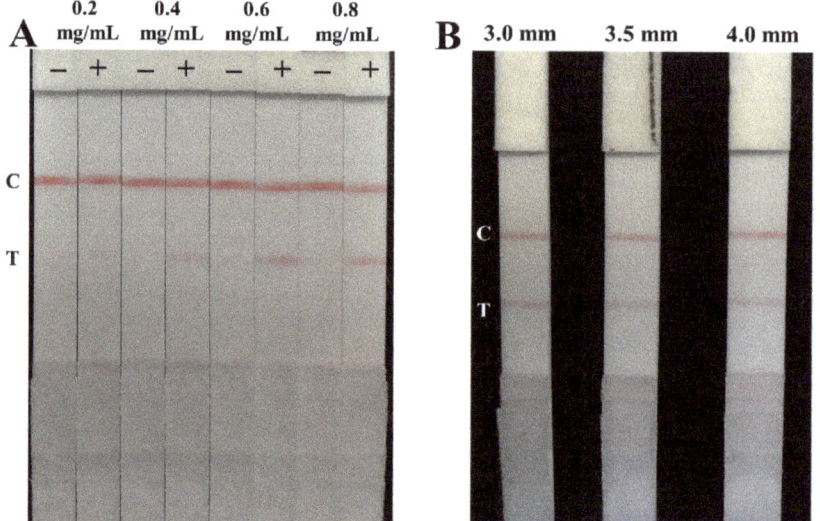

Figure 4. Optimization of the antibody II amount on the test line (**A**) and the width of LFIA test strip (**B**).

3.3. Signal Amplification for NP Antigen Detection

First, a simple and portable device for copper deposition signal amplification was fabricated by 3D printing (Figure 5A). The signal amplification of each LFIA test strip can be carried out on separate trough (Figure 5B). Subsequently, the COVID-19 NP solution reference material (GBW(E)091097) was diluted into a series of standard solutions (1.0, 0.1, 10^{-2}, 10^{-3}, 10^{-4}, 10^{-5}, 10^{-6}, and 0 μg/mL) with lysis buffer and then detected by the LFIA test strips assembled with the optimized parameters. The results are shown in Figure 5C: the signal intensity detected by the naked eye increased with the concentration increasing from 0.01 μg/mL to 1.0 μg/mL, and only a weak red band was presented on the test line when the concentration was 0.01 μg/mL, which indicates that the detection sensitivity was 0.01 μg/mL. However, the signal intensity on the test lines was enhanced after copper deposition-induced signal amplification, and a weak band was also developed in 0.01 ng/mL; the results demonstrate that the sensitivity was increased by three orders of magnitude after copper deposition. The detection limit of the developed GCNP-LFIA for the SARS-CoV-2 NP antigen was 10 pg/mL. Because the sample volume used for detection was only 10 µL, the developed method has the capability of detecting 0.1 pg NP antigen within 20 min.

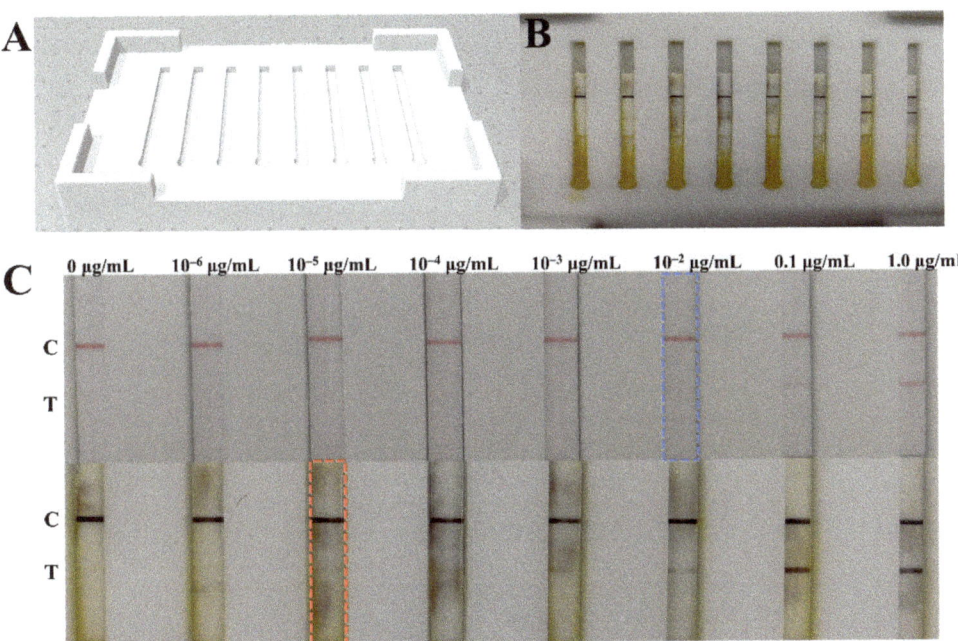

Figure 5. Simple device for copper deposition signal amplification (**A**,**B**); detection of NP antigen standard solutions before and after signal amplification (**C**).

The specificity of the proposed GCNP-LFIA was evaluated using the recombinant proteins of SARS-CoV and Middle East respiratory syndrome coronavirus. GCNP-LFIA had a cross-reactivity with SARS-CoV because of the high homology between SARS-CoV-2 and SARS-CoV (Figure S3). However, almost no SARS-CoV infection has been reported at present; therefore, the accuracy of the results obtained by GCNP-LFIA is considered reliable. As shown in Table 1, the sensitivity of the proposed LFIA is not superior to the previously reported LFIAs. However, the results prove the feasibility of copper deposition signal enhancement technology for GCNP-based LFIAs, which exhibit broad prospects for applications and social benefits. As for the SARS-CoV-2 detection, the LOD of the proposed detection method was lower, and the virus infection could be found earlier; thus, its detection capability needs to be improved in our further work. Additionally, the limitation of this work is the lack of evaluation of cultured virus or real samples, although the detection of the NP antigen in nasopharyngeal swab samples was expected. Nonetheless, the imperfection of this work does not obscure its implication for copper deposition signal enhancement.

In this work, a simple and portable device was designed to allow the copper deposition reaction to take place in an independent space for each LFIA strip, which can simplify the operational process and improve the reaction efficiency. This work extensively applied the GCNP-mediated copper deposition signal amplification to the LFIA in accordance with the research achievements of Liu's group [22]. The results indicated that the GCNP-based

LFIA combined with copper deposition is worthy of popularization and application in COVID-19 detection and even in other areas.

Table 1. Comparison of the performances among the developed method and other reported methods for SARS-CoV-2 NP antigen detection.

Method	Sensitivity	Time	Reference
Colloidal gold nanoparticle based LFIA	250 pg/mL	15 min	Mertens et al. [26]
Half-strip lateral flow assay	650 pg/mL	about 20 min	BD Grant et al. [12]
Cellulose nanobead-based LFIA	20 ng/mL	20 min	Kim et al. [14]
Fluorescent immunochromatographic assay	/	10 min	Diao et al. [15]
Fluorescent immunochromatographic assay based on multilayer quantum dot nanobeads	5.0 pg/mL	15 min	Wang et al. [18]
Dual-Mode fluorescence lateral flow immunoassay	0.5 pg/mL	10 min	Wang et al. [19]
Cotton-tipped electrochemical immunosensor	0.8 pg/mL	about 20 min	Shimaa Eissa and Mohammed Zourob [9,10]
Parallel reaction monitoring mass spectrometry assay	2×10^5 viral particles/mL	about 3 h	Cazares et al. [9]
Colloidal gold nanoparticles based LFIA with copper deposition	10 pg/mL	Within 20 min	This work

4. Conclusions

This study developed a GCNP-based LFIA for sensitive SARS-CoV-2 NP antigen detection and proved that a GCNP-mediated copper deposition technique further enhances the LFIA signal. Under the optimized parameters, the detection limit of the developed GCNP-LFIA coupled with copper deposition for SARS-CoV-2 NP antigen detection was 10 pg/mL, which indicates a better sensitivity than the reported GCNP-LFIA. It provides a convenient supplementary approach to rapidly screen the suspected population for the prevention and control of the COVID-19 pandemic. However, further investigation with real samples is warranted.

Supplementary Materials: The following supporting information can be downloaded at: https://www.mdpi.com/article/10.3390/bios12010013/s1, Figure S1: The result of antibody pair optimization; Figure S2: UV-vis spectra of the GCNPs and GCNP-antibody I detection probes; Figure S3: Evaluation of the specificity of the proposed GCNP-LFIA.

Author Contributions: Conceptualization, X.D. and X.F.; methodology, T.P., X.Y. and X.D.; validation, T.P., X.J. and Z.L.; formal analysis, T.P., X.J. and J.X.; investigation, X.J. and Z.L.; resources, Y.J., Y.Z. and H.Z.; data curation, T.P. and X.J.; writing—original draft preparation, T.P. and X.J.; writing—review and editing, T.P.; supervision, X.D.; project administration, Y.Z., T.P. and H.Z.; funding acquisition, Y.Z., T.P. and H.Z. All authors have read and agreed to the published version of the manuscript.

Funding: This work was financially supported by the Central Public-interest Scientific Institution Basal Research Fund, National Institute of Metrology (No. AKYZD2111), and the Special fund of the State Key Joint Laboratory of Environment Simulation and Pollution Control (20K10ESPCT).

Institutional Review Board Statement: Not applicable.

Informed Consent Statement: Not applicable.

Data Availability Statement: The authors confirm that the data supporting the findings of this study are available within the article.

Conflicts of Interest: The authors declare no conflict of interest.

References

1. Xu, W.Z.; Li, J.; He, X.Y.; Zhang, C.Q.; Li, C.R.; Li, Y.; Cheng, S.H.; Zhang, P.A. The diagnostic value of joint detection of serum IgM and IgG antibodies to 2019-nCoV in 2019-nCoV infection. *Chin. J. Lab. Med.* **2020**, *43*, E01–E06.
2. Ong, D.S.Y.; de Man, S.J.; Lindeboom, F.A.; Koeleman, J.G.M. Comparison of diagnostic accuracies of rapid serological tests and ELISA to molecular diagnostics in patients with suspected COVID-19 presenting to the hospital. *Clin. Microbiol. Infect.* **2020**, *26*, 1094.e7–1094.e10. [CrossRef]
3. Wang, C.W.; Yang, X.S.; Gu, B.; Liu, H.F.; Zhou, Z.H.; Shi, L.L.; Cheng, X.D.; Wang, S.Q. Sensitive and Simultaneous Detection of SARS-CoV-2-Specific IgM/IgG Using Lateral Flow Immunoassay Based on Dual-Mode Quantum Dot Nanobeads. *Anal. Chem.* **2020**, *92*, 15542–15549. [CrossRef]
4. Seo, G.; Lee, G.; Kim, M.J.; Baek, S.-H.; Choi, M.; Ku, K.B.; Lee, C.-S.; Jun, S.; Park, D.; Kim, H.G.; et al. Rapid Detection of COVID-19 Causative Virus (SARS-CoV-2) in Human Nasopharyngeal Swab Specimens Using Field-Effect Transistor-Based Biosensor. *ACS Nano* **2020**, *14*, 5135–5142. [CrossRef]
5. Cui, J.; Li, F.; Shi, Z.L. Origin and evolution of pathogenic coronaviruses. *Nat. Rev. Microbiol.* **2019**, *17*, 181–192. [CrossRef]
6. Di, B.; Hao, W.; Gao, Y.; Wang, M.; Qiu, L.; Wen, K.; Zhou, D.; Wu, X.; Lu, E. Monoclonal antibody-based antigen capture enzyme-linked immunosorbent assay reveals high sensitivity of the nucleocapsid protein in acute-phase sera of severe acute respiratory syndrome patients. *Clin. Diagn. Lab. Immunol.* **2005**, *12*, 135–140. [CrossRef] [PubMed]
7. Che, X.; Hao, W.; Wang, Y.; Di, B.; Yin, K.; Xu, Y.-C.; Feng, C.-S.; Wan, Z.-Y.; Cheng, V.C.C.; Yuen, K.-Y. Nucleocapsid protein as early diagnostic marker for SARS. *Emerg. Infect. Dis.* **2004**, *10*, 1947–1949. [CrossRef] [PubMed]
8. Wu, F.; Zhao, S.; Yu, B.; Chen, Y.M.; Zhang, Y.Z. A new coronavirus associated with human respiratory disease in China. *Nature* **2020**, *579*, 265–269. [CrossRef] [PubMed]
9. Cazares, L.H.; Chaerkady, R.; Weng, S.H.S.; Boo, C.C.; Cimbro, R.; Hsu, H.-E.; Rajan, S.; Dall'Acqua, W.; Clarke, L.; Ren, K.; et al. Development of a Parallel Reaction Monitoring Mass Spectrometry Assay for the Detection of SARS-CoV2 Spike Glycoprotein and Nucleoprotein. *Anal. Chem.* **2020**, *92*, 13813–13821. [CrossRef] [PubMed]
10. Eissa, S.; Zourob, M. Development of a Low-Cost Cotton-Tipped Electrochemical Immunosensor for the Detection of SARS-CoV-2. *Anal. Chem.* **2021**, *93*, 1826–1833. [CrossRef]
11. Eissa, S.; Alhadrami, H.A.; Al-Mozaini, M.; Hassan, A.M.; Zourob, M. Voltammetric-based immunosensor for the detection of SARS-CoV-2 nucleocapsid antigen. *Microchim. Acta* **2021**, *188*, 199. [CrossRef]
12. Grant, B.D.; Anderson, C.E.; Williford, J.R.; Alonzo, L.F.; Glukhova, V.A.; Boyle, D.S.; Weigl, B.H.; Nichols, K.P. SARS-CoV-2 Coronavirus Nucleocapsid Antigen-Detecting Half-Strip Lateral Flow Assay Toward the Development of Point of Care Tests Using Commercially Available Reagents. *Anal. Chem.* **2020**, *92*, 11305–11309. [CrossRef] [PubMed]
13. Peng, T.; Sui, Z.W.; Huang, Z.H.; Xie, J.; Wen, K.; Zhang, Y.Z.; Huang, W.F.; Mi, W.; Peng, K.; Dai, X.H.; et al. Point-of-care test system for detection of immunoglobulin-G and -M against nucleocapsid protein and spike glycoprotein of SARS-CoV-2. *Sens. Actuators B Chem.* **2021**, *331*, 129415. [CrossRef]
14. Kim, H.Y.; Lee, J.H.; Mi, J.K.; Sun, C.P.; Kim, S.I. Development of a SARS-CoV-2-specific biosensor for antigen detection using scFv-Fc fusion proteins. *Biosens. Bioelectron.* **2020**, *175*, 112868. [CrossRef] [PubMed]
15. Diao, B.; Wen, K.; Zhang, J.; Chen, J.; Han, C.; Chen, Y.W.; Wang, S.F.; Deng, G.H.; Zhou, H.W.; Wu, Y.Z. Accuracy of a nucleocapsid protein antigen rapid test in the diagnosis of SARS-CoV-2 infection. *Clin. Microbiol. Infect.* **2021**, *27*, 289.e1–289.e4. [CrossRef]
16. Corman, V.M.; Haage, V.C.; Bleicker, T.; Schmidt, M.L.; Mühlemann, B.; Zuchowski, M.; Jo, W.K.; Tscheak, P.; Möncke-Buchner, E.; Müller, M.A.; et al. Comparison of seven commercial SARS-CoV-2 rapid point-of-care antigen tests: A single-centre laboratory evaluation study. *Lancet Microbe* **2021**, *2*, e311–e319. [CrossRef]
17. Seiya, Y.; Yuko, S.T.; Michiko, K.; Osamu, A.; Yoshihiro, K. Comparison of Rapid Antigen Tests for COVID-19. *Viruses* **2020**, *12*, 1420.
18. Wang, C.W.; Cheng, X.D.; Liu, L.Y.; Zhang, X.C.; Yang, X.S.; Zheng, S.; Rong, Z.; Wang, S.Q. Ultrasensitive and Simultaneous Detection of Two Specific SARS-CoV-2 Antigens in Human Specimens Using Direct/Enrichment Dual-Mode Fluorescence Lateral Flow Immunoassay. *ACS Appl. Mater. Interfaces* **2021**, *13*, 40342–40353. [CrossRef]
19. Wang, C.W.; Yang, X.S.; Zheng, S.; Cheng, X.D.; Xiao, R.; Li, Q.J.; Wang, W.Q.; Liu, X.X.; Wang, S.Q. Development of an ultrasensitive fluorescent immunochromatographic assay based on multilayer quantum dot nanobead for simultaneous detection of SARS-CoV-2 antigen and influenza A virus. *Sens. Actuators B Chem.* **2021**, *345*, 130372. [CrossRef]
20. Liu, D.; Ju, C.H.; Han, C.; Shi, R.; Chen, X.H.; Duan, D.M.; Yan, J.H.; Yan, X.Y. Nanozyme chemiluminescence paper test for rapid and sensitive detection of SARS-CoV-2 antigen. *Biosens. Bioelectron.* **2021**, *173*, 112817. [CrossRef]
21. Shan, S.; Lai, W.H.; Xiong, Y.H.; Wei, H.; Xu, H.Y. Novel strategies to enhance lateral flow immunoassay sensitivity for detecting foodborne pathogens. *J. Agric. Food Chem.* **2015**, *63*, 745–753. [CrossRef]
22. Tian, M.L.; Lei, L.L.; Xie, W.Y.; Yang, Q.M.; Li, C.M.; Liu, Y.S. Copper deposition-induced efficient signal amplification for ultrasensitive lateral flow immunoassay. *Sens. Actuators B Chem.* **2019**, *282*, 96–103. [CrossRef]
23. Liu, Y.S.; Zhang, Z.Y.; Yu, J.; Xie, J.; Li, C.M. A concentration dependent multicolor conversion strategy for ultrasensitive colorimetric immunoassay with the naked eye. *Anal. Chim. Acta* **2017**, *963*, 129–135. [CrossRef] [PubMed]

24. Liu, Y.S.; Xie, J.; Zhang, Z.Y.; Lu, Z.S. An ultrasensitive colorimetric strategy for protein O-GlcNAcylation detection via copper deposition-enabled nonenzymatic signal amplification. *RSC Adv.* **2016**, *6*, 89484–89491. [CrossRef]
25. Berg, E.A.; Fishman, J.B. Labeling Antibodies Using Colloidal Gold. *Cold Spring Harb. Protoc.* **2020**, *4*, 099333. [CrossRef]
26. Pascal, M.; Nathalie, D.V.; Delphine, M.; Christian, J.; Ali, M.; Lize, C.; Sigi, V.W.; Vanessa, M.; Pierrette, M.; Karolien, S.; et al. Development and Potential Usefulness of the COVID-19 Ag Respi-Strip Diagnostic Assay in a Pandemic Context. *Front. Med.* **2020**, *7*, 225.

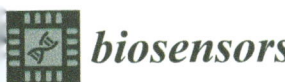

Communication

Latex Microsphere-Based Bicolor Immunochromatography for Qualitative Detection of Neutralizing Antibody against SARS-CoV-2

Zhanwei Liang [1,2,†], Tao Peng [2,†], Xueshima Jiao [1,2], Yang Zhao [2], Jie Xie [2], You Jiang [2], Bo Meng [2], Xiang Fang [2], Xiaoping Yu [1,*] and Xinhua Dai [2,*]

1 College of Life Sciences, China Jiliang University, Hangzhou 310018, China; s20090710033@cjlu.edu.cn (Z.L.); s20090710020@cjlu.edu.cn (X.J.)
2 Technology Innovation Center of Mass Spectrometry for State Market Regulation, Center for Advanced Measurement Science, National Institute of Metrology, Beijing 100029, China; pengtao@nim.ac.cn (T.P.); zhaoy@nim.ac.cn (Y.Z.); xiejie@nim.ac.cn (J.X.); jiangyou@nim.ac.cn (Y.J.); mengbo@nim.ac.cn (B.M.); fangxiang@nim.ac.cn (X.F.)
* Correspondence: yxp@cjlu.edu.cn (X.Y.); daixh@nim.ac.cn (X.D.); Tel./Fax: +86-010-645-24962 (X.D.)
† These authors contributed equally to this work.

Abstract: Neutralizing antibody (NAb) is a family of antibodies with special functions, which afford a degree of protection against infection and/or reduce the risk of clinically severe infection. Receptor binding domain (RBD) in the spike protein of SARS-CoV-2, a portion of the S1 subunit, can stimulate the immune system to produce NAb after infection and vaccination. The detection of NAb against SARS-CoV-2 is a simple and direct approach for evaluating a vaccine's effectiveness. In this study, a direct, rapid, and point-of-care bicolor lateral flow immunoassay (LFIA) was developed for NAb against SARS-CoV-2 detection without sample pretreatment, and which was based on the principle of NAb-mediated blockage of the interaction between RBD and angiotensin-converting enzyme 2. In the bicolor LFIA, red and blue latex microspheres (LMs) were used to locate the test and control lines, leading to avoidance of erroneous interpretations of one-colored line results. Under the optimal conditions, NAb against SARS-CoV-2 detection carried out using the bicolor LFIA could be completed within 9 min, and the visible limit of detection was about 48 ng/mL. Thirteen serum samples were analyzed, and the results showed that the NAb levels in three positive serum samples were equal to, or higher than, 736 ng/mL. The LM-based bicolor LFIA allows one-step, rapid, convenient, inexpensive, and user-friendly determination of NAb against SARS-CoV-2 in serum.

Keywords: neutralizing antibody; latex microspheres; lateral flow immunoassay; SARS-CoV-2; receptor binding domain

1. Introduction

Severe acute respiratory syndrome coronavirus 2 (SARS-CoV-2) has spread globally over the past two years, causing pneumonia disease since 2019 (COVID-19) and resulting in significant morbidity and mortality [1]. SARS-CoV-2 particles contain four structural proteins, namely, nucleocapsid protein, envelope protein, membrane protein, and spike (S) protein. During infection, SARS-CoV-2 entry to cells depends on the S protein, which contains the receptor binding domain (RBD), mediating binding to the viral receptor of human angiotensin-converting enzyme 2 (ACE2) [2–7]. Fortunately, a variety of vaccines have been developed and used to protect humans against SARS-CoV-2. Studies on vaccinated subjects have demonstrated that the human body has the ability to rapidly induce a protective immune response and produce neutralizing antibodies (NAb) after vaccination, which affords a degree of protection against infection and/or reduces the risk of clinically severe infection [8–17]. S protein RBD of SARS-CoV-2 is the main protein that stimulates the human immune system to produce Nab [17–19].

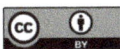

The NAb against SARS-CoV-2 detection is a direct approach to evaluating the effectiveness of vaccines. Currently, virus neutralization testing is the gold standard for NAb detection [20,21]. However, it is highly technical, often time consuming, and high risk, because live virus- or pseudovirus-based neutralization testing is restricted to biosafety level 3 and 2 facilities. Although an enzyme-linked immunosorbent assay (ELISA) has also been developed for accurate and sensitive detection of SARS-CoV-2 antibodies, its labor- and time-consuming operation limits its widespread application on site [22–24]. In practice, a direct and rapid detection method without pretreatment is deserved for point-of-care testing of NAb among vaccine recipients.

A lateral flow immunoassay (LFIA), which combines chromatography technology with conventional immunoassay and nanomaterials, is considered the most attractive point-of-care testing device, because it exhibits several advantages, including simple technical requirements, rapid detection capability, portability, affordability, high detection accuracy, and high efficiency [25]. LFIAs have been widely applied in detecting pesticide [26,27] and veterinary drugs residues [28,29], toxicants [30–32], pathogens [32,33], various diseases biomarkers, as well as SARS-CoV-2 antigen/antibody [34,35]. Usually, the results of a LFIA are presented with the test and control lines showing the same color, resulting in it not being easy for users to discern the locations of test and control zones. If only one colored line appears, the result is interpreted as a defective test with only test line signaling, or as positive/negative result with only control line staining. Therefore, test and control lines of LFIA with different colors could avoid the misinterpretation of a result with only one colored line. Gold nanoparticles in different shapes exhibiting multicolor optical properties have been used for this purpose, a universal bicolor LFIA with blue gold nanoflowers in the test zone and red gold nanospheres in the control zone was designed by Dzantiev's group [36]. In addition, latex microspheres (LMs) with rich and diverse colors can also be applied, especially, the abundant carboxyl groups on the surface of LMs that allow stable preparation of probes. In this study, a bicolor LFIA, based on red and blue LMs, was designed, in which the interaction between RBD and ACE2 can be blocked by the NAb without appearance of the red band. The LM-based bicolor LFIA allows one-step, rapid, convenient, inexpensive, and user-friendly determination of NAb against SARS-CoV-2 in serum.

2. Materials and Methods

2.1. Reagents and Instruments

ACE-2 recombinant protein and RBD recombinant protein were purchased from Okay-Bio (Nanjing, China). Polyvidone (PVP), sucrose, ProClin™ 300, and bovine serum albumin were obtained from Sigma-Aldrich (Germany). N-Hydroxysulfosuccinimide sodium salt (NHS), N-(3-Dimethylaminopropyl)-N′-ethylcarbodiimide hydrochloride (EDC), polyethylene glycol (PEG-20,000), and TWEEN-20 were purchased from Aladdin (Shanghai, China). Reference material of Nab with purity higher than 95% was provided by Suzhou novoprotein (Suzhou, China). 2-Morpholinoethanesulfonic Acid (MES) was obtained from TCI (Shanghai, China). 400 nM Carboxylated LMs (Blue/Red) were provided by Magsphere (Pasadena, CA, USA). Ultrapure water (18 MΩ cm at 25 °C) purified with a Milli-Q system from Millipore Corp. (Bedford, MA, USA) was used for solution preparation.

UniSart CN 140 nitrocellulose membranes were obtained from Sartorius (Shanghai, China). Glass fiber Pads SB-08, XYZ 3D film spraying instrument, CNC cutting machine (CTS300), and microcomputer automatic cutting machine (ZQ2402) were supplied by Kinbio Tech Co., Ltd. (Shanghai, China).

The blank serum used to optimize the parameters was purchased from Sigma. The 10 negative samples were obtained from Wuhan Jinyintan Hospital and stored at −80 °C until use. The 3 positive samples were donated by the vaccinated with informed consent.

2.2. Preparation of RBD-Labeled Red LMs and IgG-Conjugated Blue LMs

The RBD-labeled red LMs (RLM@RBD) and IgG-conjugated blue LMs (BLM@IgG) were prepared by the active ester method. With gentle stirring, 5 µL of blue or red LMs was added to 1 mL of MES buffer (50 mM, pH 6.0), then 10 µL of freshly prepared EDC solution (1 mg/mL) and 10 µL of NHS solution (1 mg/mL) were sequentially added into the above LMs solution. After activation for 15 min at room temperature, LMs were centrifuged at 10,000 rpm for 15 min at 4 °C, and the precipitate was dissolved in 1 mL of PBS buffer (0.01 M, pH 7.4). Recombinant RBD protein and mouse IgG were diluted to 0.04 mg/mL and 0.1 mg/mL with PB buffer (0.01 M, pH 7.7), respectively. Then, 100 µL of protein dilution was added into the LMs solution and mixed thoroughly. After incubation for another 30 min, 100 µL of 20%BSA (w/v) was added dropwise to block unbound sites for 15 min. Finally, the mixture was centrifuged at 10000 rpm for 15 min at 4 °C, the precipitate was resuspended with 200 µL of 0.01 M PBS buffer containing 0.5% polyvinylpyrrolidone K30, 10% sucrose, 1% BSA, and 0.05% ProClin300 and stored at 4 °C until use.

2.3. Preparation of LFIA Test Strips

The ACE2 recombinant protein and goat anti-mouse IgG with the appropriate concentration were sprayed on the NC membrane as a test line (T line) and control line (C line), respectively. The distance between the T and C lines was 5.0 mm, and then the prepared NC membranes were placed and dried at 37 °C for 12 h. The sample pad was immersed in the treatment solution (0.01 M of PBS buffer containing 0.25% PVP, 0.1% S9, 0.4% Tween-20 and 0.05% ProClin300) for 30 s, and dried at 37 °C for 10 h. Finally, the prepared sample pad, NC membrane, and absorbent pad were pasted onto the PVC bottom plate. The fabricated LFIA plate was cut into 3.0 mm-wide test strips, stored at room temperature, and kept dry.

2.4. Optimization of the LFIA Parameters

In order to obtain better performance of the bicolor LFIA, various analytical parameters were optimized: pH (4.0, 5.0, 6.0, 7.0) for RLM@RBD and BLM@IgG preparation, RBD concentration for labeling (0.01, 0.02, 0.04, and 0.08 mg/mL), and volume of RLM@RBD and BLM@IgG in each LFIA test strip (1.5, 2.0, 2.5, and 3.0 µL).

2.5. Test Procedure for Sample Testing

First, 10 µL of serum sample and 70 µL of dilution buffer (0.01 M of PBS containing 0.5% BSA and 0.01% Tween-20) were mixed with 2.5 µL of RLM@RBD and BLM@IgG, and incubated at room temperature, and then the mixture was added to the sample pad of the LFIA test strip. The results could be inspected to qualitatively detect NAb against SARS-CoV-2 after 9 min.

3. Results and Discussion

3.1. Principle and Validation of LM-Based Bicolor LFIA for NAb Detection

It is reported that SARS-COV-2 infection is accomplished through RBD targeting to the human ACE2 receptor, but the NAb is able to bind with the RBD and disturbs the virus–receptor engagement, contributing to protecting humans from SARS-CoV-2 infection [8–17]. The developed LM-based bicolor LFIA for NAb detection is principally based on NAb-mediated blockage of the interaction between RBD and ACE2. As shown in Figure 1, RLM@RBD and BLM@IgG are used as detection and control probes, in the absence of NAb, RLM@RBD detection probes are captured by the ACE2 coated on the T line with red band appearance, and the C line is presented as a blue band because of the conjugation between BLM@IgG control probes and goat anti-mouse IgG. On the contrary, RLM@RBD detection probes binding with ACE2 is prevented in the presence of NAb, resulting in no color appearing on the T line, but it has no effect on the blue color display of the C line. The red signal intensity on the T line is inversely correlated with the NAb levels, namely, the red signal intensity decreases with the increase of NAb levels. Moreover, the LFIA test strip is invalid in the case of no blue band appearing.

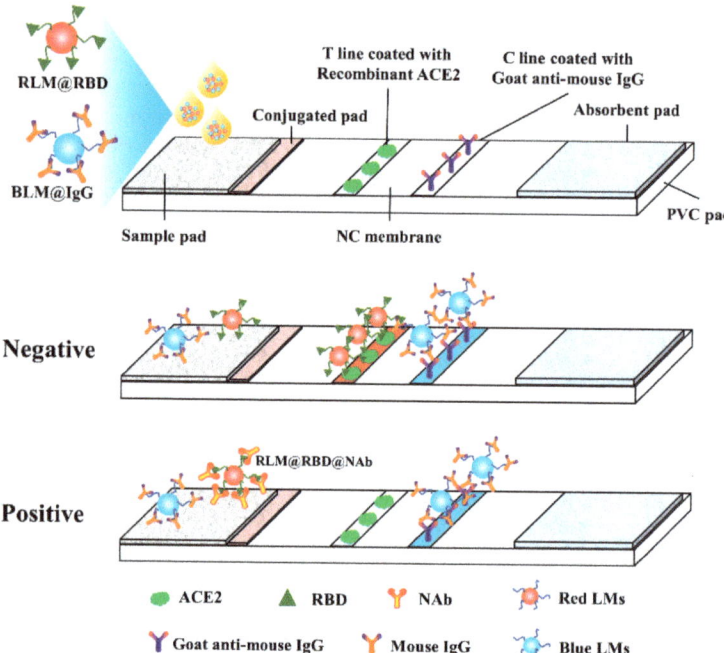

Figure 1. Schematic of the LFIA for anti-RBD neutralizing antibody rapid detection.

The RLM@RBD and BLM@IgG were applied separately on the LFIA test strip to evaluate feasibility. As displayed in Figure 2, RLM@RBD and BLM@IgG were individually captured on the T and C lines with no interference with each other, and the T and C lines were presented with clear red and blue bands on the LFIA test strip when RLM@RBD and BLM@IgG were mixed. This result demonstrated that the LM-based bicolor LFIA is capable of rapid detection.

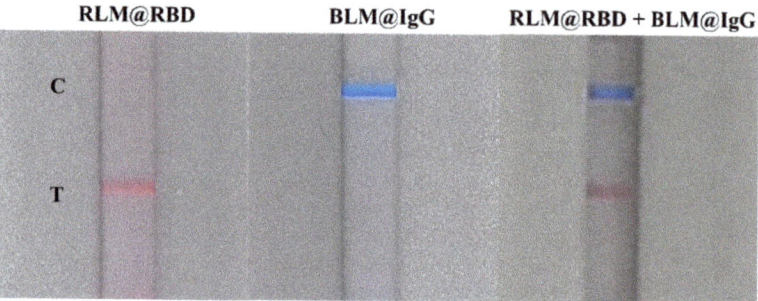

Figure 2. Evaluation of the interference between RLM@RBD and BLM@IgG probes.

3.2. Optimization of the Parameters

In order to obtain better performance for the bicolor LFIA, various analytical parameters were optimized. The active ester method was used to prepare RLM@RBD and BLM@IgG probes because of the abundant carboxy groups on the surface of LMs. pH is a key parameter for carboxyl group activation, which is relative to the couple efficiency between the LMs and protein. As shown in Figure 3, when the probes were prepared with pH 6.0, the test line of LFIA appeared as a clear red band with clean background on the

NC membrane for negative samples. Thus, pH 6.0 was selected, which is consistent with the conclusion of a previous study [37], the carboxyl groups were better activated by EDC under a weak acid condition.

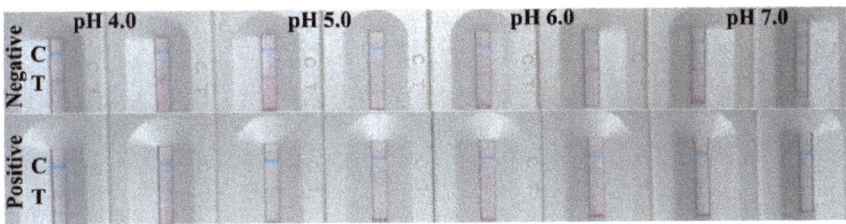

Figure 3. Optimization of pH for probe preparation, each measurement was tested in duplicate.

The amount of RBD protein labeled on the LMs plays a decisive role in the color development and inhibition effect of the LFIA test strip. The prepared RLM@RBD probes with different RBD protein amounts were evaluated using the blank serum and the spiked serum. The results indicated that the red signal intensity on the T line was promoted with the increase of RBD protein amount labeled on the red LMs when the blank serum was detected. However, when the RBD protein concentration was 0.04 mg/mL, the inhibition of spiked serum detection was the highest; thus, 100 µL of 0.04 mg/mL recombinant RBD protein was selected. In addition, giving consideration to the detection sensitivity and the signal intensity on the T and C lines, RLM@RBD and BLM@IgG were mixed with a ratio of 1:1 to prepare detection probes, and the volumes of the mixed detection probes were optimized. The blue signal intensity of the C line was independent of the BLM@IgG amount, but the T line showed the strongest red signal intensity when the volume of mixed detection probes was 2.5 µL, and it exhibited a good performance in detection of the spiked serum (Figure 4). Thus, 2.5 µL of mixed detection probes containing 1.25 µL of RLM@RBD and 1.25 µL of BLM@IgG were used in the subsequent experiments.

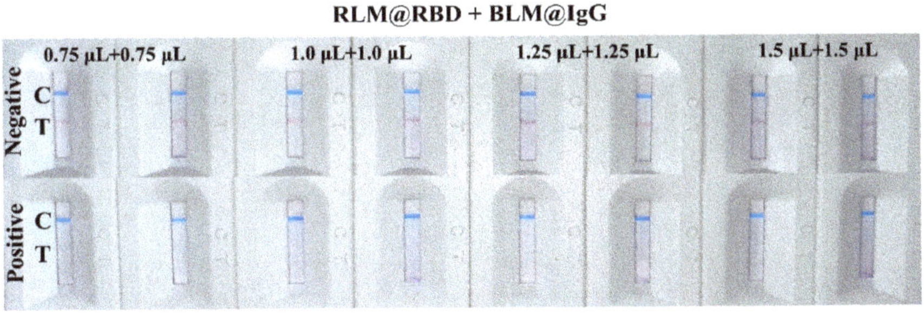

Figure 4. Result of the detection probe amount optimization, each measurement was tested in duplicate.

3.3. Performance of the Developed LM-Based Bicolor LFIA

The proposed LM-based bicolor LFIA is intended to directly and rapidly detect NAb against SARS-CoV-2 in human serum. Commonly, the reaction occurring on the LFIA is instantaneous when the sample and probes migrate through the NC membrane by capillary action. The reaction time was evaluated using the negative sample, and the result obtained by naked eye showed that the detection could be completed within 9 min. In principle, the developed bicolor LFIA involved a competitive binding immunoassay, the NAb in human serum competed with the ACE2 protein on the T line for the limited binding sites on RLM@RBD. The reference material of NAb against SARS-CoV-2 was spiked into the blank human serum with the concentrations of 1472, 736, 184, 48, 12, and 0 ng/mL, and then the spiked serum samples were tested using the developed LM-based bicolor LFIA. As the result shows in Figure 5, the red signal intensity of the T line gradually weakened with increasing NAb concentration; and when the concentration was 48 ng/mL, the red signal intensity of the T line exhibited a remarkable difference compared with that of the blank serum sample. Thus, the limit of detection (LOD) for qualitative detection by the naked eye was defined as 48 ng/mL.

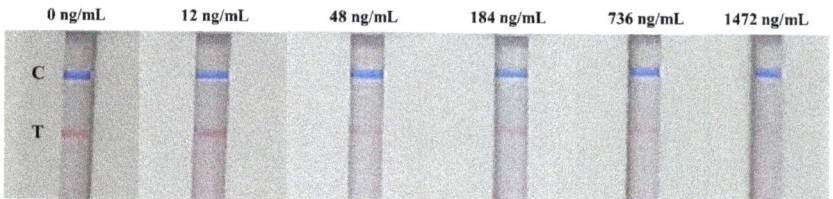

Figure 5. A series of spiked serum samples detected using the LM-based bicolor LFIA.

To validate the LM-based bicolor LFIA performance in detection of real samples, 13 serum samples from non-SARS-CoV-2 infected or vaccinated healthy donors (10 negative and 3 positive) were detected. As displayed in Figure 6, the T lines of bicolor LFIA were presented with clear red bands in the case of detecting 10 negative samples, and the red bands almost disappeared when the three positive samples were tested; however, the C lines presented distinct blue bands in both cases. Comparing with Figure 5, the red signal intensity of the positive was lower than 736 ng/mL, which indicated the NAb levels in the positive serum samples may have been equal to, or even higher than, 736 ng/mL. A limitation of this work is that the number of real samples is not sufficient to validate the method, more samples will be tested to dynamically monitor the NAb level after vaccination in further work. The results demonstrated that the developed LM-based bicolor LFIA could potentially be used to directly, rapidly, and conveniently test NAb against SARS-CoV-2, which helps to predict the acquired protective immunity in COVID-19 patients or vaccines.

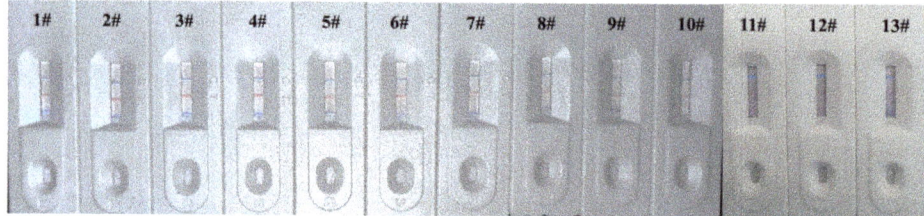

Figure 6. Results of the developed LM-based bicolor LFIA for 13 human serum samples point-of-care detection (1#–10# negative samples and 11#–13# positive samples).

4. Discussion

NAb against SARS-CoV-2 plays a pivotal role in preventing infection and clinically severe infection, thus, NAb measurement is a good choice for the prediction of protective immunity after vaccination. Live virus- or pseudovirus-based neutralization testing assays are not implemented in routine practice. Recently, ELISA based Nab that interacts with ACE2 protein in vitro has been established [24], but the operation of ELISA is tedious, time-consuming, and depends on special equipment. Finding alternative methods without cell and virus culture operation is of interest to obtain reliable NAb information for in vitro assays, which are simple, fast, high-throughput, and commercially available. Wang et al. [38] designed a track-etched membrane microplate and portable immunosensing smartphone reader platform (TEMFIS) for simply and quantitatively detecting NAb against SARS-CoV-2, and it exhibited good performance in detecting serum/plasma samples from COVID-19 patients and vaccines. In comparison with the virus neutralization testing and ELISA, the detection by TEMFIS is simple and can be completed within 45 min. In addition, immunochromatography technique is considered an attractive point-of-care testing device, with which detection results can be obtained within 30 min.

In this proof-of-principle study, a LM-based bicolor LFIA with NAb-mediated blockage of the interaction between RBD and ACE2 was developed for detecting NAb against SARS-CoV-2 after vaccination. The bicolor LFIA benefited from the red and blue LMs used to declare the locations of the T and C lines on the LFIA test strip, leading to avoidance of the misinterpretation of only one colored line result in the traditional LFIA. Moreover, point-of-care detection of NAb against SARS-CoV-2 can be completed in 9 min without using live virus and professional equipment, which remarkably reduces the cost and improves efficiency.

5. Conclusions

A fully assembled LM-based bicolor LFIA was successfully developed for rapid and direct determination of NAb against SARS-CoV-2 in human serum. The red and blue LMs were used to locate the T and C lines on the LFIA; thus, the erroneous interpretation of only one colored line result, as in traditional LFIA, can be avoided. The LOD for qualitative detection by naked eye was about 48 ng/mL, and the NAb levels in three positive serum samples were detected as higher than 736 ng/mL. This point-of-care bicolor LFIA is universal and could be applied to measure other targets in multiple areas.

Author Contributions: Conceptualization, X.D. and X.F.; Methodology, T.P., X.Y. and X.D.; Validation, T.P., Z.L. and B.M.; Formal Analysis, T.P. and Z.L.; Investigation, Z.L., X.J. and J.X.; Resources, Y.J. and Y.Z.; Data Curation, T.P. and Z.L.; Writing—Original Draft Preparation, T.P. and Z.L.; Writing—Review and Editing, T.P.; Supervision, X.D. and X.Y.; Funding Acquisition, Y.Z. and T.P. All authors have read and agreed to the published version of the manuscript.

Funding: This research was funded by [the Central Public-Interest Scientific Institution Basal Research Fund, National Institute of Metrology] grant number [AKYZD2111].

Institutional Review Board Statement: Not applicable.

Informed Consent Statement: Not applicable.

Data Availability Statement: The authors confirm that the data supporting the findings of this study are available within the article.

Acknowledgments: The work was financially supported by the Central Public-Interest Scientific Institution Basal Research Fund, National Institute of Metrology (No. AKYZD2111). And the authors appreciate the cooperation of other faculty members in the Center for Advanced Measurement Science, National Institute of Metrology, China.

Conflicts of Interest: The authors declare no conflict of interest.

References

1. Huang, C.; Wang, Y.; Li, X.; Ren, L.; Zhao, J.; Hu, Y.; Zhang, L.; Fan, G.; Xu, J.; Gu, X.; et al. Clinical features of patients infected with 2019 novel coronavirus in Wuhan, China. *Lancet* **2020**, *395*, 497–506. [CrossRef]
2. Hoffmann, M.; Kleine-Weber, H.; Schroeder, S.; Krüger, N.; Herrler, T.; Erichsen, S.; Schiergens, T.S.; Herrler, G.; Wu, N.-H.; Nitsche, A.; et al. SARS-CoV-2 Cell Entry Depends on ACE2 and TMPRSS2 and Is Blocked by a Clinically Proven Protease Inhibitor. *Cell* **2020**, *181*, 271–280.e8. [CrossRef] [PubMed]
3. Shang, J.; Ye, G.; Shi, K.; Wan, Y.; Luo, C.; Aihara, H.; Geng, Q.; Auerbach, A.; Li, F. Structural basis of receptor recognition by SARS-CoV-2. *Nature* **2020**, *581*, 221–224. [CrossRef] [PubMed]
4. Wang, Q.; Zhang, Y.; Wu, L.; Niu, S.; Song, C.; Zhang, Z.; Lu, G.; Qiao, C.; Hu, Y.; Yuen, K.Y.; et al. Structural and Functional Basis of SARS-CoV-2 Entry by Using Human ACE2. *Cell* **2020**, *181*, 894–904.e9. [CrossRef] [PubMed]
5. Wrapp, D.; Wang, N.; Corbett, K.S.; Goldsmith, J.A.; Hsieh, C.-L.; Abiona, O.; Graham, B.S.; McLellan, J.S. Cryo-EM structure of the 2019-nCoV spike in the prefusion conformation. *Science* **2020**, *367*, 1260–1263. [CrossRef] [PubMed]
6. Ke, Z.; Oton, J.; Qu, K.; Cortese, M.; Zila, V.; McKeane, L.; Nakane, T.; Zivanov, J.; Neufeldt, C.J.; Cerikan, B.; et al. Structures and distributions of SARS-CoV-2 spike proteins on intact virions. *Nature* **2020**, *588*, 498–502. [CrossRef]
7. Neuman, B.; Buchmeier, M. Supramolecular Architecture of the Coronavirus Particle. *Adv. Virus Res.* **2016**, *96*, 1–27. [CrossRef]

8. Walls, A.C.; Park, Y.-J.; Tortorici, M.A.; Wall, A.; McGuire, A.T.; Veesler, D. Structure, Function, and Antigenicity of the SARS-CoV-2 Spike Glycoprotein. *Cell* **2020**, *181*, 281–292.e6. [CrossRef]
9. Wang, C.; Li, W.; Drabek, D.; Okba, N.M.A.; van Haperen, R.; Osterhaus, A.D.M.E.; van Kuppeveld, F.J.M.; Haagmans, B.L.; Grosveld, F.; Bosch, B.-J. A human monoclonal antibody blocking SARS-CoV-2 infection. *Nat. Commun.* **2020**, *11*, 1–6. [CrossRef]
10. Kreer, C.; Zehner, M.; Weber, T.; Ercanoglu, M.S.; Gieselmann, L.; Rohde, C.; Halwe, S.; Korenkov, M.; Schommers, P.; Vanshylla, K.; et al. Longitudinal Isolation of Potent Near-Germline SARS-CoV-2-Neutralizing Antibodies from COVID-19 Patients. *Cell* **2020**, *182*, 843–854.e12. [CrossRef]
11. Zhou, G.; Zhao, Q. Perspectives on therapeutic neutralizing antibodies against the Novel Coronavirus SARS-CoV-2. *Int. J. Biol. Sci.* **2020**, *16*, 1718–1723. [CrossRef]
12. Robbiani, D.F.; Gaebler, C.; Muecksch, F.; Lorenzi, J.C.C.; Wang, Z.; Cho, A.; Agudelo, M.; Barnes, C.O.; Gazumyan, A.; Finkin, S.; et al. Convergent antibody responses to SARS-CoV-2 in convalescent individuals. *Nature* **2020**, *584*, 437–442. [CrossRef] [PubMed]
13. Liu, L.D.; Lian, C.; Yeap, L.-S.; Meng, F.-L. The development of neutralizing antibodies against SARS-CoV-2 and their common features. *J. Mol. Cell Biol.* **2020**, *12*, 980–986. [CrossRef]
14. Sharma, O.; Sultan, A.A.; Ding, H.; Triggle, C.R. A Review of the Progress and Challenges of Developing a Vaccine for COVID-19. *Front. Immunol.* **2020**, *11*, 585354. [CrossRef]
15. Kim, Y.-I.; Kim, S.-M.; Park, S.-J.; Kim, E.-H.; Yu, K.-M.; Chang, J.-H.; Kim, E.J.; Casel, M.A.B.; Rollon, R.; Jang, S.-G.; et al. Critical role of neutralizing antibody for SARS-CoV-2 reinfection and transmission. *Emerg. Microbes Infect.* **2021**, *10*, 152–160. [CrossRef] [PubMed]
16. Khoury, D.S.; Cromer, D.; Reynaldi, A.; Schlub, T.E.; Wheatley, A.K.; Juno, J.A.; Subbarao, K.; Kent, S.J.; Triccas, J.A.; Davenport, M.P. Neutralizing antibody levels are highly predictive of immune protection from symptomatic SARS-CoV-2 infection. *Nat. Med.* **2021**, *27*, 1205–1211. [CrossRef] [PubMed]
17. Yuan, M.; Wu, N.C.; Zhu, X.; Lee, C.-C.D.; So, R.T.Y.; Lv, H.; Mok, C.K.P.; Wilson, I.A. A highly conserved cryptic epitope in the receptor binding domains of SARS-CoV-2 and SARS-CoV. *Science* **2020**, *368*, 630–633. [CrossRef] [PubMed]
18. Kondo, T.; Iwatani, Y.; Matsuoka, K.; Fujino, T.; Umemoto, S.; Yokomaku, Y.; Ishizaki, K.; Kito, S.; Sezaki, T.; Hayashi, G.; et al. Antibody-like proteins that capture and neutralize SARS-CoV-2. *Sci. Adv.* **2020**, *6*, eabd3916. [CrossRef]
19. Barnes, C.O.; Jette, C.A.; Abernathy, M.E.; Dam, K.-M.A.; Esswein, S.R.; Gristick, H.B.; Malyutin, A.G.; Sharaf, N.G.; Huey-Tubman, K.E.; Lee, Y.E.; et al. SARS-CoV-2 neutralizing antibody structures inform therapeutic strategies. *Nature* **2020**, *588*, 682–687. [CrossRef]
20. Nie, J.; Li, Q.; Wu, J.; Zhao, C.; Hao, H.; Liu, H.; Zhang, L.; Nie, L.; Qin, H.; Wang, M.; et al. Establishment and validation of a pseudovirus neutralization assay for SARS-CoV-2. *Emerg. Microbes Infect.* **2020**, *9*, 680–686. [CrossRef]
21. Schmidt, F.; Weisblum, Y.; Muecksch, F.; Hoffmann, H.-H.; Michailidis, E.; Lorenzi, J.C.; Mendoza, P.; Rutkowska, M.; Bednarski, E.; Gaebler, C.; et al. Measuring SARS-CoV-2 neutralizing antibody activity using pseudotyped and chimeric viruses. *J. Exp. Med.* **2020**, *217*, e20201181. [CrossRef] [PubMed]
22. Bundschuh, C.; Egger, M.; Wiesinger, K.; Gabriel, C.; Clodi, M.; Mueller, T.; Dieplinger, B. Evaluation of the EDI enzyme linked immunosorbent assays for the detection of SARS-CoV-2 IgM and IgG antibodies in human plasma. *Clin. Chim. Acta* **2020**, *509*, 79–82. [CrossRef] [PubMed]
23. Krähling, V.; Halwe, S.; Rohde, C.; Becker, D.; Berghöfer, S.; Dahlke, C.; Eickmann, M.; Ercanoglu, M.S.; Gieselmann, L.; Herwig, A.; et al. Development and characterization of an indirect ELISA to detect SARS-CoV-2 spike protein-specific antibodies. *J. Immunol. Methods* **2021**, *490*, 112958. [CrossRef] [PubMed]
24. Wouters, E.; Verbrugghe, C.; Devloo, R.; Debruyne, I.; De Clippel, D.; Van Heddegem, L.; Van Asch, K.; Van Gaver, V.; Vanbrabant, M.; Muylaert, A.; et al. A novel competition ELISA for the rapid quantification of SARS-CoV-2 neutralizing antibodies in convalescent plasma. *Transfusion* **2021**, *61*, 2981–2990. [CrossRef]
25. Mahmoudi, T.; de la Guardia, M.; Baradaran, B. Lateral flow assays towards point-of-care cancer detection: A review of current progress and future trends. *TrAC Trends Anal. Chem.* **2020**, *125*, 115842. [CrossRef]
26. Sheng, E.; Lu, Y.; Xiao, Y.; Li, Z.; Wang, H.; Dai, Z. Simultaneous and ultrasensitive detection of three pesticides using a surface-enhanced Raman scattering-based lateral flow assay test strip. *Biosens. Bioelectron.* **2021**, *181*, 113149. [CrossRef]
27. Tian, Y.; Bu, T.; Zhang, M.; Sun, X.; Jia, P.; Wang, Q.; Liu, Y.; Bai, F.; Zhao, S.; Wang, L. Metal-polydopamine framework based lateral flow assay for high sensitive detection of tetracycline in food samples. *Food Chem.* **2020**, *339*, 127854. [CrossRef]
28. Xu, Y.; Ma, B.; Chen, E.; Yu, X.; Sun, C.; Zhang, M. Functional Up-Conversion Nanoparticle-Based Immunochromatography Assay for Simultaneous and Sensitive Detection of Residues of Four Tetracycline Antibiotics in Milk. *Front. Chem.* **2020**, *8*, 759. [CrossRef]
29. Wang, Z.; Wu, X.; Liu, L.; Xu, L.; Kuang, H.; Xu, C. Rapid and sensitive detection of diclazuril in chicken samples using a gold nanoparticle-based lateral-flow strip. *Food Chem.* **2019**, *312*, 126116. [CrossRef]
30. Li, Y.; Xu, X.; Liu, L.; Kuang, H.; Xu, L.; Xu, C. A gold nanoparticle-based lateral flow immunosensor for ultrasensitive detection of tetrodotoxin. *Analyst* **2020**, *145*, 2143–2151. [CrossRef]
31. Mousseau, F.; Tarisse, C.F.; Simon, S.; Gacoin, T.; Alexandrou, A.; Bouzigues, C.I. Luminescent lanthanide nanoparticle-based imaging enables ultra-sensitive, quantitative and multiplexed in vitro lateral flow immunoassays. *Nanoscale* **2021**, *13*, 14814–14824. [CrossRef] [PubMed]

32. Nuntawong, P.; Ochi, A.; Chaingam, J.; Tanaka, H.; Sakamoto, S.; Morimoto, S. The colloidal gold nanoparticle-based lateral flow immunoassay for fast and simple detection of plant-derived doping agent, higenamine. *Drug Test. Anal.* **2020**, *13*, 762–769. [CrossRef]
33. Chen, K.; Ma, B.; Li, J.; Chen, E.; Xu, Y.; Yu, X.; Sun, C.; Zhang, M. A Rapid and Sensitive Europium Nanoparticle-Based Lateral Flow Immunoassay Combined with Recombinase Polymerase Amplification for Simultaneous Detection of Three Food-Borne Pathogens. *Int. J. Environ. Res. Public Health* **2021**, *18*, 4574. [CrossRef]
34. Wang, Z.; Zheng, Z.; Hu, H.; Zhou, Q.; Liu, W.; Li, X.; Liu, Z.; Wang, Y.; Ma, Y. A point-of-care selenium nanoparticle-based test for the combined detection of anti-SARS-CoV-2 IgM and IgG in human serum and blood. *Lab Chip* **2020**, *20*, 4255–4261. [CrossRef]
35. Peng, T.; Jiao, X.; Liang, Z.; Zhao, H.; Zhao, Y.; Xie, J.; Jiang, Y.; Yu, X.; Fang, X.; Dai, X. Lateral Flow Immunoassay Coupled with Copper Enhancement for Rapid and Sensitive SARS-CoV-2 Nucleocapsid Protein Detection. *Biosensors* **2021**, *12*, 13. [CrossRef]
36. Petrakova, A.V.; Urusov, A.E.; Zherdev, A.; Dzantiev, B.B. Gold nanoparticles of different shape for bicolor lateral flow test. *Anal. Biochem.* **2018**, *568*, 7–13. [CrossRef] [PubMed]
37. Mao, X.; Wang, W.; Du, T.E. Dry-reagent nucleic acid biosensor based on blue dye doped latex beads and lateral flow strip. *Talanta* **2013**, *114*, 248–253. [CrossRef] [PubMed]
38. Wang, C.; Wu, Z.; Liu, B.; Zhang, P.; Lu, J.; Li, J.; Zou, P.; Li, T.; Fu, Y.; Chen, R.; et al. Track-etched membrane microplate and smartphone immunosensing for SARS-CoV-2 neutralizing antibody. *Biosens. Bioelectron.* **2021**, *192*, 113550. [CrossRef]

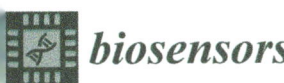

Review

Microfluidics-Based Biosensing Platforms: Emerging Frontiers in Point-of-Care Testing SARS-CoV-2 and Seroprevalence

Elda A. Flores-Contreras [1], Reyna Berenice González-González [1], Iram P. Rodríguez-Sánchez [2], Juan F. Yee-de León [3], Hafiz M. N. Iqbal [1,*] and Everardo González-González [2,*]

1. Tecnologico de Monterrey, School of Engineering and Sciences, Monterrey 64849, Nuevo León, Mexico; eldafc@tec.mx (E.A.F.-C.); reyna.g@tec.mx (R.B.G.-G.)
2. Laboratorio de Fisiología Molecular y Estructural, Facultad de Ciencias Biológicas, Universidad Autónoma de Nuevo León, San Nicolás de los Garza 66455, Nuevo León, Mexico; iram.rodriguezsa@uanl.edu.mx
3. Delee Corp., Mountain View, CA 94041, USA; juan.felipe@delee.bio
* Correspondence: hafiz.iqbal@tec.mx (H.M.N.I.); e.gzz@tec.mx (E.G.-G.)

Abstract: Severe acute respiratory syndrome coronavirus 2 (SARS-CoV-2) caused the ongoing COVID-19 (coronavirus disease-2019) outbreak and has unprecedentedly impacted the public health and economic sector. The pandemic has forced researchers to focus on the accurate and early detection of SARS-CoV-2, developing novel diagnostic tests. Among these, microfluidic-based tests stand out for their multiple benefits, such as their portability, low cost, and minimal reagents used. This review discusses the different microfluidic platforms applied in detecting SARS-CoV-2 and seroprevalence, classified into three sections according to the molecules to be detected, i.e., (1) nucleic acid, (2) antigens, and (3) anti-SARS-CoV-2 antibodies. Moreover, commercially available alternatives based on microfluidic platforms are described. Timely and accurate results allow healthcare professionals to perform efficient treatments and make appropriate decisions for infection control; therefore, novel developments that integrate microfluidic technology may provide solutions in the form of massive diagnostics to control the spread of infectious diseases.

Keywords: SARS-CoV-2; COVID-19; microfluidic; chip; biosensors; diagnostics

1. Introduction

The World Health Organization (WHO) has reported that, up to January 2022, the number of confirmed COVID-19 infections exceeded 340 million cases worldwide. Moreover, consequences in terms of public health have been severely exacerbated due to the viral evolution over time, which is causing the emergence of new variants. These mutations can give rise to substitutions in the amino acids of the viral proteins, affecting properties such as the propagation of the virus and the severity of symptoms post-infection, causing changes in public health measures and a loss in the effectiveness of drugs, vaccines, and diagnostic methods [1].

Therefore, massive diagnostic tests for detecting SARS-CoV-2 have been suggested by the WHO to decrease the spread of the virus and its consequences on populations' health and the global economy. In this manner, accessible, affordable, and accurate diagnostic devices are urgently required for SARS-CoV-2 and its emerging variants, both for controlling the spread of COVID-19 and for the resumption of economic activities [2]. In this regard, quantitative reverse-transcription–polymerase chain reaction (RT-qPCR) has been reported to be the most reliable method for the screening and diagnosis of COVID-19 [3,4], and is the most predominantly used method through the analysis of respiratory samples [3,4]. Although this method is highly sensitive, it requires expensive instruments and reagents, extensive sample processing, and specialized personnel, limiting its large-scale application outside equipped clinical laboratories [2,5].

To overcome these challenges, microfluidics for point-of-care (POC) testing devices have been recently applied for COVID-19 [2,6]. In this work, we review and discuss the different types of microfluidic-based tests relevant to COVID-19. We divide the tests into three categories based on their detection targets: nucleic acid, antigens, and anti-SARS-CoV-2 antibodies. This review examines the emerging role of microfluidics in a pandemic context that demands a reduction in costs and the substitution of sophisticated equipment, massifying and democratizing diagnosis for the entire population.

2. Microfluidics Applied to COVID-19

Microfluidics is an emerging technology that studies the behavior, control, and manipulation of fluids, either gases or liquids, constrained into micrometer- or nanometer-sized structures or channels [7]. The behavior of the fluids in such microchannels is different in comparison to the macroscale. Consequently, microfluidic systems exhibit apparent advantages such as: (i) less sample is required, (ii) lower consumption of reagents, (iii) the ability for simultaneous sample processing, (iv) accelerated reaction rates, (v) enhanced precision and sensitivity, and (vi) reductions in the quantities of waste products [8,9].

Due to the ability of microfluidics to accurately handle small quantities of samples and its use of well-controlled environments, it has been effectively applied in different applications such as nanofabrication [10], energy generation [11], and optofluidic reactors for water treatment [12]. Moreover, microfluidic systems have been successfully applied as diagnostic devices, motivated by the inaccessibility, impracticality, unaffordability, and high costs of fully equipped laboratories for a large part of the population [13].

Microfluidics forms the basis of technologies such as lab-on-a-chip, which allows any sample analysis procedure—separation, concentration, dosing, mixing, incubation, reaction, and detection—to be integrated on a microfluidic chip [9]. Moreover, the operation of microfluidic platforms can be completely automated, thus reducing human errors and improving repeatability [14]. In this sense, microfluidic research on diagnosis has been rapidly increasing in recent times (Figure 1).

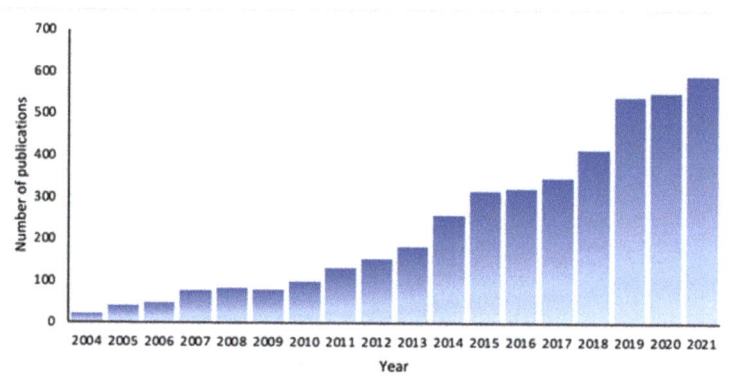

Figure 1. The number of publications per year on microfluidics applied in diagnosis. Note: Scopus database using a combination of the keywords "microfluidics" and "diagnosis".

Microfluidics diagnostic systems are integrated by detection components and fluid regulatory elements that can detect different molecules such as nucleic acid, antigens, or antibodies, producing an optical, electrical, or electrochemical signal with a diagnostic result [15] (Figure 2). In addition, their portability, convenience, and connectivity allow for the rapid examination of diagnostic results near the patient site (point-of-care devices) [16]. Therefore, research efforts in microfluidics have been focused on the diagnosis of different infectious diseases, such as dengue [17,18], Malaria [19], Zika [18], and more recently, SARS-CoV-2 [2].

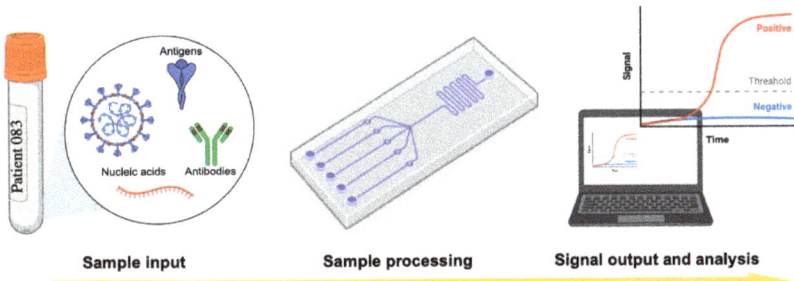

Figure 2. Schematic representation of a basic workflow using a microfluidic platform capable of sensing molecules such as nucleic acid, antigens, and anti-SARS-CoV-2 antibodies, producing a signal output. Created with Biorender.com (accessed on 11 February 2022) and extracted under premium membership.

3. Nucleic Acid Detection

The first sequence of the SARS-CoV-2 virus was obtained at the end of 2019. This achievement enabled the possibility of accessing its genetic code in databases, which is the most critical information for developing diagnostic techniques based on nucleic acid detection. SARS-CoV-2 is a single-stranded positive RNA virus with several genes such as the ORF1ab, RdRP, E, N, and S genes. The first diagnostic tests approved and used in this pandemic were designed to detect the N gene. Currently, researchers have developed different tests with multiple-gene detection to increase the certainty and ability to identify viral variants [20,21]. RT-qPCR is the gold standard for COVID diagnosis and the test recommended by the WHO due to its relatively elevated sensitivity and specificity. In addition, RT-qPCR tests have been extensively studied, showing significant advances in understanding the technology and infrastructure necessary to implement protocols worldwide [22]. However, the pandemic requires better techniques to manage the outbreak efficiently; thus, research efforts are imperative to develop new diagnostic tools that meet the current demands. We present several proposals regarding nucleic acid detection by means of microfluidics, divided into three main sections depending on the technology used: PCR, isothermal amplification, and clustered regularly interspaced short palindromic repeats (CRISPR)/biosensors. Figure 3 presents a graphical overview of microfluidic techniques used to detect nucleic acid from SARS-CoV-2.

3.1. Based on PCR

Millions of RT-qPCR tests have been performed worldwide, which have significantly helped to diagnose COVID-19. However, the severity of the pandemic makes the traditional PCR method insufficient to control the problem. The most important limitations are shortages of reagents, limited staff, the analysis time, and the massive sample processing requirements [22]. Several proposals have recently been reported in scientific journals to solve those challenges. For example, a portable microfluidic-chip qPCR method that can detect the SARS-CoV-2 virus directly from saliva samples has been recently reported. This technique utilized a microfluidic chip where the sample is placed, and all the reaction stages (heat, mix, and detection) are performed; this device can perform multiplex assays detecting up to three targets, showing a virus detection of 1000 copies/mL in saliva samples [23].

An essential approach in microfluidics is high-throughput sample processing. Fassy et al. and Xie et al. have reported the use of a qPCR method with the potential to perform massive assays to detect the SARS-CoV-2 virus [24,25]. The reported technology is based on a nanofluidic qPCR method using the 192.24 IFC chip (Fluidigm, CA, USA) (Figure 3), which can process 4608 samples in a single run. This technology also performs multiplex assays with 24 different probe sets, which is very convenient for identifying SARS-CoV-2 variants or confirming the diagnosis with the amplification of other targets. Moreover, the reaction volume was reported to be as low as 10 nL, which is an important characteristic in terms of reducing the amount of reagents used and the consequent decrease in the price of tests [24,25].

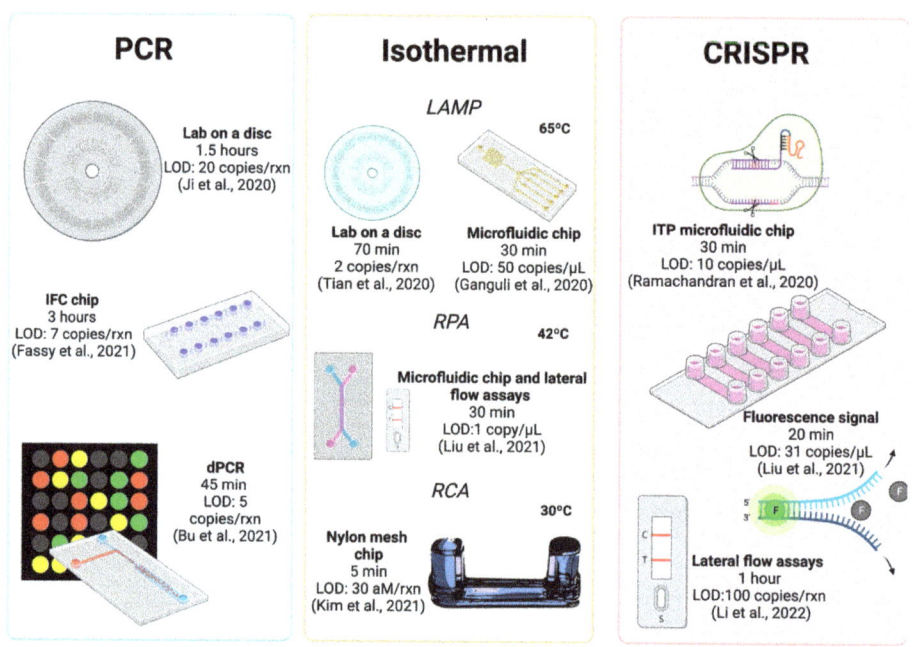

Figure 3. Graphical summary of microfluidic techniques used to detect nucleic acid from SARS-CoV-2 and its main characteristics. Created with Biorender.com (accessed on 11 February 2022) and extracted under premium membership.

Using this technology, Fassy et al. proposed an optimized protocol for SARS-CoV-2 RNA detection without the need for viral RNA extraction, which reduces the processing time [24]. Through microfluidics, researchers have pursued volume reduction with the aim of producing low-cost tests. For example, Cojocaru et al. reported a PCR test based on a disposable microchip with lyophilized primers and probes capable of providing results in less than 30 min using a volume of 1.2 µL per reaction. They determined a limit of detection (LOD) of one copy per reaction with clinical samples from Canadian patients [26]. Moreover, another microfluidic form of PCR is the lab-on-a-disc, applied to COVID-19, including the multi-detection of Influenza A and B. The LOD of this device was 20 viral copies, with a test time of 1.5 h [27]. Another recent and novel development is a microfluidic nanoplasmonic qPCR method based on a microfluidic chip that integrates glass nanopillar arrays with Au nanoislands and microfluidic channels, in which the PCR reaction amplifies the E gene from SARS-CoV-2. The main characteristic of the reported microfluidic system is its rapid capacity to detect the presence of SARS-CoV-2, requiring around five minutes with an LOD of 259 copies/µL [28]. Overall, these microfluidic PCR platforms have demonstrated the potential for optimal and rapid virus detection.

In addition, one of the objectives of microfluidics is to integrate molecular techniques in microfluidic chips, developing complete laboratories on a chip that provide relevant information for a more precise diagnosis. Li et al. [29] reported the synergistic potential of combined technologies and proposed a workflow using a microfluidic platform to detect SARS-CoV-2 and then performing whole-genome sequencing. These devices could be responsible for controlling the pandemic in the future due to the possibility of increasing the sensitivity of the tests and reducing the costs and time of the tests [29].

Digital PCR (dPCR) is an emergent and highly precise PCR test, which has received increasing research attention since it provides absolute quantification of nucleic acid molecules from very small samples [30]. The most crucial difference between traditional qPCR and dPCR is the reaction preparation and the equipment required; dPCR requires, as the first step, the preparation of the sample to be separated in the dispensed reaction, mainly by means of micropores and droplets. In this way, the overall response can be divided into multiple compartmentalized reactions, generating small reactors to amplify nucleic acid independently with a Poisson distribution, leading to analysis based on fluorescent signals in each compartment. dPCR has shown potential for its use in the clinical field. Thus, several research groups have employed it to diagnose COVID-19. Bu et al. developed a microfluidic system that generates programmable on-demand droplets, with the viral detection of 4.68 copies/µL, amplifying the ORF1ab and N genes [31]. A similar SARS-CoV-2 dPCR test was reported by Yin et al., which showed equivalent results in viral detection (five copies/reaction), amplifying the same two genes with the ability to detect the virus in less than 5 min [32] (Figure 3). Recently, Sun et al. reported a dPCR test composed of a microfluidic chamber manufactured using a wet-etching process and silicon-glass bonding. Some interesting features of this microfluidic chip are the low-cost fabrication method, the generation of microdroplets of uniform volume, and higher stability, with the authors reporting an LOD of 10 copies/µL, using the ORF1ab gene as the target [33].

3.2. Based on Isothermal Amplification

The use of a thermocycler is essential to perform PCR tests. However, infrastructure deficits in underdeveloped places is one of the most critical limitations. Therefore, there is an urgent need to develop strategies that do not require expensive equipment, thus achieving a diagnosis that is accessible to the entire population, regardless of their economic context. For example, there is an approach based on the isothermal amplification of nucleic acid, which avoids the use of a thermocycler, replacing it with a simple water bath or incubator. Several isothermal techniques have been developed and deployed, such as loop-mediated isothermal amplification (LAMP), rolling circle amplification (RCA), and recombinase polymerase amplification (RPA) [34]. The isothermal COVID-19 diagnosis method has attracted worldwide attention due to its potential to massify the diagnosis in places where there are no laboratories or expensive facilities.

LAMP is a technology that employs four to six primers to recognize different regions from a target sequence; it is distinguished by requiring a temperature reaction around 65 °C and having shorter reaction times compared to other techniques such as PCR. To date, the FDA has approved ten COVID-19 tests based on LAMP, and this technology has been widely applied for the development of COVID-19 microfluidic devices. One of the first developments was an automated microfluidic disc that is able to perform the entire process—sample treatment, LAMP reaction, and fluorescence signal detection—after injecting samples into the disc. The estimated LOD is two copies per reaction, enabling the processing of up to 21 samples per microfluidic disc in 70 min [35]. Another successful example of this technology is a device integrated within an aluminum block, detecting fluorescence emission using a camera controlled by a single-board computer. The authors demonstrated the ability to detect 100 copies of viral RNA within 10 to 20 min, estimating the device's cost at around 150 USD [36]. Ganguli et al. created a platform that includes a microfluidic chip and a smartphone-based reader that demonstrated an LOD of 50 copies/µL within 30 min [37]. Similarly, de Oliveira et al. employed a cell phone as a reader; they printed a polyester-toner microfluidic device controlled by a fidget spinner using centrifugal force. The microfluidic chip contains chambers with a 5 µL of volume capacity, and to perform the LAMP reaction, the sample is incubated using a thermoblock. They reported a time assay of 10 min, with an LOD of 10^{-3} copies of viral RNA and an estimated cost of 5 USD per test [38].

Recently, colorimetric LAMP tests based on changes in pH values have been developed, which have also been implemented in microfluidics. Davidson et al. prepared microfluidic paper-based analytical devices (µPADs) to detect SARS-CoV-2 via colorimetry. They demonstrated direct viral detection from saliva samples (without sample processing), obtaining results that were visible to the naked eye. The microfluidic device could detect up to 200 copies/µL from saliva samples within 60 min, with an estimated cost of 10 USD per test [39]. Furthermore, Deng et al. developed a portable device that employs a colorimetric LAMP with an LOD of 300 copies/reaction within 35 min [40]. On the other hand, Kim et al. reported a microfluidic device using RCA, which is another isothermal technique that employs a short primer and is amplified to form long single-stranded nucleic acid using a circular template and polymerases. This test is based on a device integrated with a nylon mesh with multiple microfluidic pores and an immobilized primer. Its operation is based on the fact that RCA amplification occurs when the viral target is present, causing DNA gelation and, consequently, a blockage of the micropores, preventing the flow of microfluidics. This device was able to detect SARS-SoV-2 within 5 min at a concentration of 30 aM [41] (Figure 3).

The RPA isothermal assay has also been applied in microfluidic testing for COVID-19; this technology has interesting features such as high sensitivity, fast reaction times, lower temperatures (37 °C to 42 °C), and simple protocols and primer design. RPA is based on recombinase enzymes to facilitate primer binding to templates and the synthesis of strands. As in other methods, it is also possible to quantify the amplification process via fluorescence or colorimetry using lateral flow assays. For example, Liu et al. developed a microfluidic chip and combined RPA and lateral flow assays to diagnose COVID-19. They fabricated a PMMA (polymethyl methacrylate) microfluidic chip with two reservoirs, in which the reactants are mixed, and the reaction is conducted. It also includes a strip with the conjugated antibodies to perform the colorimetric detection. The chip is incubated at 42 °C for 15 min using a thermoblock; after the amplification time, the chip is inverted to start the reveal process with the lateral flow assay. They reported an LOD of 1 copy/µL within 30 min [42] (Figure 3). Interestingly, a microfluidic disc combining LAMP and RPA technologies was recently developed, demonstrating the ability to detect multiple targets of SARS-CoV-2 and measles virus via fluorescence, with an LOD as low as 10 copies within one hour of the reaction [43].

3.3. Based on CRISPR

CRISPR is an emerging and powerful technique that has also been applied to detect nucleic acid, exhibiting high versatility, sensitivity, and specificity. The use of CRISPR in diagnostics is based on the reaction of "collateral cleavage" induced by a nuclease, such as Cas12 and Cas13. These CRISPR-Cas nucleases can be directed to a guide RNA (gRNA)-specific target sequence. Furthermore, this reaction can be analyzed through fluorescence signals, a practical approach to detecting pathogens.

Several research groups have integrated CRISPR into microfluidic technology to detect SARS-CoV-2, developing novel devices to improve diagnosis. One of the first CRISPR microfluidic chips developments applied to the diagnosis of COVID-19 used an electrokinetic microfluidic technique termed "isotachophoresis" (ITP) (Figure 3). Using this technology, Ramachandran et al. developed a microfluidic chip to extract nucleic acid from raw biological samples. Furthermore, the chip can mix the reagents and accelerate enzymatic reactions with the viral target. The authors reported multiple benefits obtained using this technique, such as lower consumption of reagents in comparison to traditional methods (lower than 0.2 µL), a decrease in the sample processing time (30–40 min from sample to results), and an LOD as low as 10 copies/µL [44].

Li et al. proposed a microfluidic system combining RPA amplification, CRISPR cleavage, and lateral flow detection. Their developed microfluidic chip was integrated with a reaction chamber that stored lyophilized reagents and a portable hand warmer to incubate the reactions to amplify SARS-CoV-2 nucleic acid, avoiding the use of electricity; this portable microfluidic system displayed an LOD as low as 100 copies [45] (Figure 3). Similarly, a CRISPR assay that is able to detect SARS-CoV-2 was implemented in a microfluidic chip with reaction chambers, a heating module to incubate the reactions at 37 °C, and a compact fluorescence imaging system for monitoring the fluorescence signal; an LOD of 31 copies/µL within 20 min of reaction was reported [46].

3.4. Other Microfluidic Developments

The detection of SARS-CoV-2 nucleic acid has also been achieved using other types of microfluidic biosensors. For example, Zhao et al. developed an automated microfluidic platform based on nanotechnology to detect the S gene from the SARS-CoV-2 virus. This technology, known as the "electrochemical system integrating reconfigurable enzyme-DNA nanostructures" (eSIREN), integrates multiple responsive molecular nanostructures to form a catalytic molecular circuit with the aim of sensing the viral presence. It presented an LOD of 7 copies/µL after approximately 20 min of reaction at room temperature [2].

Another example of technologies not frequently explored is the one developed by Hwang et al., which consists of interdigitated platinum/titanium electrodes to detect SARS-CoV-2 nucleic acid. In this technique, the detection is based on sensing the hybridization from the viral analyte with probe DNA, and using physicochemical analytical techniques such as Fourier-transform infrared (FTIR) spectrometry, contact-angle analysis, and capacitance-frequency measurements. This approach allowed the detection of the RdRp gene with a sensitivity of 0.843 nF/nM [47]. Finally, Iwanaga reported the development of a microfluidic chip using a biosensor based on an all-dielectric metasurface fabricated with silicon-on-insulator nanorod arrays to enhance the fluorescence signal and demonstrated an LOD of 250 amol/mL within 30 min of the reaction [48]. Table 1 summarizes the diverse microfluidic assays used for the detection of SARS-CoV-2 nucleic acid.

Table 1. Microfluidic assays for the detection of SARS-CoV-2 nucleic acid.

Type of Technique	LOD	Target Gene	Detection Method	Processing Time (Minutes)	Reference
qPCR	9 copies/rxn	N	Fluorescence	NR	[23]
qPCR	7 copies/rxn	N, E, ORF1ab, S and NSP6	Fluorescence	<120	[24]
qPCR	7 copies/µL	N	Fluorescence	<120	[25]
qPCR	1 copy/rxn	N	Fluorescence	30	[26]
qPCR	20 copies/rxn	N	Fluorescence	90	[27]
qPCR	259 copies/µL	E	Nanoplasmonic	5	[28]
dPCR	4.68 copies/µL	N and ORF1ab	Fluorescence	45	[31]
dPCR	5 copies/rxn	N and ORF1ab	Fluorescence	5	[32]
dPCR	10 copies/µL	ORF1ab	Fluorescence	<60	[33]
LAMP	2 copies/rxn	N, E and ORF1ab	Fluorescence	70	[35]
LAMP	100 copies/rxn	ORF1ab	Fluorescence	20	[36]
LAMP	50 copies/µL	N, ORF1ab and ORF8	Fluorescence	30	[37]
LAMP	<1 copy/µL	N	Fluorescence	10	[38]
LAMP	200 copies/µL	N and ORF1ab	Colorimetric	60	[39]
LAMP	300 copies/rxn	N and E	Colorimetric	35	[40]
RCA	30 aM/rxn	ORF1ab	Gelation	5	[41]
RPA-LFA	1 copy/µL	N	Colorimetric	30	[42]
RPA-LAMP	10 copies/rxn	S	Fluorescence	60	[43]
CRISPR	10 copies/µL	N and E	Fluorescence	40	[44]
CRISPR-LFA	100 copies/rxn	N	Colorimetric	NR	[45]
CRISPR	31 copies/µL	N, S and ORF1ab	Fluorescence	20	[46]

Abbreviations: LOD (limit of detection); NR (not reported); rxn (reaction); LFA (lateral flow assay).

4. Antigen Detection

Currently, there are a few reports on microfluidic immunoassays for the detection of SARS-CoV-2 viral proteins, despite their multiple benefits such as their low cost and the rapid processing of samples compared to PCR tests that use nucleic acid detection. In addition, antigen immunoassays can perform more convenient detection since they can detect the presence of the virus when the person can transmit it, unlike serological immunoassays that identify IgG and IgM antibodies against SARS-CoV-2, which require at least a few weeks for their detection. Therefore, immunoassays of antigens allow effective measurements of viral proteins, obtaining results in less than an hour with detection ranges from fg to µg (Table 2).

The most relevant antigens for detecting SARS-CoV-2 in clinical samples are the nucleocapsid protein (N) and the spike protein (S). The S protein is a glycoprotein on the virus's surface, composed of S1 and S2. In addition, S1 contains a region known as the receptor-binding domain (RBD), which facilitates the entry of SARS-CoV-2 into the host cells [49,50]. The N protein is an immunogenic protein that packages the genome RNA of the virus, forming helical nucleocapsids [50,51]; it is used as an early indicator since it allows the identification of SARS-CoV-2 up to one day before symptoms appear [52]. Furthermore, the N protein is considered a better target than the S protein because the latter is less abundant and, under selective pressure, is more prone to mutations [53]. The detection of SARS-CoV-2 proteins by means of microfluidic immunoassays consists mainly of flow-through assays [54]. The sample obtained from serum or nasopharyngeal or oropharyngeal swabs [55] is subjected to this flow to identify viral SARS-CoV-2 proteins via direct or sandwich immunoassays. Direct immunoassays consist of immobilized anti-SARS-CoV-2 antibodies or nanomaterials (polymers and fibronectin) on a sensor's surface, which allows one to identify the presence of proteins such as S, RBD, and N [56–59]. In contrast, sandwich-type immunoassays consist of the formation of complexes between anti-SARS-CoV-2 antibodies anchored to microspheres, nanobeads, or microbeads that interact with SARS-CoV-2 viral proteins such as S, RBD, and N. These complexes are subsequently captured by aptamers or a second anti-SARS-CoV-2 antibody, either immobilized (on a gold electrode or silica) or free (attached to fluorescent reporters or colored nanobeads) [53,57,60,61]. The identification of SARS-CoV-2 virus in samples of interest by means of direct or sandwich microfluidic immunoassays is performed after the interaction of the anti-SARS-CoV-2 antibodies, nanomaterials, or aptamers with the viral proteins, which produes a fluorescence signal, or changes in electric current, absorbance, or color [62–64].

The primary type of microfluidic immunoassays is based on the interaction of viral proteins with anti-SARS-CoV-2 antibodies or nanomaterials immobilized on a sensor (which detects changes in the electric current) or an electrode, typically covered with graphene, aluminum, fluorine-doped tin oxide electrode (FTO), screen-printed carbon electrode (SPE), or gold nanoparticles (AuNPs). These materials allow the identification of electrical conductivity changes when the antibodies interact with the antigens [57,59,65]. As a representative work of this type of immunoassay, Seo et al. developed a direct microfluidic immunoassay that uses a field-effect transistor (FET) coated with graphene sheets conjugated with anti-SARS-CoV-2-Spike antibodies that cause a voltage change when interacting with the viral particles. This chip did not require the processing or labeling of samples obtained from a nasopharyngeal swab and presented an LOD of 2.42×10^2 copies/mL in less than 5 min [66]. Another important type of microfluidic immunoassay is generating a redox reaction caused by anti-SARS-CoV-2 antibodies conjugated with enzymes (that interact with their substrate) or redox probes (electron transfer) in the presence of the SARS-CoV-2 viral proteins. Li and Lillehoj reported an immunoassay using this type of signal, which consumes minimum quantities of reagents and enhances the detection sensitivity. Their immunosensor comprises a novel sandwich immunoassay. It uses dually-labeled magnetic nanobeads tagged with HRP (horseradish peroxidase). It is covered with anti-SARS-CoV-2 antibodies that interact with the viral proteins, forming a complex captured by a second anti-SARS-CoV-2 antibody immobilized on a gold electrode. In the presence of a TMB substrate, this complex produces an electrochemical signal that can be detected by smartphones or electronic devices, with an LOD of 50 pg/mL in whole serum samples, providing results in less than an hour [60].

Interestingly, Yousefi et al. designed a direct immunoassay that integrates an antibody conjugated with a negatively charged DNA linker, labeled with a redox probe (ferrocene), which binds to the surface of the positively charged sensor when it interacts with an S protein, thus generating a redox reaction that the sensor detects. This immunosensor has an LOD of 4×10^3 viral particles/mL in unprocessed saliva samples, generating results in approximately five minutes [58]. On the other hand, Raziq et al. proposed an electrochemical sensor using molecularly imprinted polymers (MIPs) acting as the antibodies; they were interfaced with a thin film electrode and connected to a portable potentiostat, providing high sensitivity and the ability to discriminate between molecules to exclusively detect N proteins from nasopharyngeal samples with an LOD of 15 fM [63].

Microfluidic immunoassays that use fluorescence signals to detect SARS-CoV-2 consist of antibodies or aptamers labeled with fluorescent reporters (probes, fluorophores, or submicron particles) that emit a signal that is directly proportional to the viral particles dispersed in the analyzed sample [56,67]. Stambaugh et al. presented a successful example of this technique, creating a photonic chip-based sandwich immunoassay. Basically, the anti-SARS-CoV-2 antibody is linked to a fluorescent DNA probe that has a photo-cleavable spacer, which interacts with the SARS-CoV-2 viral proteins, forming a complex. This complex is captured by a second antibody, which emits a fluorescence signal when is exposed to UV radiation. This compact device allows the simultaneous detection of Influenza A and SARS-CoV-2 with an LOD of 30 ng/mL from nasopharyngeal samples [68]. Alternatively, Ge et al. developed a test for the effective detection of the SARS-CoV-2 virus at the femtoliter scale. The device confined magnetic beads covered with anti-SARS-CoV-2-N antibodies and biotin-labeled aptamers interacting with the N protein, forming a sandwich immunoassay. The fluorescence signal was observed in the presence of the SARS-CoV-2 virus and streptavidin-B-galactosidase. This device had an LOD of 33.28 pg/mL, which is 300 times lower than that of the traditional ELISA sandwich method [61].

Optical techniques have also been used to detect SARS-CoV-2 proteins, in which antibodies anchored to AuNPs, enzymes, or colored nanobeads are used; their interaction with viral proteins leads to changes in the absorbance or the observation of a color signal in the visible spectrum. An excellent example of this technique was reported by Xu et al., who prepared a handheld microfluidic hydrodynamic filtration device based on a sandwich immunoassay, in which the N protein of SARS-CoV-2 interacts with anti-SARS-CoV-2-N antibodies, binding to white microbeads and to a second antibody anchored to a red nanobead, forming a complex. Then, the complex enters the observation zone (OZ) via microfluidic filtration; a red color is observed when the antigen is present, whereas a white color is observed in the absence of the antigen since free red nanobeads pass through the pillar gaps, leaving the white beads in the OZ. This device had an LOD of <100 copies/mL in nasal samples, with outstanding sensitivity and specificity of 95.4% and 100%, respectively. In addition, they reported an estimated cost of 0.98 USD per test and the possibility of reusing the device more than 50 times [53].

Regarding the use of conjugated enzymes, Sun et al. proposed a paper-based microfluidic sandwich immunoassay, which consists of an antibody conjugated to HRP and a second anti-SARS-CoV-2-N antibody immobilized on the chitosan-glutaraldehyde surface of the immunosensor. In the presence of the N protein, this biosensor generates a black spot observed with the naked eye with an LOD of 8 µg/mL [64]. On the other hand, Murugan et al. reported a biosensor based on absorbance changes. The authors created a plasmonic fiber-optic absorbance biosensor (P-FAB) on a U-bent optical fiber probe. In their work, two different types of design were proposed: a direct immunoassay and a sandwich immunoassay. In the direct immunoassay, antibodies were immobilized to AuNPs placed on the biosensor's surface. In contrast, the sandwich immunoassay consisted of antibodies anchored to the biosensor's surface and secondary antibodies conjugated with AuNPs. In both designs, the interaction of the N proteins with the antibodies resulted in absorbance changes. This portable device had an LOD of 10^{-8} M for saliva samples (using a volume of 25 µL) with minimal pre-processing procedures, obtaining results within 15 min [62]. These types of microfluidic immunoassays allow the rapid detection of SARS-CoV-2 proteins (<1 h) and involve minimum or null sample processing, compared to ELISA. However, this traditional technique involves time-consuming processes ranging from several hours to days. Another emergent method to detect viral antigens is through Raman spectroscopy. Recently, Huang et al. reported a rapid assay combing Raman spectroscopy and a deep learning model to detect the S protein from COVID-19 patients within 20 min [69].

Table 2. Microfluidic immunoassays for the detection of SARS-CoV-2 proteins.

Type Immunoassay	Specimen	LOD	Target Protein	Detection Method	Processing Time (Minutes)	Reference
Sandwich Immunoassay	Serum	33.28 pg/mL	N	Fluorescence	<120	[61]
Direct Immunoassay	Saliva	NR	VP	Fluorescence	<30	[56]
Sandwich Immunoassay	Serum, Saliva, Nasopharyngeal and urine	8 µg/mL	N	Colorimetric	>30	[64]
Direct and sandwich Immunoassay	Saliva	NR	N	Absorbance	15	[62]
Direct Immunoassay	Blood	1 fg/mL	S	Voltage	0.05	[57]
Direct Immunoassay	Saliva	4000 viral particles/mL	S	Electrochemical	5	[58]
Direct Immunoassay	Food	2.29×10^{-6} ng/mL	S	Voltage	0.33	[59]
Direct immunoassay	Saliva	90 fM	S	Electrochemical	0.5	[65]
Sandwich immunoassay	Serum	230 pg/mL	N	Electrochemical	<60	[60]
Sandwich immunoassay	Nasopharyngeal and serum	NR	VP	Fluorescence	15	[67]
Sandwich immunoassay	Nasopharyngeal	<100 copies/mL	N	Colorimetric	>30	[53]
Sandwich immunoassay	Nasopharyngeal	30 ng/mL	N	Fluorescence	<120	[68]
Direct immunoassay	Nasopharyngeal	2.42×10^2 copies/mL	S	Voltage	>1	[66]
Direct immunoassay	Serum	1 pg/mL	S	Voltage	15	[70]
Direct immunoassay	Nasopharyngeal	15 fM	N	Electrochemical	>30	[63]

Abbreviations: LOD (limit of detection); N (nucleocapsid protein); S (spike protein); VP (unspecified SARS-CoV-2 viral proteins); NR (not reported).

5. Anti-SARS-CoV-2 Antibody Detection

Serological tests for SARS-CoV-2 are highly relevant since they not only provide information on the existence of a viral infection but also on the severity of the disease (which is correlated with age and antibody expression), as well as information on the success of vaccination in people not infected with SARS-CoV-2 [71,72]. Antibody expression occurs as a reaction to the SARS-CoV-2 virus, secreted by B lymphocytes. There are various antibodies involved; however, IgG and IgM isotypes are the most relevant for developing serological tests since these isotypes are found more frequently in the blood and are expressed during different periods [73–75]. IgM antibodies appear between the fourth and tenth day post-infection, whereas IgG antibodies are expressed during the second week post-infection [74,76–78]. Microfluidic immunoassays for detecting antibodies against SARS-CoV-2 consist mainly of antigens (S, RBD, or N proteins) that capture IgM or IgG antibodies depending on the post-inoculation time of SARS-CoV-2 via direct, indirect, and sandwich immunoassays (Table 3) [79–81].

Direct immunoassays consist of an immobilized antigen on a sensor or electrode that captures IgG or IgM antibodies. In contrast, indirect immunoassays consist of an antigen immobilized on the surface of the microfluidic chip, sensor, or electrode (glass/polydimethylsiloxane, polystyrene, silicon, or paper) that binds to IgG and IgM antibodies. However, it is necessary to use a second antibody, either label-free or labeled by an enzyme or fluorophore, in the microfluidic environment emitting a signal (fluorescence, voltage change, electrochemical, or colorimetric) in the presence of antibodies against the SARS-CoV-2 virus [81]. On the other hand, sandwich-type immunoassays consist of an antigen fixed on the surface of the microfluidic device. They require a second antigen that is labeled (not immobilized); if the antibodies are against SARS-CoV-2, they will interact with both antigens producing a fluorescent signal [82].

The signals produced by microfluidic immunoassays to detect anti-SARS-CoV-2 antibodies (IgG or IgM) include fluorescence, colorimetry, and electrochemical signals. Thus, microfluidic immunoassays can be classified as label-based or label-free assays [83–85]. Label-based microfluidic biosensors for detecting antibodies are usually indirect or sandwich immunoassays. They typically consist of secondary antibodies (anti IgG or IgM) linked to enzymes (in the presence of their substrates) and fluorophores producing color changes and fluorescence signals, respectively, when they interact with antibodies against SARS-CoV-2. They can reach low LODs in the range of pg/mL to ng/mL, providing results in less than one hour [82,86,87].

Regarding microfluidic assays based on colorimetry changes, González-González et al. reported an automated ELISA on-chip of polystyrene with four straight channels (with a capacity of 50 µL/channel). This device is based on an indirect immunoassay that is able to detect anti-SARS-CoV-2 antibodies against the S protein from serum samples, either from vaccinated or COVID-19 patients. This microfluidic device consists of S proteins immobilized on the surface of a microfluidic chip that, using a secondary antibody labeled with HRP (in the presence of the substrate TMB), detects anti-SARS-CoV-2 (IgG) antibodies. A colorimetric signal is visible through the use of a smartphone or a microplate reader. In addition, processes can be programmed using Zen lab software, avoiding sample manipulation and human error [80]. Tripathi and Agrawal developed a semi-automated on-chip ELISA to detect anti-SARS-CoV-2 antibodies and were able to separate 10 µL of serum from 1 mL of whole blood in approximately 3 min. They used a microfluidic chip fabricated out of polydimethylsiloxane (PDMS) and glass covered with the S protein [81].

Tan et al. developed a microfluidic immunoassay that detects anti-SARS-CoV-2 (IgG) antibodies using portable microfluidic chemiluminescent ELISA technology. The device is made of polystyrene and has 12 channels, with an inner diameter of 0.8 mm, requiring only 8 µL of serum. This immunoassay consists of an anti-polyhistidine antibody that immobilizes the S and N proteins that interact with anti-SARS-CoV-2 antibodies, which in turn bind to the secondary antibody (anti-IgG) labeled with HRP. This immunosensor has an LOD of 0.06 ng/mL and 1 ng/mL for the N and S proteins, respectively. This microfluidic chip also allows the detection of antigens (S and N proteins) by immobilizing a captured antibody on the surface of the chip [88].

On the other hand, the devices that use fluorescence signals to identify anti-SARS-CoV-2 antibodies consist of antigens or secondary anti-IgG or anti-IgM antibodies labeled with fluorophores (phycoerythrin and Dylight 550). An example of their successful application for the detection of SARS-CoV-2 is a polydimethylsiloxane (PDMS) microfluidic chip developed by Lee et al., which comprises carboxylate polystyrene beads that immobilize the RBD protein on the microfluidic chip and conjugated secondary antibodies with Dylight 550 (not immobilized) that release a fluorescence signal when they bind to anti-SARS-CoV-2 antibodies. Furthermore, this microfluidic chip allows the detection of Zika, Dengue, and Chikungunya viruses within 30 min [86]. Another example of fluorescence immunoassays was proposed by Rodriguez-Moncayo et al., who used a multiplex format on a semi-automated platform made of PDMS/glass that allows the identification of the affinity of anti-SARS-CoV-2 antibodies (IgG or IgM) towards different viral proteins (S, N, RBD, and S1). This device can process up to 50 samples with an LOD of 1.6 ng/mL, and a sensitivity and specificity of 95% and 91%, respectively [87].

Similarly, Heggestad et al. reported a microfluidic immunoassay that determines the affinity of different SARS-CoV-2 viral proteins (S1, N, and RBD). They used labeled antigens with fluorophores on a platform that consisted of a completely autonomous immunoassay. All the reagents were added to the surface of the platform via inkjet printing. The reported sensitivity of this device was 100% for antibodies that recognize S1 and RBD proteins and 96.3% for antibodies that interact with the N protein. The specificity for the S1, RBD, and N proteins was 100% two weeks after the appearance of symptoms [82].

On the other hand, label-free microfluidic assays detect changes in the electrical current and refractive index. They are typically used in direct or indirect immunoassays to detect the presence of anti-SARS-CoV-2 antibodies (IgG or IgM). These types of immunoassays have an LOD for antibodies (IgG or IgM) against SARS-CoV-2 in the range of ng/mL in diluted serum samples. Qualitative microfluidic chips have also been reported, indicating only the presence of anti-SARS-CoV-2 antibodies. Sample processing and collection for label-free-type immunoassays require less than an hour [84,89,90]. An example of this type of biosensor was proposed by Li et al., consisting of a direct immunoassay on a working electrode of pieces of paper and carbon ink and zinc oxide nanowires (ZnO NWs), with an LOD of 10 ng/mL in serum samples. The RBD protein was immobilized, detecting a current change via electrochemical impedance spectroscopy (EIS) when it interacts with the anti-SARS-CoV-2 antibodies (IgG) [84]. Another novel immunoassay was reported by Djaileb et al., detecting IgG antibodies specific for the N and S proteins of infected or vaccinated patients in serum, plasma, and dried blood spot samples. The immobilized viral proteins on the surface of the plasmon resonance instrument produced a shift in the refractive index when they interacted with anti-SARS-CoV-2 antibodies. The LOD was 2 nM for indirect immunoassays and 3 nM for direct immunoassays [89].

Funari et al. developed an indirect immunoassay based on a localized surface plasmon in an opto-microfluidic chip. The S protein was immobilized on gold nanostructures, causing a change in the refractive index after interacting with anti-SARS-CoV-2 (IgG) antibodies and a secondary anti-IgG antibody. This immunoassay has an LOD of approximately 0.08 ng/mL (0.5 pM), and the results are obtained in 30 min [79]. Xu et al. developed an all-fiber Fresnel reflection microfluidic (FRMB) that detects IgG and IgM antibodies against the S protein through a secondary antibody (anti IgG or IgM) acting as a transducer and biorecognition element. The quantification is achieved according to the relationship of the intensity of Fresnel reflection light. This biosensor provided results in 7 min and presented an LOD of 0.82 ng/mL for IgM and 0.45 ng/mL for IgG antibodies [90].

Overall, these microfluidic chips have a lower LOD and higher specificity than traditional ELISA methods [91]. Furthermore, these devices are highly useful for evaluating the success of vaccination programs, estimating the affinity of anti-SARS-CoV-2 antibodies for new variants, and finding plasma donors for patients severely affected by SARS-CoV-2. However, there are still limitations, such as the production time required for the antibodies, on which the sensitivity depends, to avoid false negatives. Therefore, further research is still required to achieve accurate results and practical application.

Table 3. Microfluidic immunoassays for the detection of anti-SARS-CoV-2 antibodies.

Type Immunoassay	Specimen	LOD	Target Antibodies	Detection Method	Processing Time (Minutes)	Reference
Indirect immunoassay	Serum	NR	Anti-S	Colorimetric	<150	[80]
Sandwich immunoassay	Blood	NR	Anti-S	Colorimetric	<5	[81]
Indirect immunoassay	Serum	0.06–1 ng/mL	Anti-N and S	Chemiluminescent	15	[88]
Indirect immunoassay	Serum, nasopharyngeal	NR	Anti-RBD	Fluorescence	30	[86]
Indirect immunoassay	Serum	1.6 ng/mL	Anti-N, S and RBD	Fluorescence	<90	[87]
Sandwich immunoassay	Blood	0.12 ng/mL	Anti-N, S and RBD	Fluorescence	60	[82]
Direct immunoassay	Serum	10 ng/mL	Anti-RBD	Electrochemical	30	[84]
Direct and indirect immunoassay	Blood	2–3 nM	Anti-N and S	Absorbance	30	[89]
Indirect immunoassay	Blood	0.08 ng/mL	Anti-S	Absorbance	30	[79]
Indirect immunoassay	Serum	0.82–0.45 ng/mL	Anti-S	Absorbance	7	[90]
Indirect immunoassay	Serum	NR	Anti-S and RBD	Absorbance	NR	[83]

Abbreviations: LOD (limit of detection); N (nucleocapsid protein); S (spike protein); RBD (receptor-binding domain); NR (not reported).

6. Commercially Available Microfluidic Tests for SARS-CoV-2

The ongoing COVID-19 outbreak has led to high demand for diagnostic tests and their development; thus, some companies have launched different microfluidic products on the market. These devices can provide a qualitative diagnosis of the presence of nucleic acid [91–97] or viral antigens [98–100] of SARS-CoV-2; however, most of them are highly specialized and exclusive to laboratory use [91–93,95–100]. In addition, these platforms can be fully automated without requiring sample processing, minimizing contamination or human error due to manual handling [91–94,96]. Semi-automated modalities can also be found. However, the processing of the sample plays a fundamental role since purification and extraction are required to obtain nucleic acid [95,97] or proteins [98,99] before they are loaded into the equipment.

The microfluidic equipment used to identify SARS-CoV-2 nucleic acid is based on assays using RT-qPCR, multiplex RT-qPCR (identifying pathogens and respiratory viruses), RT-LAMP, and isothermal amplification, and in the presence of SARS-CoV-2. These devices release signals that are directly proportional to the number of viral particles present in the sample, detected by fluorescence, voltage, or colorimetric sensors (Table 4). On the other hand, a few commercial microfluidic tests identify SARS-CoV-2 antigens. These are mainly based on sandwich-type immunoassays, which are released in the presence of SARS-CoV-2 fluorescence, electrochemical signals, or resonance frequency changes (Table 4).

Table 4. Commercially available microfluidic tests for SARS-CoV-2.

Product	Manufacturer Name	Type of Platform	Target	Detection Method	Processing Time (Minutes)	Reference
ePlex SARS-CoV-2 Test	GenMark Diagnostics, Inc.	RT-qPCR	Nucleic Acid	Voltage	~120	[92]
BioFire COVID-19 test	BioFire Defense, LLC	Multiplex RT-qPCR	Nucleic Acid	Fluorescence	50	[93]
QIAstat-Dx Respiratory SARS-CoV-2 panel	QIAGEN GmbH	Multiplex RT-qPCR	Nucleic Acid	Fluorescence	~60	[94]
Lucira COVID-19 All-In-One Test Kit	Lucira Health, Inc.	RT-LAMP	Nucleic Acid	Colorimetric	30	[95]
Respiratory Virus Nucleic Acid Detection kit	CapitalBio Technology	Isothermal amplification	Nucleic Acid	Fluorescence	90	[96]
Xpert Xpress SARS-CoV-2 test	Cepheid	RT-qPCR	Nucleic Acid	Fluorescence	45	[97]
Microchip RT-PCR COVID-19 detection system	Lumex Instruments Canada	RT-qPCR	Nucleic Acid	Fluorescence	50	[98]
Omnia SARS-CoV-2	Qorvo Biotechnologies	Antigen immunoassay	Proteins	Resonance frequency	~20	[99]
LumiraDx SARS-CoV-2 Ag test	LumiraDx	Antigen immunoassay	Proteins	Fluorescence	12	[100]
Sampinute COVID-19	Celltrion	Antigen immunoassay	Proteins	Electrochemical	30–45	[101]

Overall, these diagnostic tests provide results within a few minutes, representing a valuable benefit in contrast to technologies that require a long time from sample processing to obtaining the result, allowing the immediate implementation of preventive measures.

7. Limitations and Perspectives

An upward trend related to microfluidics, mainly applied for diagnostics, has recently emerged; unfortunately, most of the microfluidic-based diagnostic devices are in a proof-of-concept or prototype stage, which is why more microchips are reported in the literature than are commercially available. Therefore, there is an evident necessity to mature this technology for its practical application in diagnosing infectious diseases. Such microfluidic devices would involve multidisciplinary expertise, compatibility in biological aspects, and feasible manufacturing at a large scale. For example, the materials used for the fabrication of microfluidic chips must be designed for final applications to achieve the optimal performance; a microfluidic chip that requires functionalizing an antibody to detect a viral antigen will use different materials than those used in a microfluidic device capable of performing qPCR to detect a viral gene.

Commonly used materials for the fabrication of microfluidic chips that allow the detection of nucleic acid, antibodies, and proteins of SARS-CoV-2 are based on glass, silicon, polymers (e.g., PDMS), paper, and metal. With respect to glass, this material is ideal for chemical reactions in extreme conditions. One of the significant advantages of silicon is that it allows the molecular diagnosis of biomolecules from diverse samples. However, its high cost for large-scale production is a disadvantage that hinders its application.

On the other hand, microfluidic assays using polymers, paper, or metal have accessible costs for large-scale production; however, they have other drawbacks. The sample should be selected appropriately in the case of platforms that use polymers since this material can present a high or low capacity to adsorb diverse molecules. In comparison, paper-based microfluidic assays are characterized by low cost and small mechanical resistance. A significant limitation is that if the microfluidic device uses passive pumping, it can be a considerable challenge to design the fluid circuit's hydrodynamic resistance properly. Microfluidic devices made from metal are incompatible with optical detection [102].

Therefore, for large-scale production, it is important to consider the materials to be used, since the transition from the "proof-of-concept" stage to the "final product" stage, especially in microfluidics, can result in drastic changes to the original microfluidic chip design, such as modifications to microfluidic chip materials, dimensions, and structures. Profitability and large-scale manufacturing capacity are the main factors involved in launching a microfluidic product to the market, mainly when it is intended to be widely distributed in a pandemic situation.

Another important factor is the type of biomolecules to be detected. For example, microfluidic assays that detect SARS-CoV-2 nucleic acid have advantages such as high sensitivity compared to microfluidic platforms for antigens or antibodies, requiring up to two viral copies and volumes up to 10 nL due to the exponential amplification [24,25], indicating the presence of the virus in the early stages of infection [103]. These microfluidic devices are the market leaders; however, their high costs compared to immunoassays and the fast degradation of nucleic acids if the samples are not processed immediately or properly stored represent significant disadvantages.

Microfluidic assays for SARS-CoV-2 antigens are used due to the excellent stability that the proteins present compared with the nucleic acid. This type of microfluidic assays can detect SARS-CoV-2 proteins in concentration ranges from fg/mL to µg/mL [57,64].

To avoid false negatives, the proper detection of SARS-CoV-2 proteins should be performed approximately on the fifth day after the infection, which is typically accompanied by tests of nucleic acid to confirm the results [49,50]. On the other hand, microfluidic platforms based on immunoassays to detect antibodies identify the severity of the disease depending on age and levels of expression of anti-SARS-CoV-2 antibodies. They also allow the identification of asymptomatic patients and the evaluation of or the success of vaccination against SARS-CoV-2 with LODs of ng/mL. However, they cannot provide early diagnosis since the production of antibodies takes approximately two weeks post-inoculation [70,71].

The commercially available microfluidic equipment is based on the analysis of nucleic acid or viral antigens of SARS-CoV-2. Currently, there are no commercial microfluidic platforms for identifying anti-SARS-CoV-2 antibodies, for which ELISA is the main method used [90]. In addition, most microfluidic devices are highly specialized and require laboratories to handle them, making them inaccessible in rural areas. In this manner, a significant limitation is the transportation of samples from the collection site to the laboratories, which can cause degradation of the nucleic acid or proteins.

Therefore, the different microfluidic platforms used for diagnosing SARS-CoV-2 and seroprevalence are equally important and complementary to each other, since each one offers valuable results that will indicate the presence or absence of the virus or the state of health of the patient. Furthermore, these devices require similar test times for sample processing and obtaining results and their costs will depend on the material used for their design.

To achieve progress in microfluidic diagnosis, it is also fundamental to consider that some microfluidic chips require pumps or fluid controllers to supply the necessary reagents, which are specialized instruments that many laboratories do not possess. Therefore, one of the main approaches regarding microfluidics in diagnosis is to simplify or avoid using specialized or expensive equipment. This will lead to a greater adaptation of microfluidic systems in different research groups worldwide, improving accessibility to this technology. Consequently, a greater understanding of microfluidics would broaden its applications. The microfluidic proposals applied to COVID-19 reviewed in this work show that a search is evidently occurring in the scientific community for means of reducing test times and costs, improving sensitivity, and simplifying or automating the processing of a test through the employment of microfluidics.

8. Conclusions

This review article describes the diagnostic tools that have emerged to detect nucleic acid, viral antigens, and anti-SARS-CoV-2 antibodies, using several techniques such as PCR, isothermal amplification, CRISPR, and immunoassays on microfluidic platforms. Most of these devices are innovative and portable, with the capacity to be stored for months, allowing them to reach communities or places without access to laboratories or hospitals. Furthermore, the microfluidic tests reviewed in this work use minimal amounts of reagents, reducing the total cost and the need for highly qualified personnel. Compared to conventional techniques, microfluidic tests can take minutes to a few hours to obtain accurate results, enabling healthcare professionals to implement efficient treatments and more appropriate infection control decisions. Microfluidic technology can gradually change the course of diagnosis in infectious diseases, especially in successive contagious disease outbreaks. COVID-19 has highlighted the importance of having sufficient supplies and technology that can to be applied directly to the clinical area. The pandemic has left us with several interesting proposals for microfluidic chips that may provide solutions in the near future to enable massive diagnosis, replacing qPCR as the gold standard.

Author Contributions: E.A.F.-C. and R.B.G.-G.—conceptualization, revision, and writing of the manuscript; J.F.Y.-d.L., and I.P.R.-S.—manuscript writing; E.G.-G. and H.M.N.I.—conceptualization, revision, and writing and editing of the manuscript. All authors have read and agreed to the published version of the manuscript.

Funding: This research received no external funding.

Institutional Review Board Statement: Not applicable.

Informed Consent Statement: Not applicable.

Data Availability Statement: Not applicable.

Acknowledgments: This work was supported by Consejo Nacional de Ciencia y Tecnología (CONACYT) and Tecnológico de Monterrey under Sistema Nacional de Investigadores (SNI) program to Hafiz M. N. Iqbal (CVU. 735340) and Everardo González-González (CVU. 635891).

Conflicts of Interest: The authors declare no conflict of interest.

References

1. WHO Coronavirus (COVID-19) Dashboard | WHO Coronavirus (COVID-19) Dashboard with Vaccination Data. Available online: https://covid19.who.int/ (accessed on 22 January 2022).
2. Zhao, H.; Zhang, Y.; Chen, Y.; Ho, N.R.Y.; Sundah, N.R.; Natalia, A.; Liu, Y.; Miow, Q.H.; Wang, Y.; Tambyah, P.A.; et al. Accessible detection of SARS-CoV-2 through molecular nanostructures and automated microfluidics. *Biosens. Bioelectron.* **2021**, *194*, 113629–113638. [CrossRef]
3. Das, P.; Mondal, S.; Pal, S.; Roy, S.; Vidyadharan, A.; Dadwal, R.; Bhattacharya, S.; Mishra, D.K.; Chandy, M. COVID diagnostics by molecular methods: A systematic review of nucleic acid based testing systems. *Indian J. Med. Microbiol.* **2021**, *39*, 271–278. [CrossRef]
4. Udugama, B.; Kadhiresan, P.; Kozlowski, H.N.; Malekjahani, A.; Osborne, M.; Li, V.Y.C.; Chen, H.; Mubareka, S.; Gubbay, J.B.; Chan, W.C.W. Diagnosing COVID-19: The disease and tools for detection. *ACS Nano* **2020**, *14*, 3822–3835. [CrossRef]
5. Esbin, M.N.; Whitney, O.N.; Chong, S.; Maurer, A.; Darzacq, X.; Tjian, R. Overcoming the bottleneck to widespread testing: A rapid review of nucleic acid testing approaches for COVID-19 detection. *RNA* **2020**, *26*, 771–783. [CrossRef]
6. Dong, X.; Liu, L.; Tu, Y.; Zhang, J.; Miao, G.; Zhang, L.; Ge, S.; Xia, N.; Yu, D.; Qiu, X. Rapid PCR powered by microfluidics: A quick review under the background of COVID-19 pandemic. *Trends Analyt. Chem.* **2021**, *143*, 116377–116386. [CrossRef]
7. Tarn, M.D.; Pamme, N. Microfluidics. *Ref. Modul. Chem. Mol. Sci. Chem. Eng.* **2014**, 1–7. [CrossRef]
8. Wang, R.; Wang, X. Sensing of inorganic ions in microfluidic devices. *Sens. Actuators B Chem.* **2021**, *329*, 129171–129188. [CrossRef]

9. Shi, H.; Jiang, S.; Liu, B.; Liu, Z.; Reis, N.M. Modern microfluidic approaches for determination of ions. *Microchem. J.* **2021**, *171*, 106845–106857. [CrossRef]
10. Lin, L.; Yin, Y.; Starostin, S.A.; Xu, H.; Li, C.; Wu, K.; He, C.; Hessel, V. Microfluidic fabrication of fluorescent nanomaterials: A review. *Chem. Eng. J.* **2021**, *425*, 131511–131525. [CrossRef]
11. Safdar, M.; Jänis, J.; Sánchez, S. Microfluidic fuel cells for energy generation. *Lab Chip* **2016**, *16*, 2754–2758. [CrossRef]
12. Lei, L.; Wang, N.; Zhang, X.M.; Tai, Q.; Tsai, D.P.; Chan, H.L.W. Optofluidic planar reactors for photocatalytic water treatment using solar energy. *Biomicrofluidics* **2010**, *4*, 043004. [CrossRef]
13. Weigl, B.; Domingo, G.; LaBarre, P.; Gerlach, J. Towards non- and minimally instrumented, microfluidics-based diagnostic devices. *Lab Chip* **2008**, *8*, 1999–2014. [CrossRef]
14. Saez, J.; Catalan-Carrio, R.; Owens, R.M.; Basabe-Desmonts, L.; Benito-Lopez, F. Microfluidics and materials for smart water monitoring: A review. *Anal. Chim. Acta* **2021**, *1186*, 338392–338405. [CrossRef]
15. Mejía-Salazar, J.R.; Cruz, K.R.; Vásques, E.M.M.; de Oliveira, O.N. Microfluidic point-of-care devices: New trends and future prospects for eHealth diagnostics. *Sensors* **2020**, *20*, 1951. [CrossRef]
16. Sachdeva, S.; Davis, R.W.; Saha, A.K. Microfluidic point-of-care testing: Commercial landscape and future directions. *Front. Bioeng. Biotechnol.* **2021**, *8*, 1537. [CrossRef]
17. Lee, W.C.; Lien, K.Y.; Lee, G.B.; Lei, H.Y. An integrated microfluidic system using magnetic beads for virus detection. *Diagn. Microbiol. Infect. Dis.* **2008**, *60*, 51–58. [CrossRef]
18. Seok, Y.; Batule, B.S.; Kim, M.G. Lab-on-paper for all-in-one molecular diagnostics (LAMDA) of zika, dengue, and chikungunya virus from human serum. *Biosens. Bioelectron.* **2020**, *165*, 112400–1124228. [CrossRef]
19. Fraser, L.A.; Kinghorn, A.B.; Dirkzwager, R.M.; Liang, S.; Cheung, Y.W.; Lim, B.; Shiu, S.C.C.; Tang, M.S.L.; Andrew, D.; Manitta, J.; et al. A portable microfluidic Aptamer-Tethered Enzyme Capture (APTEC) biosensor for malaria diagnosis. *Biosens. Bioelectron.* **2018**, *100*, 591–596. [CrossRef]
20. Alves, P.A.; de Oliveira, E.G.; Franco-Luiz, A.P.M.; Almeida, L.T.; Gonçalves, A.B.; Borges, I.A.; de Rocha, F.; Rocha, R.P.; Bezerra, M.F.; Miranda, P.; et al. Optimization and clinical validation of colorimetric reverse transcription loop-mediated isothermal amplification, a fast, highly sensitive and specific COVID-19 molecular diagnostic tool that is robust to detect SARS-CoV-2 variants of concern. *Front. Microbiol.* **2021**, *12*, 713713. [CrossRef]
21. Yaniv, K.; Ozer, E.; Shagan, M.; Lakkakula, S.; Plotkin, N.; Bhandarkar, N.S.; Kushmaro, A. Direct RT-qPCR assay for SARS-CoV-2 variants of concern (Alpha, B.1.1.7 and Beta, B.1.351) detection and quantification in wastewater. *Environ. Res.* **2021**, *201*, 111653–1116661. [CrossRef]
22. Mercer, T.R.; Salit, M. Testing at scale during the COVID-19 pandemic. *Nat. Rev. Genet.* **2021**, *22*, 415–426. [CrossRef]
23. Yang, J.; Kidd, M.; Nordquist, A.R.; Smith, S.D.; Hurth, C.; Modlin, I.M.; Zenhausern, F. A Sensitive, portable microfluidic device for SARS-CoV-2 detection from self-collected saliva. *Infect. Dis. Rep.* **2021**, *13*, 1061–1077. [CrossRef]
24. Fassy, J.; Lacoux, C.; Leroy, S.; Noussair, L.; Hubac, S.; Degoutte, A.; Vassaux, G.; Leclercq, V.; Rouquié, D.; Marquette, C.H.; et al. Versatile and flexible microfluidic qPCR test for high-throughput SARS-CoV-2 and cellular response detection in nasopharyngeal swab samples. *PLoS ONE* **2021**, *16*, e0243333. [CrossRef]
25. Xie, X.; Gjorgjieva, T.; Attieh, Z.; Dieng, M.M.; Arnoux, M.; Khair, M.; Moussa, Y.; Al Jallaf, F.; Rahiman, N.; Jackson, C.A.; et al. Microfluidic nano-scale qPCR enables ultra-sensitive and quantitative detection of SARS-CoV-2. *Process* **2020**, *8*, 1425. [CrossRef]
26. Cojocaru, R.; Yaseen, I.; Unrau, P.J.; Lowe, C.F.; Ritchie, G.; Romney, M.G.; Sin, D.D.; Gill, S.; Slyadnev, M. Microchip RT-PCR detection of nasopharyngeal SARS-CoV-2 samples. *J. Mol. Diagn.* **2021**, *23*, 683–690. [CrossRef]
27. Ji, M.; Xia, Y.; Loo, J.F.C.; Li, L.; Ho, H.P.; He, J.; Gu, D. Automated multiplex nucleic acid tests for rapid detection of SARS-CoV-2, influenza A and B infection with direct reverse-transcription quantitative PCR (dirRT-qPCR) assay in a centrifugal microfluidic platform. *RSC Adv.* **2020**, *10*, 34088–34098. [CrossRef]
28. Kang, B.H.; Lee, Y.; Yu, E.S.; Na, H.; Kang, M.; Huh, H.J.; Jeong, K.H. Ultrafast and real-time nanoplasmonic on-chip polymerase chain reaction for rapid and quantitative molecular diagnostics. *ACS Nano* **2021**, *15*, 10194–10202. [CrossRef]
29. Li, T.; Chung, H.K.; Pireku, P.K.; Beitzel, B.F.; Sanborn, M.A.; Tang, C.Y.; Hammer, R.D.; Ritter, D.; Wan, X.F.; Berry, I.M.; et al. Rapid high-throughput whole-genome sequencing of SARS-CoV-2 by using one-step reverse transcription-PCR amplification with an integrated microfluidic system and next-generation sequencing. *J. Clin. Microbiol.* **2021**, *59*, e02784-20. [CrossRef]
30. Millier, M.J.; Stamp, L.K.; Hessian, P.A. Digital-PCR for gene expression: Impact from inherent tissue RNA degradation. *Sci. Rep.* **2017**, *7*, 17235. [CrossRef]
31. Bu, W.; Li, W.; Li, J.; Ao, T.; Li, Z.; Wu, B.; Wu, S.; Kong, W.; Pan, T.; Ding, Y.; et al. A low-cost, programmable, and multi-functional droplet printing system for low copy number SARS-CoV-2 digital PCR determination. *Sens. Actuators B Chem.* **2021**, *348*, 130678–130689. [CrossRef]
32. Yin, H.; Wu, Z.; Shi, N.; Qi, Y.; Jian, X.; Zhou, L.; Tong, Y.; Cheng, Z.; Zhao, J.; Mao, H. Ultrafast multiplexed detection of SARS-CoV-2 RNA using a rapid droplet digital PCR system. *Biosens. Bioelectron.* **2021**, *188*, 113282–113290. [CrossRef]
33. Sun, Y.; Huang, Y.; Qi, T.; Jin, Q.; Jia, C.; Zhao, J.; Feng, S.; Liang, L. Wet-etched microchamber array digital PCR chip for SARS-CoV-2 virus and ultra-early stage lung cancer quantitative detection. *ACS Omega* **2022**, *7*, 1819–1826. [CrossRef]
34. De Oliveira, K.G.; Estrela, P.F.N.; Mendes, G.D.M.; Dos Santos, C.A.; Silveira-Lacerda, E.D.P.; Duarte, G.R.M. Rapid molecular diagnostics of COVID-19 by RT-LAMP in a centrifugal polystyrene-toner based microdevice with end-point visual detection. *Analyst* **2021**, *146*, 1178–1187. [CrossRef]

35. Tian, F.; Liu, C.; Deng, J.; Han, Z.; Zhang, L.; Chen, Q.; Sun, J. A fully automated centrifugal microfluidic system for sample-to-answer viral nucleic acid testing. *Sci. China Chem.* **2020**, *63*, 1498–1506. [CrossRef]
36. Sreejith, K.R.; Umer, M.; Dirr, L.; Bailly, B.; Guillon, P.; von Itzstein, M.; Soda, N.; Kasetsirikul, S.; Shiddiky, M.J.A.; Nguyen, N.T. A portable device for LAMP based detection of SARS-CoV-2. *Micromachines* **2021**, *12*, 1151. [CrossRef]
37. Ganguli, A.; Mostafa, A.; Berger, J.; Aydin, M.Y.; Sun, F.; Stewart de Ramirez, S.A.; Valera, E.; Cunningham, B.T.; King, W.P.; Bashir, R. Rapid isothermal amplification and portable detection system for SARS-CoV-2. *Proc. Natl. Acad. Sci. USA* **2020**, *117*, 22727–22735. [CrossRef]
38. Oliveira, B.B.; Veigas, B.; Baptista, P.V. Isothermal amplification of nucleic acids: The race for the next "Gold Standard". *Front. Sens.* **2021**, *14*, 35. [CrossRef]
39. Davidson, J.L.; Wang, J.; Maruthamuthu, M.K.; Dextre, A.; Pascual-Garrigos, A.; Mohan, S.; Putikam, S.V.S.; Osman, F.O.I.; McChesney, D.; Seville, J.; et al. A paper-based colorimetric molecular test for SARS-CoV-2 in saliva. *Biosens. Bioelectron. X* **2021**, *9*, 100076. [CrossRef]
40. Deng, H.; Jayawardena, A.; Chan, J.; Tan, S.M.; Alan, T.; Kwan, P. An ultra-portable, self-contained point-of-care nucleic acid amplification test for diagnosis of active COVID-19 infection. *Sci. Rep.* **2021**, *11*, 15176. [CrossRef]
41. Kim, H.S.; Abbas, N.; Shin, S. A rapid diagnosis of SARS-CoV-2 using DNA hydrogel formation on microfluidic pores. *Biosens. Bioelectron.* **2021**, *177*, 113005–113012. [CrossRef]
42. Liu, D.; Shen, H.; Zhang, Y.; Shen, D.; Zhu, M.; Song, Y.; Zhu, Z.; Yang, C. A microfluidic-integrated lateral flow recombinase polymerase amplification (MI-IF-RPA) assay for rapid COVID-19 detection. *Lab Chip* **2021**, *21*, 2019–2026. [CrossRef] [PubMed]
43. Huang, Q.; Shan, X.; Cao, R.; Jin, X.; Lin, X.; He, Q.; Zhu, Y.; Fu, R.; Du, W.; Lv, W.; et al. Microfluidic chip with two-stage isothermal amplification method for highly sensitive parallel detection of SARS-CoV-2 and Measles Virus. *Micromachines* **2021**, *12*, 1582. [CrossRef] [PubMed]
44. Ramachandran, A.; Huyke, D.A.; Sharma, E.; Sahoo, M.K.; Huang, C.; Banaei, N.; Pinsky, B.A.; Santiago, J.G. Electric field-driven microfluidics for rapid CRISPR-based diagnostics and its application to detection of SARS-CoV-2. *Proc. Natl. Acad. Sci. USA* **2020**, *117*, 29518–29525. [CrossRef] [PubMed]
45. Li, Z.; Ding, X.; Yin, K.; Avery, L.; Ballesteros, E.; Liu, C. Instrument-free, CRISPR-based diagnostics of SARS-CoV-2 using self-contained microfluidic system. *Biosens. Bioelectron.* **2022**, *199*, 113865–113872. [CrossRef] [PubMed]
46. Liu, T.Y.; Knott, G.J.; Smock, D.C.J.; Desmarais, J.J.; Son, S.; Bhuiya, A.; Jakhanwal, S.; Prywes, N.; Agrawal, S.; Díaz de León Derby, M.; et al. Accelerated RNA detection using tandem CRISPR nucleases. *Nat. Chem. Biol.* **2021**, *17*, 982–988. [CrossRef]
47. Hwang, C.; Park, N.; Kim, E.S.; Kim, M.; Kim, S.D.; Park, S.; Kim, N.Y.; Kim, J.H. Ultra-fast and recyclable DNA biosensor for point-of-care detection of SARS-CoV-2 (COVID-19). *Biosens. Bioelectron.* **2021**, *185*, 113177–113182. [CrossRef]
48. Iwanaga, M. High-sensitivity high-throughput detection of nucleic acid targets on metasurface fluorescence biosensors. *Biosensors* **2021**, *11*, 33. [CrossRef]
49. Hoffmann, M.; Kleine-Weber, H.; Schroeder, S.; Krüger, N.; Herrler, T.; Erichsen, S.; Schiergens, T.S.; Herrler, G.; Wu, N.H.; Nitsche, A.; et al. SARS-CoV-2 cell entry depends on ACE2 and TMPRSS2 and is blocked by a clinically proven protease inhibitor. *Cell* **2020**, *181*, 271–280.e8. [CrossRef]
50. Ji, T.; Liu, Z.; Wang, G.Q.; Guo, X.; Akbar Khan, S.; Lai, C.; Chen, H.; Huang, S.; Xia, S.; Chen, B.; et al. Detection of COVID-19: A review of the current literature and future perspectives. *Biosens. Bioelectron.* **2020**, *166*, 112455–112472. [CrossRef]
51. Masters, P.S. Coronavirus genomic RNA packaging. *Virology* **2019**, *537*, 198–207. [CrossRef]
52. Diao, B.; Wen, K.; Zhang, J.; Chen, J.; Han, C.; Chen, Y.; Wang, S.; Deng, G.; Zhou, H.; Wu, Y. Accuracy of a nucleocapsid protein antigen rapid test in the diagnosis of SARS-CoV-2 infection. *Clin. Microbiol. Infect.* **2021**, *27*, 289.e1–289.e4. [CrossRef] [PubMed]
53. Xu, J.; Suo, W.; Goulev, Y.; Sun, L.; Kerr, L.; Paulsson, J.; Zhang, Y.; Lao, T. Handheld microfluidic filtration platform enables rapid, low-cost, and robust self-testing of SARS-CoV-2 virus. *Small* **2021**, *17*, 2104009. [CrossRef] [PubMed]
54. Liu, Y.; Tan, Y.; Fu, Q.; Lin, M.; He, J.; He, S.; Yang, M.; Chen, S.; Zhou, J. Reciprocating-flowing on-a-chip enables ultra-fast immunobinding for multiplexed rapid ELISA detection of SARS-CoV-2 antibody. *Biosens. Bioelectron.* **2021**, *176*, 112920–112927. [CrossRef] [PubMed]
55. Kyosei, Y.; Yamura, S.; Namba, M.; Yoshimura, T.; Watabe, S.; Ito, E. Antigen tests for COVID-19. *Biophys. Physicobiol.* **2021**, *18*, 28–39. [CrossRef] [PubMed]
56. Kim, S.; Akarapipad, P.; Nguyen, B.T.; Breshears, L.E.; Sosnowski, K.; Baker, J.; Uhrlaub, J.L.; Nikolich-Zugich, J.; Yoon, J.-Y. Direct capture and smartphone quantification of airborne SARS-CoV-2 on a paper microfluidic chip. *Biosens. Bioelectron.* **2022**, *200*, 956–5663. [CrossRef] [PubMed]
57. Sharma, P.K.; Kim, E.S.; Mishra, S.; Ganbold, E.; Seong, R.S.; Kaushik, A.K.; Kim, N.Y. Ultrasensitive and reusable graphene oxide-modified double-interdigitated capacitive (DIDC) sensing chip for detecting SARS-CoV-2. *ACS Sensors* **2021**, *6*, 3468–3476. [CrossRef] [PubMed]
58. Yousefi, H.; Mahmud, A.; Chang, D.; Das, J.; Gomis, S.; Chen, J.B.; Wang, H.; Been, T.; Yip, L.; Coomes, E.; et al. Detection of SARS-CoV-2 viral particles using direct, reagent-free electrochemical sensing. *J. Am. Chem. Soc.* **2021**, *143*, 1722–1727. [CrossRef] [PubMed]
59. Zhang, J.; Fang, X.; Mao, Y.; Qi, H.; Wu, J.; Liu, X.; You, F.; Zhao, W.; Chen, Y.; Zheng, L. Real-time, selective, and low-cost detection of trace level SARS-CoV-2 spike-protein for cold-chain food quarantine. *NPJ Sci. Food* **2021**, *5*, 2–7. [CrossRef]

60. Li, J.; Lillehoj, P.B. Microfluidic magneto immunosensor for rapid, high sensitivity measurements of SARS-CoV-2 nucleocapsid protein in serum. *ACS Sens.* **2021**, *6*, 1270–1278. [CrossRef]
61. Ge, C.; Feng, J.; Zhang, J.; Hu, K.; Wang, D.; Zha, L.; Hu, X.; Li, R. Aptamer/antibody sandwich method for digital detection of SARS-CoV2 nucleocapsid protein. *Talanta* **2022**, *236*, 122847–122854. [CrossRef]
62. Murugan, D.; Bhatia, H.; Sai, V.V.R.; Satija, J. P-FAB: A fiber-optic biosensor device for rapid detection of COVID-19. *Trans. Indian Natl. Acad. Eng.* **2020**, *5*, 211–215. [CrossRef]
63. Raziq, A.; Kidakova, A.; Boroznjak, R.; Reut, J.; Öpik, A.; Syritski, V. Development of a portable MIP-based electrochemical sensor for detection of SARS-CoV-2 antigen. *Biosens. Bioelectron.* **2021**, *178*, 113029–113035. [CrossRef] [PubMed]
64. Sun, M.; Han, M.; Xu, S.; Yan, K.; Nigal, G.; Zhang, T.; Song, B. Paper-based microfluidic chip for rapid detection of SARS-CoV-2 N protein. *Bioengineered* **2022**, *13*, 876–883. [CrossRef] [PubMed]
65. Mahari, S.; Roberts, A.; Shahdeo, D.; Gandhi, S. Ecovsens-ultrasensitive novel in-house built printed circuit board based electrochemical device for rapid detection of nCovid-19 antigen, a spike protein domain 1 of SARS-CoV-2. *bioRxiv* **2020**, 1–20. [CrossRef]
66. Seo, G.; Lee, G.; Kim, M.J.; Baek, S.H.; Choi, M.; Ku, K.B.; Lee, C.S.; Jun, S.; Park, D.; Kim, H.G.; et al. Rapid detection of COVID-19 causative virus (SARS-CoV-2) in human nasopharyngeal swab specimens using field-effect transistor-based biosensor. *ACS Nano* **2020**, *14*, 5135–5142. [CrossRef] [PubMed]
67. Lin, Q.; Wen, D.; Wu, J.; Liu, L.; Wu, W.; Fang, X.; Kong, J. Microfluidic immunoassays for sensitive and simultaneous detection of IgG/IgM/Antigen of SARS-CoV-2 within 15 min. *Anal. Chem.* **2020**, *92*, 9454–9458. [CrossRef] [PubMed]
68. Stambaugh, A.; Parks, J.W.; Stott, M.A.; Meena, G.G.; Hawkins, A.R.; Schmidt, H. Optofluidic multiplex detection of single SARS-CoV-2 and influenza A antigens using a novel bright fluorescent probe assay. *Proc. Natl. Acad. Sci. USA* **2021**, *118*, 2–7. [CrossRef]
69. Huang, J.; Wen, J.; Zhou, M.; Ni, S.; Le, W.; Chen, G.; Wei, L.; Zeng, Y.; Qi, D.; Pan, M.; et al. On-site detection of SARS-CoV-2 antigen by deep learning-based surface-enhanced raman spectroscopy and its biochemical foundations. *Anal. Chem.* **2021**, *93*, 9174–9182. [CrossRef]
70. Cui, T.-R.; Qiao, Y.-C.; Gao, J.-W.; Wang, C.-H.; Zhang, Y.; Han, L.; Yang, Y.; Ren, T.-L.; Wang, J.-W.; Zhang, C.-H.; et al. Ultrasensitive detection of COVID-19 causative virus (SARS-CoV-2) spike protein using laser induced graphene field-effect transistor. *Molecules* **2021**, *26*, 6947. [CrossRef]
71. Ou, J.; Tan, M.; He, H.; Tan, H.; Mai, J.; Long, Y.; Jiang, X.; He, Q.; Huang, Y.; Li, Y.; et al. SARS-CoV-2 Antibodies and associated factors at different hospitalization time points in 192 COVID-19 cases. *J. Appl. Lab. Med.* **2021**, *6*, 1133–1142. [CrossRef]
72. Schneider, M.M.; Emmenegger, M.; Xu, C.K.; Condado Morales, I.; Meisl, G.; Turelli, P.; Zografou, C.; Zimmermann, M.R.; Frey, B.M.; Fiedler, S.; et al. Microfluidic characterisation reveals broad range of SARS-CoV-2 antibody affinity in human plasma. *Life Sci. Alliance* **2022**, *5*, 1–12. [CrossRef] [PubMed]
73. Qu, J.; Wu, C.; Li, X.; Zhang, G.; Jiang, Z.; Li, X.; Zhu, Q.; Liu, L. Profile of IgG and IgM antibodies against severe acute respiratory syndrome coronavirus 2 (SARS-CoV-2). *Clin. Infect. Dis. An Off. Publ. Infect. Dis. Soc. Am.* **2020**, *71*, 2255–2258. [CrossRef] [PubMed]
74. Shaffaf, T.; Ghafar-Zadeh, E. COVID-19 diagnostic strategies. Part i: Nucleic acid-based technologies. *Bioengineering* **2021**, *8*, 49. [CrossRef] [PubMed]
75. Tahmasebi, S.; Khosh, E.; Esmaeilzadeh, A. The outlook for diagnostic purposes of the 2019-novel coronavirus disease. *J. Cell. Physiol.* **2020**, *235*, 9211–9229. [CrossRef] [PubMed]
76. Fang, X.; Mei, Q.; Yang, T.; Li, L.; Wang, Y.; Tong, F.; Geng, S.; Pan, A. Low-dose corticosteroid therapy does not delay viral clearance in patients with COVID-19. *J. Infect.* **2020**, *81*, 147–178. [CrossRef] [PubMed]
77. Morales-Narváez, E.; Dincer, C. The impact of biosensing in a pandemic outbreak: COVID-19. *Biosens. Bioelectron.* **2020**, *163*, 112274–112279. [CrossRef]
78. Poghossian, A.; Jablonski, M.; Molinnus, D.; Wege, C.; Schöning, M.J. Field-effect sensors for virus detection: From Ebola to SARS-CoV-2 and plant viral enhancers. *Front. Plant Sci.* **2020**, *11*, 1792. [CrossRef]
79. Funari, R.; Chu, K.Y.; Shen, A.Q. Detection of antibodies against SARS-CoV-2 spike protein by gold nanospikes in an opto-microfluidic chip. *Biosens. Bioelectron.* **2020**, *169*, 112578–112584. [CrossRef]
80. González-González, E.; Garcia-Ramirez, R.; Díaz-Armas, G.G.; Esparza, M.; Aguilar-Avelar, C.; Flores-Contreras, E.A.; Rodríguez-Sánchez, I.P.; Delgado-Balderas, J.R.; Soto-García, B.; Aráiz-Hernández, D.; et al. Automated ELISA on-chip for the detection of anti-SARS-CoV-2 antibodies. *Sensors* **2021**, *21*, 6785. [CrossRef]
81. Tripathi, S.; Agrawal, A. Blood plasma microfluidic device: Aiming for the detection of COVID-19 antibodies using an on-chip ELISA platform. *Trans. Indian Natl. Acad. Eng.* **2020**, *5*, 217–220. [CrossRef]
82. Heggestad, J.T.; Kinnamon, D.S.; Olson, L.B.; Liu, J.; Kelly, G.; Wall, S.A.; Oshabaheebwa, S.; Quinn, Z.; Fontes, C.M.; Joh, D.Y.; et al. Multiplexed, quantitative serological profiling of COVID-19 from blood by a point-of-care test. *Sci. Adv.* **2021**, *7*, eabg4901. [CrossRef] [PubMed]
83. Cognetti, J.S.; Steiner, D.J.; Abedin, M.; Bryan, M.R.; Shanahan, C.; Tokranova, N.; Young, E.; Klose, A.M.; Zavriyev, A.; Judy, N.; et al. Disposable photonics for cost-effective clinical bioassays: Application to COVID-19 antibody testing. *Lab Chip* **2021**, *21*, 2913–2921. [CrossRef]

84. Li, X.; Qin, Z.; Fu, H.; Li, T.; Peng, R.; Li, Z.; Rini, J.M.; Liu, X. Enhancing the performance of paper-based electrochemical impedance spectroscopy nanobiosensors: An experimental approach. *Biosens. Bioelectron.* **2021**, *177*, 112672–112679. [CrossRef] [PubMed]
85. Murillo, A.M.M.; Tomé-Amat, J.; Ramírez, Y.; Garrido-Arandia, M.; Valle, L.G.; Hernández-Ramírez, G.; Tramarin, L.; Herreros, P.; Santamaría, B.; Díaz-Perales, A.; et al. Developing an optical interferometric detection method based biosensor for detecting specific SARS-CoV-2 immunoglobulins in Serum and Saliva, and their corresponding ELISA correlation. *Sens. Actuators B Chem.* **2021**, *345*, 130394–130403. [CrossRef] [PubMed]
86. Lee, W.; Kim, H.; Bae, P.K.; Lee, S.; Yang, S.; Kim, J. A single snapshot multiplex immunoassay platform utilizing dense test lines based on engineered beads. *Biosens. Bioelectron.* **2021**, *190*, 113388–113398. [CrossRef]
87. Rodriguez-Moncayo, R.; Cedillo-Alcantar, D.F.; Guevara-Pantoja, P.E.; Chavez-Pineda, O.G.; Hernandez-Ortiz, J.A.; Amador-Hernandez, J.U.; Rojas-Velasco, G.; Sanchez-Muñoz, F.; Manzur-Sandoval, D.; Patino-Lopez, L.D.; et al. A high-throughput multiplexed microfluidic device for COVID-19 serology assays. *Lab Chip* **2021**, *21*, 93–104. [CrossRef] [PubMed]
88. Tan, X.; Krel, M.; Dolgov, E.; Park, S.; Li, X.; Wu, W.; Sun, Y.L.; Zhang, J.; Khaing Oo, M.K.; Perlin, D.S.; et al. Rapid and quantitative detection of SARS-CoV-2 specific IgG for convalescent serum evaluation. *Biosens. Bioelectron.* **2020**, *169*, 112572–112580. [CrossRef]
89. Djaileb, A.; Jodaylami, M.H.; Coutu, J.; Ricard, P.; Lamarre, M.; Rochet, L.; Cellier-Goetghebeur, S.; Macaulay, D.; Charron, B.; Lavallée, É.; et al. Cross-validation of ELISA and a portable surface plasmon resonance instrument for IgG antibody serology with SARS-CoV-2 positive individuals. *Cite Anal.* **2021**, *146*, 4905–4917. [CrossRef]
90. Xu, W.; Liu, J.; Song, D.; Li, C.; Zhu, A.; Long, F. Rapid, label-free, and sensitive point-of-care testing of anti-SARS-CoV-2 IgM/IgG using all-fiber Fresnel reflection microfluidic biosensor. *Microchim. Acta* **2021**, *188*, 161–271. [CrossRef]
91. Mou, L.; Jiang, X.; Mou, L.; Jiang, X. Materials for microfluidic immunoassays: A Review. *Adv. Healthc. Mater.* **2017**, *6*, 1601403–1601412. [CrossRef]
92. Detection of Variant SARS-CoV-2 Strains on the ePlex® Respiratory Panel 2. Available online: https://www.genmarkdx.com/detection-of-variant-sars-cov-2-strains-on-eplex-rp2-panel/ (accessed on 11 February 2022).
93. BioFire COVID-19 Testing Solutions I BioFire Diagnostics. Available online: https://www.biofiredx.com/covid-19/ (accessed on 11 February 2022).
94. QIAstat-Dx SARS-CoV-2. Available online: https://www.qiagen.com/ca/products/diagnostics-and-clinical-research/infectious-disease/qiastat-dx-syndromic-testing/qiastat-dx-ca/ (accessed on 11 February 2022).
95. Lucira COVID-19 All-In-One Test Kit + PDF Report (Good For Travel)—Plus PDF Results (Good for Travel). Available online: https://www.meenta.io/product/lucira-covid-19-all-in-one-test/ (accessed on 11 February 2022).
96. Respiratory Virus Nucleic Acid Detection Kit (Isothermal Amplification Chip Meth—FIND. Available online: https://www.finddx.org/product/respiratory-virus-nucleic-acid-detection-kit-isothermal-amplification-chip-meth/ (accessed on 11 February 2022).
97. Cepheid I Cepheid I Xpert® Xpress SARS-CoV-2—FDA Emergency Use Authorization. Available online: https://www.cepheid.com/en/coronavirus (accessed on 11 February 2022).
98. Microchip RT-PCR COVID-19 (SARS-CoV-2) Detection Test System by rt PCR. Available online: https://www.lumexinstruments.com/applications/covid-19_detection_system.php (accessed on 11 February 2022).
99. Qorvo Biotechnologies Omnia SARS-CoV-2 Antigen Test Detects Delta and Other Circulating Variants in Two Studies—Qorvo. Available online: https://www.qorvo.com/newsroom/news/2021/qorvo-biotechnologies-omnia-sars-cov-2-antigen-test-detects-delta-and-other-circulating-variants (accessed on 11 February 2022).
100. The LumiraDx SARS-CoV-2 Ag Test Is a Rapid Microfluidic Immunoassay Detecting SARS-CoV-2 Antigen. Available online: https://www.lumiradx.com/uk-en/test-menu/antigen-test (accessed on 10 February 2022).
101. SAMPINUTE™. Available online: https://www.celltrion.com/en-us/kit/sampinute (accessed on 10 February 2022).
102. Niculescu, A.G.; Chircov, C.; Bîrcă, A.C.; Grumezescu, A.M. Fabrication and Applications of Microfluidic Devices: A Review. *Int. J. Mol. Sci.* **2021**, *22*, 2011. [CrossRef] [PubMed]
103. Jia, Y.; Sun, H.; Tian, J.; Song, Q.; Zhang, W. Paper-Based Point-of-Care Testing of SARS-CoV-2. *Front. Bioeng. Biotechnol.* **2021**, *9*, 773304. [CrossRef] [PubMed]

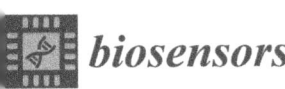

Article

Rapid Detection of Anti-SARS-CoV-2 Antibodies with a Screen-Printed Electrode Modified with a Spike Glycoprotein Epitope

Wilson A. Ameku [1,2], David W. Provance [1,2], Carlos M. Morel [1] and Salvatore G. De-Simone [1,2,3,*]

1. Oswaldo Cruz Foundation (FIOCRUZ), Center for Technological Development in Health (CDTS)/National Institute of Science and Technology for Innovation in Neglected Populations Diseases (INCT-IDPN), Rio de Janeiro 21040-900, RJ, Brazil; akira.ameku@gmail.com (W.A.A.); bill.provance@fiocruz.br (D.W.P.); carlos.morel@fiocruz.br (C.M.M.)
2. Laboratory of Epidemiology and Molecualr Systematics (LESM), Oswaldo Cruz Institute, FIOCRUZ, Rio de Janeiro 21040-900, RJ, Brazil
3. Cellular and Molecular Department, Biology Institute, Federal Fluminense University, Niterói 24020-141, RJ, Brazil
* Correspondence: salvatore.simone@fiocruz.br; Tel.: +55-21-3865-8183

Abstract: Background: The coronavirus disease of 2019 (COVID-19) is caused by an infection with severe acute respiratory syndrome coronavirus 2 (SARS-CoV-2). It was recognized in late 2019 and has since spread worldwide, leading to a pandemic with unprecedented health and financial consequences. There remains an enormous demand for new diagnostic methods that can deliver fast, low-cost, and easy-to-use confirmation of a SARS-CoV-2 infection. We have developed an affordable electrochemical biosensor for the rapid detection of serological immunoglobulin G (IgG) antibody in sera against the spike protein. Materials and Methods: A previously identified linear B-cell epitope (EP) specific to the SARS-CoV-2 spike glycoprotein and recognized by IgG in patient sera was selected for the target molecule. After synthesis, the EP was immobilized onto the surface of the working electrode of a commercially available screen-printed electrode (SPE). The capture of SARS-CoV-2-specific IgGs allowed the formation of an immunocomplex that was measured by square-wave voltammetry from its generation of hydroquinone (HQ). Results: An evaluation of the performance of the EP-based biosensor presented a selectivity and specificity for COVID-19 of 93% and 100%, respectively. No cross-reaction was observed to antibodies against other diseases that included Chagas disease, Chikungunya, Leishmaniosis, and Dengue. Differentiation of infected and non-infected individuals was possible even at a high dilution factor that decreased the required sample volumes to a few microliters. Conclusion: The final device proved suitable for diagnosing COVID-19 by assaying actual serum samples, and the results displayed good agreement with the molecular biology diagnoses. The flexibility to conjugate other EPs to SPEs suggests that this technology could be rapidly adapted to diagnose new variants of SARS-CoV-2 or other pathogens.

Keywords: SARS-CoV-2; COVID-19; spike glycoprotein; epitope; electrochemical biosensor; point of care; immunological diagnostic

1. Introduction

Severe acute respiratory syndrome coronavirus 2 (SARS-CoV-2) has led to a global pandemic of coronavirus disease 2019 (COVID-19) [1]. Citizens of many countries were compelled to stay under partial or complete lockdown for months due to high transmissibility and disease severity [2]. Driven by the uncertainty concerning the effectiveness of rapidly deployed vaccines against severe disease, an absence of adequate therapies and appearance of new variants [1], diagnosis has played an important role in decision making. Case detection, monitoring, infection prevention, and supportive care are all tools for fighting the SARS-CoV-2 pandemic [1,3].

To keep up with our healthcare needs, it is crucial to develop a rapid point-of-care test to detect potential carriers of COVID-19 and those who have recovered as disease dynamics change at the speed of its spread [1]. While the gold standard technique for the diagnosis of the initial phase of an infection is the detection of viral genomic nucleic acid through reverse transcription-polymerase chain reactions (RT-PCR) from nasal and mouth swabs, its implementation in resource-limited settings is restricted due to infrastructure, skilled personnel, and time restrictions [1]. Serological assays for the presence of COVID-19-related immunoglobulin M (IgM) or IgG antibodies have provided a cost-effective and accurate method of tracking virus transmission to implement socio-political strategies against the spread of the contagion [1,4,5].

As a platform, electrochemical biosensors stand out to meet the demands for serological diagnostics through their characteristics: rapid, simple, portable, sensitive, easy-to-use, miniaturized, and compatible with portable instruments [6–9]. They can be combined with a wide range of biological recognition elements to detect clinically relevant compounds such as enzymes, nucleic acid, antibodies, epitopes, and others [10–15]. Among these choices, epitopes (EPs) hold a high interest since they represent the minimum amino acid sequences in a pathogen's proteome that are bound by antibodies generated in a patient in response to an infection [7]. Their use can improve selectivity by the elimination of cross-reactivity based on sequence similarity to other pathogens, which is a major concern when whole antigens are used due to the presence of non-specific epitopes that can react with antibodies [16].

Here, the sensitivity of electrochemical measurements was combined with the specificity of EPs to develop an affordable biosensor for a serological assay to detect the presence of anti-SARS-CoV-2 antibodies as a diagnosis of COVID-19. A commercially available screen-printed electrode (SPE) was employed, while an epitope in SARS-CoV-2 spike (S) glycoprotein was employed as a binding target for antibody capture. The high performance in identifying infected patients and the absence of cross-reactivity suggests that his platform could be a viable solution for screening a large number of people. The flexibility of the proposed technology also presents the advantage of being rapidly adaptable to var-iants along with wide range of diseases by altering only the binding target.

2. Materials and Methods

2.1. Patient Samples and Project Approval

Positive controls consisted of fourteen serum samples from patients confirmed with COVID-19 by RT-PCR tests on nasopharyngeal or oropharyngeal swabs. Negative controls consisted of serum samples from blood bank donors (HEMORIO, Rio de Janeiro) collected before the pandemic (pre-November, 2019). For cross-reactivity, serum samples from patients diagnosed with Chagas disease, Dengue, Leshmaniose, and Chikungunya were used. For performance evaluations, a panel of 14 sera was used, collected from individuals who had suspected contact with individuals with COVID-19 and who were subsequently diagnosed by RT-PCR on nasopharyngeal or oropharyngeal swabs. Patient privacy was preserved by disassociating identifying information from the samples. The study was conducted following the International Coordinating Council for Clinical Trials and the Helsinki Declaration and was approved by the Local Ethics Committee UNIGRANRIO (No. 21362220.1.0000.5283) and Estacio de Sá University (No. 33090820. 8.0000.5284).

2.2. Chemicals and Reagents

Reagent-grade chemicals and peptide synthesis reagents were purchased from Sigma-Merck (St. Louis, MO, USA). Secondary antibodies were purchased from ThermoFisher (São Paulo, SP, Brazil). Hydroquinone diphosphate (diPho-HQ) salt was purchased from Metrohm Dropsens (Astúrias, Astúrias, Spain). All solutions were prepared with deionized water (>18.1 MΩ cm) obtained from a Nanopure Diamond system (Barnstead, Dubuque, IA, USA).

2.3. Solid-Phase Peptide Synthesis

Epitopes in the SARS-CoV-2 spike protein were prepared as amidated peptides on a Multipep-1 automated synthesizer (CEM Corp., Charlotte, NC, USA), as previously described [17]. Peptides were synthesized in a solid state on sintered glass filters containing Rink amide AM resin using the 9-fluorenylmethoxy carbonyl (F-moc) strategy. Finally, resin-bound peptides were deprotected and cleaved using trifluoroacetic acid and triisopropylsilane precipitated with diethyl ether and then lyophilized. Stock solutions were prepared with PBS and their concentration was determined by optical density and the theoretical molar extinction coefficient generated by the PROTPARAM software package (http://www.expasy.ch; accessed on 21 October 2021). Peptide sequences were confirmed by matrix-assisted laser desorption ionization time-of-flight mass spectrometry (MALDI-TOF MS).

2.4. Modification of the SPE's Working Electrode

Carbon SPE working electrodes (DRP-110, Metrohm DropSend, Oviedo, Spain) were sensitized with peptides by a drop-casting method. First, the SPE was electrochemically treated in 0.1 mol L^{-1} of phosphate buffer solution (PBS), pH 7.4, applying +2 V (vs. Ag) for 60 s using a CompactState portable potentiostat (Ivium Technologies B.V., Eindhoven, Netherlands), rinsed with PBS, and allowed to dry at room temperature. Next, 2 µL of EP (100 µg mL^{-1} in PBS) was placed onto the surface of the SPE, followed by 10 µL of 2.5% (w/w) glutaraldehyde. After 30 min at room temperature, the peptide-modified SPEs were blocked overnight at 4 °C with 1% (w/w) BSA prepared in 0.1 mol L^{-1} PBS (pH 7.4).

2.5. Electrochemical Assay to Detect Antibodies COVID-19 Antibody IgG

The detection of anti-SARS-CoV-2 IgG antibodies was based on an indirect immunoassay wherein the subsequent binding of anti-human IgG conjugated with alkaline phosphatase (AP) hydrolyzed diPho-HQ to hydroquinone (HQ) that could be measured as electrochemical signals, shown schematically in Figure 1. Briefly, EP-specific IgGs (COVID-19 antibodies) present in 4 µL of diluted patient serum (1:100 in PBS with 1% BSA) were captured onto the sensitized working electrode surface of the SPE after a minimum 10 min incubation at 37 °C for complete drying. Then, SPEs were rinsed in PBS, and 4 µL of anti-human IgG secondary antibody solution conjugated with AP was added for another incubation to dry at 37 °C before rinsing in reaction buffer (0.1 mol L^{-1} Tris-HCl and 20 mmol L^{-1} $MgCl_2$, pH 9.8). Next, the reaction buffer with 5 mM diPho-HQ was placed onto the SPE. After brief incubation (2 min), the presence of HQ was measured by square-wave voltammetry (SWV) with the following parameters: amplitude, 10 mV; frequency, 6.3 Hz; step, 10 mV; applied potential window, −0.5 to 0.2 V vs. Ag. Each cycle required 11 s, and a stable measurement was observed after the twentieth cycle (3.7 min total time).

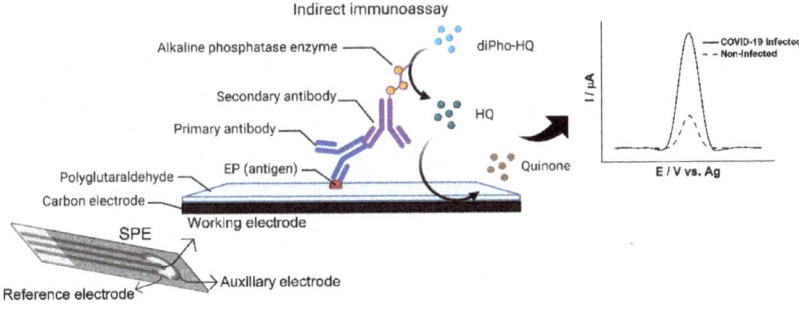

Figure 1. Schematic representation of a positive indirect immunoassay to detect COVID-19. Anti-SARS-CoV-2 IgG antibody (primary antibody) in patient serum samples is captured onto the surface

of the SPE's peptide-modified working electrode. Retained human antibodies are bound by AP-conjugated anti-human antibodies (Secondary antibodies). Enzymatic activity converts diPho-HQ into HQ, which can be measured by square-wave voltammetry.

2.6. Analysis of Blood Serum Samples

Electrochemical signals from positive and negative serum control samples were recorded to determine the cut-off value from Equation (1) (described in item 3.3) that was used to normalize all data as a reactivity index. A gray zone was defined as 1.0 ± 0.1. Next, sera were analyzed from persons with suspected contact with individuals diagnosed with COVID-19. Patient serum dilutions of 1:100 with PBS were used to perform the indirect immunoassays. The optimal dilution of 1:50,000 was employed for the secondary. Both incubations with antibodies were 8 min at 37 °C, which was sufficient to allow full evaporation of the applied solution. Differentially elevated currents were associated with serum from persons infected with SARS-CoV-2.

2.7. Statistical Analysis

One-way ANOVA tests were performed to evaluate the variation between prepared SPEs. Two-tailed Student's t-tests with a confidence level of 95% were performed for pairwise comparisons [7,17,18].

3. Results

3.1. Development of Electrochemical Immunosensor

Previously, IgG linear B-cell epitopes (EPs) in the spike protein of SARS-CoV-2 were mapped by spot synthesis analysis [16]. Four of these were chosen to serve as antibody capture molecules on the surface of screen-printed electrodes. The intention was to develop an immunosensor utilizing a drop-casting approach with glutaraldehyde (GA) to sensitize the electrode surface. GA has been widely used to modify electrode surfaces due to its introduction of aldehyde functional groups that allow the covalent bonding of compounds containing terminal amino moieties such as EPs [19]. Single-use SPEs were fabricated by mixing PBS solutions containing a prospective EP and GA onto the surface of the electrode. After drying and washing, its ability to differentially detect anti-SARS-CoV-2 antibodies as a diagnosis for COVID-19 was evaluated. The formation of immunocomplexes with AP-conjugated sec-IgG antibodies allowed enzymatic reduction of diPho-HQ to generate HQ, a redox molecule measurable by square-wave voltammetry (SWV) [7].

Initially, the performance of SPEs conjugated to peptides EP1 (GPLQSYGFQPTG), EP2 (LPPLLTDEMIAQYTS), EP3 (GLDSKVGGNYNYG), and EP4 (RSYTPGDSSSGWTAG), which represent different EPs in the spike protein, was evaluated. The peak currents were recorded from measurements of an SWV while exposed to diluted serum samples from patients who tested positive and negative for COVID-19 (Figure 2A). From the ratio of the positive to negative peak currents (Figure 2B), the most robust measurement was obtained with EP2 as it demonstrated a significantly higher positive/negative signal ratio (p-value < 0.001) than the others. Therefore, EP2 was chosen for additional optimization.

Next, the production of the SPE was optimized. Figure 2B shows that the EP concentration on the SPE surface affected the current measured from the immunoreaction (Figure 2B). The ratio between SWV signals obtained after incubation in positive and negative samples significantly rose as increasing concentrations of EP were used ($p < 0.01$, Figure 2D), reaching a plateau at 100 µg mL^{-1} ($p = 0.08$). This suggested that antibodies were increasingly captured until reaching electrode surface saturation. Therefore, the most suitable EP concentration was 100 µg mL^{-1} and was used to produce all subsequent SPEs.

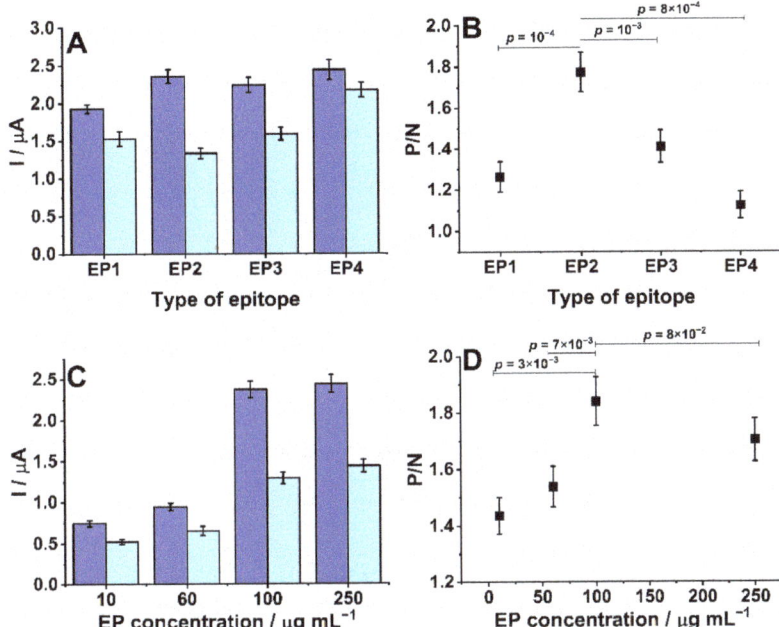

Figure 2. Target choice for conjugation to SPE and measurement optimization. SPEs were sensitized with peptides that represented four EPs identified in the SARS-CoV-2 spike protein. Next, SPEs were incubated with patient sera diluted 1:100 in PBS for 10 min at 37 °C before rinsing. SPEs were similarly incubated with an AP-labeled anti-human secondary (1:30,000), rinsed and presented with 5 mM diPho-HQ in 100 mM Tris-HCl and 20 mM MgCl2 (pH 9.8) for its enzymatic conversion to HQ. (**A**) Peak currents measured by SWV from positive (blue) or negative (light blue) sera using SPE sensitized with EP1–EP4. (**B**) Ratio between positive and negative signals (P/N) from graph A. (**C**) Peak currents measured from positive (blue) and negative (light blue) sera with SPEs sensitized over a range of EP2 peptide concentrations (10–250 µg mL^{-1}). (**D**) Ratio between positive and nega-tive signals (P/N) for data in graph C. All experiments were performed in duplicate. Solution vol-umes were 2 µL for antibody solutions and 50 µL for washes. Antibody incubations were for 8 min at 37 °C. The parameters of SWVs for amplitude, frequency, step, and applied potential window were 10 mV, 6.3 Hz, 10 mV, −0.6–0.6 V (vs. Ag), respectively.

3.2. Optimization of Experimental Parameters, Reproducibility, and Stability

To optimize the analytical signal, the level of dilution for patient serum and secondary antibodies was evaluated. A fixed time of 16 min for the incubation times was chosen for antibodies. As the dilution of the positive serum sample was increased, there was a decrease in the signal from the positive samples (Figure 3A). Similarly, the non-specific binding of antibodies to the surface of the EP-sensitized SPE, represented by the negative controls, showed decreasing signals with higher dilutions. A maximum difference in the ratio of the SWV measurements obtained from positive and negative control sera was observed for sample dilutions of 1:100 ($p < 0.001$, Figure 3B), which was subsequently chosen as the optimal dilution factor. Differential signals between positive and negative samples were detectable up to a dilution factor of 1000 ($p < 0.02$), which suggested that the dynamic range of the approach was greater than 10-fold and could permit the detection of antibodies of low titers.

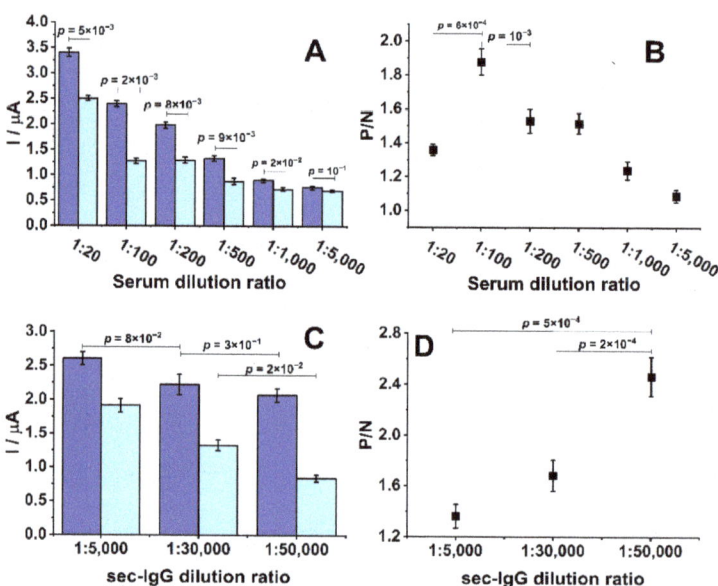

Figure 3. Optimization of primary and secondary antibody dilutions. All SPEs were sensitized with 100 µg/mL of EP2. (**A**) Peak currents measured over a dilution range of positive (blue) and negative (light blue) patient sera. (**B**) Ratio between positive and negative signals (P/N) from graph A. (**C**) Peak currents measured from positive (blue) and negative (light blue) patient sera diluted 1:100 in combination with a range of dilutions of the secondary antibody. (**D**) Ratio between positive and negative signals (P/N) from graph C. All experiments were performed in duplicate.

Another critical factor for detecting EP/IgG immunocomplexes was the concentration of the secondary antibodies. Small decreases in the positive signals over the range of secondary antibody concentrations suggested that its presence is not a limiting factor to the measurement (Figure 3C). However, a large difference in the measurement of negative sera suggests there is a potential for non-specific background signals at higher concentrations. The background signal significantly decreased to the lowest levels at a dilution of 1:50,000 ($p < 0.02$), which did not meaningfully impact the signal from the positive control (comparison between 1:5000 and 1:30,000 and between 1:30,000 and 1:50,000 provided $p = 0.08$ and 0.30, respectively) and provided the most prominent signal-to-noise ratio (Figure 3D).

3.3. Biosensor Performance

The reproducibility of the SPEs was analyzed by evaluating electrodes prepared on different days using the same protocol. A relative standard deviation (RSD) of 5% in the SWV HQ response was calculated from three measurements of a 1:100 diluted positive serum on the electrodes prepared on different days, which demonstrated the practical reproducibility of the method (Figure 4B). SPEs prepared on the same day were stored at 4 °C in PBS to test stability. After 14 days of storage, the signal obtained from a positive sample diluted at 1:100 showed an RSD of 7% ($n = 3$) and decay in the average response of 10% compared to using an SPE prepared on the same day. The measurements showed that the response was preserved statistically ($p = 0.1$) (Figure 4B). However, the SWV current decreased by 20% and presented an RSD of 8% ($n = 3$) after 30 days of storage. These levels suggested that the performance of the SPE was significantly decreased compared to the same day as prepared ($p = 0.01$). Thus, these biosensors had only a 14-day shelf life at 4 °C.

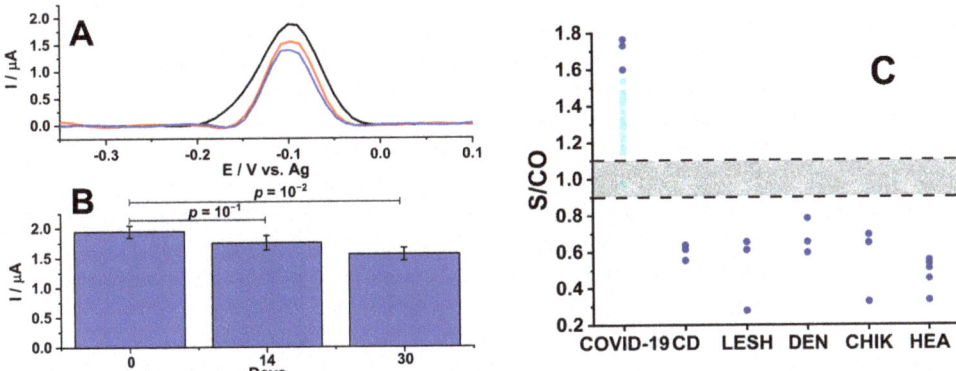

Figure 4. Stability, performance, and cross-reactivity of EP2 conjugated SPEs. (**A**) SPE reproducibility was evaluated by fabricating multiple SPEs according to the optimized protocol and performing SWVs in positive serum (1:100) on the day of fabrication (black line, $n = 3$), after 14 days of storage at 4 °C (red line, $n = 3$) and 30 days of storage at 4 °C (blue line, $n = 3$). (**B**) The graph shows the variations in recordings. (**C**) For real-world applications, the cut-off was determined using positive and negative controls (dark blue). Multiple serum samples from persons suspected of having COVID-19 (light blue); individuals with Chagas disease (CD; *Trypanosoma cruzi*), leishmaniosis (LESH), dengue (DEN), and chikungunya (CHIK); and healthy (HEA) patients were assayed. The gray region represents ±10%.

To evaluate the performance of the EP2-sensitized SPEs, a confirmed panel of positive ($n = 14$) and negative ($n = 17$) patient samples (1:100 in PBS) previously assayed by a commercial assay for COVID-19 (DiaPro Diagnostic Bioprobes Srl, Mi, Italy) was measured (Figure 4B). Using Equation (1), a cut-off was calculated as 1.4 µA for detecting COVID-19.

$$Cut - off = a \cdot X + f \cdot SD \tag{1}$$

where X is the mean and SD is the standard deviation of independent negative control readings, and a and f are two arbitrary multipliers, which were 1 and 3 in the present case, respectively [20,21]. The final results were normalized as the ratio of the sampled signal to the cut-off value (S/co). A gray zone was defined between ±10% of 1.0 wherein results between 0.9–1.1 were considered indeterminate, >1.1 as positive, and <0.9 as negative. Cross-reactivity was evaluated with sera collected from patients diagnosed with Chagas disease, dengue, leishmaniose, and chikungunya. Each presented a S/CO value of less than 0.9 which corresponds to a specificity of 100%. Positive controls collected from those confirmed with COVID-19 analyzed previously by RT-PCR demonstrated a median S/CO ratio near 1.7 (Figure 4B, dark blue). To simulate a real-world application for the diagnosis of COVID-19, 14 samples from persons with suspected contacts were assayed with the SPE. From these, 13 volunteers were considered positive and 1 was in the gray zone for selectivity of 93%.

4. Discussion

Serological diagnostic tests that utilize the presence of antibodies as the definition of whether an individual was infected by a pathogen detect antibodies in their serum or blood. This can be conducted as a lab-based assay such as an enzyme-linked immunosorbent assay (ELISA) [7] or chemiluminescent immunoassay [22], which are time-consuming and expensive, or a point-of-care test based on lateral flow technology that can show limited sensitivity [23,24]. We propose an electrochemical assay based on commercially available SPEs that can be easily sensitized to capture diagnostic antibodies. We began with the diagnosis of COVID-19 by choosing to sensitize the SPE with a peptide that represents an epitope in the spike protein to capture anti-SARS-CoV-2 IgG antibodies. The S protein is a highly exposed part of the viral structure [3] and contains several immunodominant epitopes [1,23]. The use of a single epitope allows for the development of highly specific serological assays. Furthermore, a focus on IgG antibodies, which are more prevalent than IgM antibodies [1,3], enabled improvements in sensitivity and specificity [1]. Ultimately, sensitized SPEs can be easily fabricated at a low cost that is compatible with portable equipment to provide rapid results in non-laboratory settings.

Generally, an electrochemical immunosensor consists of an electron-conducting solid surface where the molecule of interest (antibody or antigen) can be selectively captured, and its presence detected by the amplification [7] or suppression [25] of an electrochemical signal. A key element of the biosensor is the biological component that can be immobilized onto its surface, such as an antigen [25] or EP [7]. Here, the SPE was modified with a peptide representing an EP specific to the S protein of SARS-CoV-2. No cross-reactivity was displayed against serum from patients with Chagas, chikungunya, leishmaniosis, and dengue (Figure 3B), all pathogens endemic to Rio de Janeiro, Brazil [26]. The single sample that presented a S/CO ratio in the gray zone was from an individual whose blood sample was collected soon after presenting symptoms that may not have been seroconverted. Overall, within the electrochemical platform, the biosensor showed high specificity and sensitivity of 100% and 93%, respectively.

The requirement of a small patient sample combined with a low cost could make it economically viable to perform multiple assays to ensure a confident result [1,3]. The diagnostic accuracy of different assays is variable [27–30] and a recent work compared the performance of ten assays. Sensitivities of 40–77% (65–81% considering IgG plus IgM) were found [31], making our electrochemical platform a competitive methodology for the diagnosis of COVID-19. In addition, the proposed device provided a reliable method for detecting COVID-19 IgG in serum and was rapid (22 min compared to >90 min required for an ELISA), even though the time spent to modify the substrates with antigens and block them was comparable in both mentioned techniques. Notably, the measurements can be performed in volumes lesser than 100 µL, the required volume for an ELISA assay, which translates to 2 nL of serum that can be easily acquired from a single finger prick sample of blood. Furthermore, the simplicity of electrode preparation, ease of use, accuracy, and low cost all suggest that this platform could be utilized as a point-of-care diagnostic assay to detect infected individuals for observation and to track the spread of disease, as well as identify high titer samples for recruiting potential donors to provide convalescent plasma therapy [32,33]. Considering that the relevance of the information obtained from the measurements was defined by the peptide used to sensitize the SPE, this platform has a high potential to be modified towards other pathogens and aspects of the COVID-19 pandemic, such as antibody titer post-vaccination, temporal changes in antibody response, and altered reactivity to variants.

5. Conclusions

We developed a portable and affordable biosensor to rapidly detect COVID-19 infection by detecting anti-SARS-CoV-2-specific IgG antibodies in patient serum. Based on electrochemical reactivity, it showed a sensitivity of 93% and a specificity of 100%. Single-use electrodes were fabricated by the surface modification of commercially available SPE with a peptide that represents an epitope-specific SARS-CoV-2 spike glycoprotein. The immobilized peptide could capture COVID-19-specific IgG antibodies for measurement by an indirect immunoassay using an enzyme-conjugated secondary IgG that hydrolyzed diPho-HQ into HQ, a redox molecule detectable by SWV. Under optimized conditions, it differentiates infected and non-infected individuals that correlated with RT-PCR diagnosis. No cross-reactivity was displayed to other pathogens such as *Trypanosoma cruzi* (Chagas disease), chikungunya, leishmaniosis, and dengue. The biosensor platform has the flexibility to meet the demands of other pathogens and their respective diseases

6. Patents

The peptide described in this study is protected under Brazilian and US provisional patent applications BR 10.2019.017792.6 and PCT/BR2020/050341, respectively, filed by FIOCRUZ, and may serve as a future source of funding.

Author Contributions: Conceptualization, W.A.A.; methodology, W.A.A.; software, W.A.A.; formal analysis and data curation, W.A.A. and S.G.D.-S.; writing—original draft preparation, W.A.A.; writing—review and editing, D.W.P. and S.G.D.-S.; project administration, C.M.M.; S.G.D.-S.; funding acquisition, C.M.M. and S.G.D.-S. All authors have read and agreed to the published version of the manuscript.

Funding: This research was funded by Carlos Chagas Filho Foundation for Research Support of the State of Rio de Janeiro/FAPERJ (#110.198-13) and the Brazilian Council for Scientific Research (CNPq, #467.488/2014-2 and 301744/2019-0). Funding was also provided by FAPERJ (#210.003/2018) through the National Institutes of Science and Technology Program (INCT) to Carlos M. Morel (INCT-IDPN).

Institutional Review Board Statement: The study was approved by the University of Estacio de Sá (CAAE: 33090820.8.0000.5284) and UNIGRANRIO (CAAE: 21362220.1.0000.5283) study center ethics committee and conducted under good clinical practice and applicable regulatory requirements, including the Declaration of Helsinki.

Informed Consent Statement: Not applicable.

Data Availability Statement: The data presented in this study are available upon request from the corresponding author.

Acknowledgments: We are grateful to the National Institute of Quality Control, FIOCRUZ, RJ, Brazil for the MALDI-TOF analysis. Figure 1 was prepared using the Bio render drawing toolkit.

Conflicts of Interest: The authors declare no conflict of interest involving the research reported. The funding agencies had no role in the study design, data collection, data analysis, decision to publish, or preparation of the manuscript.

References

1. Ejazi, S.A.; Ghosh, S.; Ali, N. Antibody detection assays for COVID-19 diagnosis: An early overview. *Immunol. Cell Biol.* **2021**, *99*, 21–33. [CrossRef] [PubMed]
2. Karim, S.S.A.; Karim, Q.A. Omicron SARS-CoV-2 variant: A new chapter in the COVID-19 pandemic. *Lancet* **2021**, *398*, 2126–2128. [CrossRef]
3. Kudr, J.; Michalek, P.; Ilieva, L.; Adam, V.; Zitka, O. COVID-19: A challenge for electrochemical biosensors. *Trends Anal. Chem.* **2021**, *136*, 116192. [CrossRef] [PubMed]
4. Noce, A.; Santoro, M.L.; Marrone, G.; D'Agostini, C.; Amelio, I.; Duggento, A.; Tesauro, M.; Di Daniele, N. Serological determinants of COVID-19. *Biol. Direct* **2020**, *15*, 21. [CrossRef] [PubMed]
5. Harvala, H.; Mehew, J.; Robb, M.L.; Ijaz, S.; Dicks, S.; Patel, M.; Watkins, N.; Simmonds, P.; Brooks, T.; Johnson, R.; et al. Blood and transplant convalescent plasma testing group. convalescent plasma treatment for SARS-CoV-2 infection: Analysis of the first 436 donors in England, 22 April to 12 May 2020. *Euro Surveill.* **2020**, *25*, 2001260, Erratum in *Euro Surveill.* **2021**, *26*, 210325d. https://doi.org/10.2807/1560-7917.ES.2021.26.12.210325d. [CrossRef] [PubMed]
6. Romanholo, P.V.V.; Razzino, C.A.; Raymundo-Pereira, P.A.; Prado, T.M.; Machado, S.A.S.; Sgobbi, L.F. Biomimetic electrochemical sensors: New horizons and challenges in biosensing applications. *Biosens. Bioelectron.* **2021**, *185*, 113242. [CrossRef]
7. Ameku, W.A.; Ataide, V.N.; Costa, E.T.; Gomes, L.R.; Napoleão-Pêgo, P.; William Provance, D.; Paixão, T.R.L.C.; Salles, M.O.; De-Simone, S.G. A pencil-lead immunosensor for the rapid electrochemical measurement of anti-diphtheria toxin antibodies. *Biosensors* **2021**, *11*, 489. [CrossRef]
8. Hughes, G.; Westmacott, K.; Honeychurch, K.C.; Crew, A.; Pemberton, R.M.; Hart, J.P. Recent advances in the fabrication and application of screen-printed electrochemical (bio)sensors based on carbon materials for biomedical, agri-food, and environmental analyses. *Biosensors* **2016**, *6*, 50. [CrossRef]
9. Ameku, W.A.; De Araujo, W.R.; Rangel, C.J.; Ando, R.A.; Paixão, T.R.L.C. Gold nanoparticle paper-based dual-detection device for forensics applications. *ACS Appl. Nano Mater.* **2019**, *9*, 5460–5468. [CrossRef]
10. Orzari, L.O.; Cristina de Freitas, R.; Aparecida de Araujo Andreotti, I.; Gatti, A.; Janegitz, B.C. A novel disposable self-adhesive inked paper device for electrochemical sensing of dopamine and serotonin neurotransmitters and glucose biosensing. *Biosens. Bioelectron.* **2019**, *138*, 111310. [CrossRef]

11. Núnez-Bajo, E.; Carmen Blanco-López, M.; Costa-García, A.; Teresa Fernández-Abedul, M. Integration of gold-sputtered electrofluidic paper on wire-included analytical platforms for glucose biosensing. *Biosens. Bioelectron.* **2017**, *91*, 824–832. [CrossRef] [PubMed]
12. Torres, M.D.T.; de Araujo, W.R.; de Lima, L.F.; Ferreira, A.L.; de la Fuente-Nunez, C. Low-cost biosensor for rapid detection of SARS-CoV-2 at the point-of-care. *Matter* **2021**, *4*, 2403–2416. [CrossRef] [PubMed]
13. Yakoh, A.; Pimpitak, U.; Rengpipat, S.; Hirankarn, N.; Chailapakul, O.; Chaiyo, S. Paper-based electrochemical biosensor for diagnosing COVID-19: Detection of SARS-CoV-2 antibodies and antigen. *Biosens. Bioelectron.* **2021**, *176*, 112912. [CrossRef] [PubMed]
14. Ataide, V.N.; Ameku, W.A.; Bacil, R.P.; Angnes, L.; De Araujo, W.R.; Paixão, T.R.L.C. Enhanced performance of pencil-drawn paper-based electrodes by laser-scribing treatment. *RSC Adv.* **2021**, *11*, 1644–1653. [CrossRef]
15. de Araujo, W.R.; Frasson, C.M.R.; Ameku, W.A.; Silva, J.R.; Angnes, L.; Paixão, T.R. Single-step reagentless laser scribing fabrication of electrochemical paper-based analytical devices. *Angew. Chem. Int.* **2017**, *129*, 15113–15117. [CrossRef] [PubMed]
16. Bottino, C.G.; Gomes, L.P.; Pereira, J.B.; Coura, J.R.; Provance, D.W.; De-Simone, S.G. Chagas disease-specific antigens: Characterization of epitopes in CRA/FRA by synthetic peptide mapping and evaluation by ELISA-peptide assay. *BMC Infect. Dis.* **2013**, *13*, 568. [CrossRef] [PubMed]
17. Souza, A.L.; Faria, R.X.; Calabrese, K.S.; Hardoim, D.J.; Taniwaki, N.; Alves, L.A.; De-Simone, S.G. Temporizin and temporizin-1 peptides as novel candidates for eliminating *Trypanosoma cruzi*. *PLoS ONE* **2016**, *11*, e0157673. [CrossRef]
18. Doughty, P.T.; Hossain, I.; Gong, C.; Ponder, K.A.; Pati, S.; Arumugam, P.U.; Murray, T.A. Novel microwire-based biosensor probe for simultaneous real-time measurement of glutamate and GABA dynamics in vitro and in vivo. *Sci. Rep.* **2020**, *10*, 12777. [CrossRef]
19. Ahmad, H.M.N.; Dutta, G.; Csoros, J.; Si, B.; Yang, R.; Halpern, J.M.; Seitz, W.R.; Song, E. Stimuli-responsive templated polymer as a target receptor for a conformation-based electrochemical sensing platform. *ACS Appl. Polym. Mater.* **2021**, *3*, 329–341. [CrossRef]
20. Ternynck, T.; Avrameas, S. Polymerization and immobilization of proteins using ethyl chloroformate and glutaraldehyde. *Scand. J. Immunol.* **1976**, *5*, 29–35. [CrossRef]
21. Lardeux, F.; Torrico, G.; Aliaga, C. Calculation of the ELISA's cut-off based on the change-point analysis method for detection of *Trypanosoma cruzi* infection in Bolivian dogs in the absence of controls. *Mem. Inst. Oswaldo Cruz* **2016**, *111*, 501–504. [CrossRef] [PubMed]
22. Dopico, E.; Del-Rei, R.P.; Espinoza, B.; Ubillos, I.; Zanchin, N.I.T.; Sulleiro, E.; Moure, Z.; Celedon, P.A.F.; Souza, W.V.; Da Silva, E.D.; et al. Immune reactivity to *Trypanosoma cruzi* chimeric proteins for Chagas disease diagnosis in immigrants living in a non-endemic setting. *BMC Infect. Dis.* **2019**, *19*, 251. [CrossRef] [PubMed]
23. Fan, F.; Shen, H.; Zhang, G.; Jiang, X.; Kang, X. Chemiluminescence immunoassay based on microfluidic chips for α-fetoprotein. *Clin. Chim. Acta* **2014**, *431*, 113–117. [CrossRef]
24. Michel, M.; Bouam, A.; Edouard, S.; Fenollar, F.; Di Pinto, F.; Mège, J.L.; Drancourt, M.; Vitte, J. Evaluating ELISA, immunofluorescence, and lateral flow assay for SARS-CoV-2 serologic assays. *Front. Microbiol.* **2020**, *11*, 597529. [CrossRef] [PubMed]
25. Dowlatshahi, S.; Shabani, E.; Abdekhodaie, M.J. Serological assays and host antibody detection in coronavirus-related disease diagnosis. *Arch. Virol.* **2021**, *166*, 715–731. [CrossRef] [PubMed]
26. De Lima, L.F.; Ferreira, A.L.; Torres, M.D.T.; Araujo, W.R. Minute-scale detection of SARS-CoV-2 using a low-cost biosensor composed of pencil graphite electrodes. *Proc. Natl. Acad. Sci. USA* **2021**, *118*, e2106724118. [CrossRef]
27. Nicol, T.; Lefeuvre, C.; Serri, O.; Pivert, A.; Joubaud, F.; Dubée, V.; Kouatchet, A.; Ducancelle, A.; Lunel-Fabiani, F.; Le Guillou-Guillemette, H. Assessment of SARS-CoV-2 serological tests for the diagnosis of COVID-19 through the evaluation of three immunoassays: Two automated immunoassays (Euroimmun and Abbott) and one rapid lateral flow immunoassay (NG Biotech). *J. Clin. Virol.* **2020**, *129*, 104511. [CrossRef]
28. Beavis, K.G.; Matushek, S.M.; Abeleda, A.P.F.; Bethel, C.; Hunt, C.; Gillen, S.; Moran, A.; Tesic, V. Evaluation of the EUROIMMUN anti-SARS-CoV-2 ELISA assay for detection of IgA and IgG antibodies. *J. Clin. Virol.* **2020**, *129*, 104468. [CrossRef]
29. Guevara-Hoyer, K.; Fuentes-Antrás, J.; De la Fuente-Muñoz, E.; Rodríguez de la Peña, A.; Viñuela, M.; Cabello-Clotet, N.; Estrada, V.; Culebras, E.; Delgado-Iribarren, A.; Martínez-Novillo, M.; et al. Serological tests in the detection of SARS-CoV-2 Antibodies. *Diagnostics* **2021**, *11*, 678. [CrossRef]
30. Mekonnen, D.; Mengist, H.M.; Derbie, A.; Nibret, E.; Munshea, A.; He, H.; Li, B.; Jin, T. Diagnostic accuracy of serological tests and kinetics of severe acute respiratory syndrome coronavirus 2 antibody: A systematic review and meta-analysis. *Rev. Med. Virol.* **2021**, *31*, e2181. [CrossRef]
31. Gutiérrez-Cobos, A.; Gómez de Frutos, S.; Domingo García, D.; Navarro Lara, E.; Yarci Carrión, A.; Fontán García-Rodrigo, L.; Fraile Torres, A.M.; Cardeñoso Domingo, L. Evaluation of diagnostic accuracy of 10 serological assays for detection of SARS-CoV-2 antibodies. *Eur. J. Clin. Microbiol. Infect. Dis.* **2021**, *40*, 955–961. [CrossRef] [PubMed]
32. Gomes, L.R.; Durans, A.M.; Napole, P.; Waterman, J.A.; Freitas, M.S.; De Sá, N.B.; Pereira, L.V.; Furtado, J.S.; Aquino, G.; Machado, M.C.R.; et al. Multiepitope proteins for the differential detection of IgG antibodies against RBD of the spike protein and non-RBD regions of SARS-CoV-2. *Vaccines* **2021**, *9*, 986. [CrossRef] [PubMed]
33. Ji, T.; Liu, Z.; Wang, G.; Guo, X.; Akbar Khan, S.; Lai, C.; Chen, H.; Huang, S.; Xia, S.; Chen, B.; et al. Detection of COVID-19: A review of the current literature and future perspectives. *Biosens Bioelectron.* **2020**, *166*, 112455. [CrossRef] [PubMed]

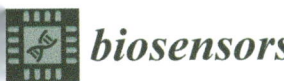

Review

Plasmonic Approaches for the Detection of SARS-CoV-2 Viral Particles

Sabine Szunerits *, Hiba Saada, Quentin Pagneux and Rabah Boukherroub

University of Lille, CNRS, Centrale Lille, University Polytechnique Hauts-de-France, UMR 8520-IEMN, F-59000 Lille, France; hiba.saada@univ-lille.fr (H.S.); quentin.pagneux@univ-lille.fr (Q.P.); rabah.boukherroub@univ-lille.fr (R.B.)
* Correspondence: sabine.szunerits@univ-lille.fr; Tel.: +33-3-62-53-17-25

Abstract: The ongoing highly contagious Coronavirus disease 2019 (COVID-19) pandemic, caused by severe acute respiratory syndrome coronavirus 2 (SARS-CoV-2), underlines the fundamental position of diagnostic testing in outbreak control by allowing a distinction of the infected from the non-infected people. Diagnosis of COVID-19 remains largely based on reverse transcription PCR (RT-PCR), identifying the genetic material of the virus. Molecular testing approaches have been largely proposed in addition to infectivity testing of patients via sensing the presence of viral particles of SARS-CoV-2 specific structural proteins, such as the spike glycoproteins (S1, S2) and the nucleocapsid (N) protein. While the S1 protein remains the main target for neutralizing antibody treatment upon infection and the focus of vaccine and therapeutic design, it has also become a major target for the development of point-of care testing (POCT) devices. This review will focus on the possibility of surface plasmon resonance (SPR)-based sensing platforms to convert the receptor-binding event of SARS-CoV-2 viral particles into measurable signals. The state-of-the-art SPR-based SARS-CoV-2 sensing devices will be provided, and highlights about the applicability of plasmonic sensors as POCT for virus particle as well as viral protein sensing will be discussed.

Keywords: SARSC-CoV-2; diagnostics; surface plasmonic resonance (SPR); spike protein; point-of-care testing

Citation: Szunerits, S.; Saada, H.; Pagneux, Q.; Boukherroub, R. Plasmonic Approaches for the Detection of SARS-CoV-2 Viral Particles. *Biosensors* **2022**, *12*, 548. https://doi.org/10.3390/bios12070548

Received: 27 June 2022
Accepted: 19 July 2022
Published: 21 July 2022

Publisher's Note: MDPI stays neutral with regard to jurisdictional claims in published maps and institutional affiliations.

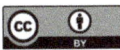

Copyright: © 2022 by the authors. Licensee MDPI, Basel, Switzerland. This article is an open access article distributed under the terms and conditions of the Creative Commons Attribution (CC BY) license (https://creativecommons.org/licenses/by/4.0/).

1. Introduction

Infection with the recent coronavirus COVID-19 leads to severe illness, which derives from the host's immune response, especially the release of a storm of pro-inflammatory cytokines. This cytokine storm produces extreme inflammatory and immune responses, especially in the lungs, leading to acute respiratory distress. Hope that SARS-CoV-2, the virus that causes COVID-19, becomes endemic over time is still pending. Widespread vaccination has contributed to fewer people becoming infected and hospitalized, ultimately alleviating the burden of COVID-19. Vaccines play a critical role in preventing deaths and hospitalization caused by this infectious disease and are contributing to controlling the spread of the disease. However, both vaccinated and nonvaccinated people need to remain aware of the additional protective behaviors required to control the pandemic. Several strategies were implemented to combat COVID-19, including wearing masks, hand hygiene and social distancing [1]. The impact of these strategies on COVID-19 remains largely unclear. However, a recent meta-analysis demonstrated that face mask use was associated with an 85% reduced risk of developing clinical symptoms of the viral infection causing COVID-19 [2].

Next to vaccination and protection strategies, the implementation of an early diagnostics of people infected with COVID-19 has proven to be crucial to the COVID-19 pandemic management. There are mainly three major methods for the detection of SARS-CoV-2 infection [3]. Molecular tests, such as polymerase chain reaction (PCR) approaches, are highly sensitive and specific for detecting viral RNA and are recommended for those symptomatic and for activating public health measures. Lateral-flow-based antigen rapid detection assays [4] detect viral proteins and, although less sensitive than the molecular tests, have the advantages of being cheap, fast and easy to be performed by any individual. Antigen rapid detection tests, mainly in the form of lateral flow devices, can be used as a public health tool for screening individuals at enhanced risk of infection, to protect people who are clinically vulnerable, to ensure safe travel and the resumption of schooling and social activities, and to enable economic recovery [3]. Realistically, the expansion of regular testing relies on the development of fast, low-infrastructure testing or self-testing, such as antigenic rapid tests with a sensitivity comparable to that of PCR [5]. Such COVID-19 diagnostic tests will continue to play a crucial role in the transition from pandemic response to pandemic control.

Concerns about the reduced sensitivity of lateral flow antigenic tests in comparison to PCR have resulted in the consideration of alternative approaches and concepts [6,7]. To evaluate the quality of these new diagnostic concepts, it is primordial to define a target sensitivity in terms of the minimal viral particles per mL concentration to be sensed, how this value correlates to plaque-forming units per mL (PFU mL^{-1}) and what the correction to cycle threshold (C_t) values from RT-PCR could be. It is believed that infectiousness begins 2–3 days prior to symptoms onset, with people being most infectious around the time of symptom onset (Figure 1a) [8]. Asymptomatic and symptomatic SARS-CoV-2 infections can have different characteristic time scales of transmission, with a mean infectious period of about 9–10 days for asymptomatic individuals [9–11] compared to symptomatic ones of about 1–4 days [12].

One fundamental issue in considering viral diagnostics sensitivity is consequently related to the question of how to compare/relate cycle threshold (Ct) values form RT-PCR obtained from different protocols and viral samples [13]. This exercise remains complex, as Ct values can only be interpreted correctly by having an idea about the health history of the patient [14]. The uncertainty about the range of viral loads that constitute a transmission risk is an additional factor when considering Ct cut-off values and diagnostic sensitivity [15]. People are most infectious around the time of symptom onset (Figure 1a), for whom the viral load in the upper respiratory tract is the highest [8]. Asymptotic individuals follow a similar dynamic and contribute in the same manner as pre-symptomatic individuals to the viral spread. There is a general agreement that Ct values are linked to SARS-CoV-2 viral load, with Ct of 33–35 being associated with low infectivity, Ct value < 20 being linked to high viral load and Ct = 40 being the cut-off between positively and negatively identified individuals. The timeline of SARS-CoV-2 RNA was lately confirmed by some of us [16] using data from 520 COVID-19 patients (Figure 1b). The lowest Ct values, corresponding to the highest virus loads, were recorded early after symptom onset, followed by a decline in virus load with increasing time after symptom onset.

To correlate Ct values with the absolute number of virions, the number of viral RNA copies can be determined in parallel (Figure 1c). As expected, a linear relation between RT-PCR Ct values and viral RNA copies mL^{-1} was observed. A Ct value thus corresponds to 2.1×10^3 viral RNA mL^{-1}, while a Ct = 12 correlates with 7.1×10^9 viral RNA mL^{-1}. The presence of viral RNA does not necessarily imply the presence of infectious virions. Virions could be defective (e.g., by mutation) or might have been deactivated by environmental conditions. Therefore, the use of viral RNA copies as an approximation for the number of infectious viral particles leads to an overestimation. It is important to keep this caveat in mind when interpreting the data about viral loads. Nevertheless, for many viruses, even a small dose of virions can lead to infection. For the common cold, for example, ~0.1 TCID$_{50}$ is sufficient to infect half of the exposed people [17]. To assess the concentration of infectious viruses, the 50% tissue-culture infectious dose with 1 PFU mL^{-1} = TCID$_{50}$/mL $\times$ 0.7 has to be determined by infecting replicate cultures of susceptible cells with dilutions of the virus and noting the dilution at which half the replicate dishes become infected. Figure 1d indicates that 2.1×10^3 viral particles mL^{-1} results in no palatable virus. The onset for forming 1 PFU mL^{-1} corresponds with a minimal viral particle load of

$(4.0 \pm 1.9) \times 10^4$ viral particles mL^{-1}. This correlates with about Ct = 32 ± 1. In a recent wok by Pickering et al. [6], Ct values of 30 were correlated to 1 PFU mL^{-1} and 5×10^4 RNA viral particles mL^{-1}. The viral particle load correlates extremely well with our findings. The difference in Ct values is linked to the different fragments being used, i.e., the N gene by Pickering et al. [6] and IP targets by us [18]. Such benchmarking is of high importance for evaluating novel sensing approaches and their performance level. For RT-PCR, 100 copies of viral RNA per mL corresponds with a positive result. In addition, serological tests can provide valuable information on the immune response and are a good complement to SARS-CoV-2 RNA test. In fact, as a patient recovers, the viral load starts to decrease, and immunoglobulin levels increase until about 10 days after symptom onset. Serological tests can be performed at this timepoint.

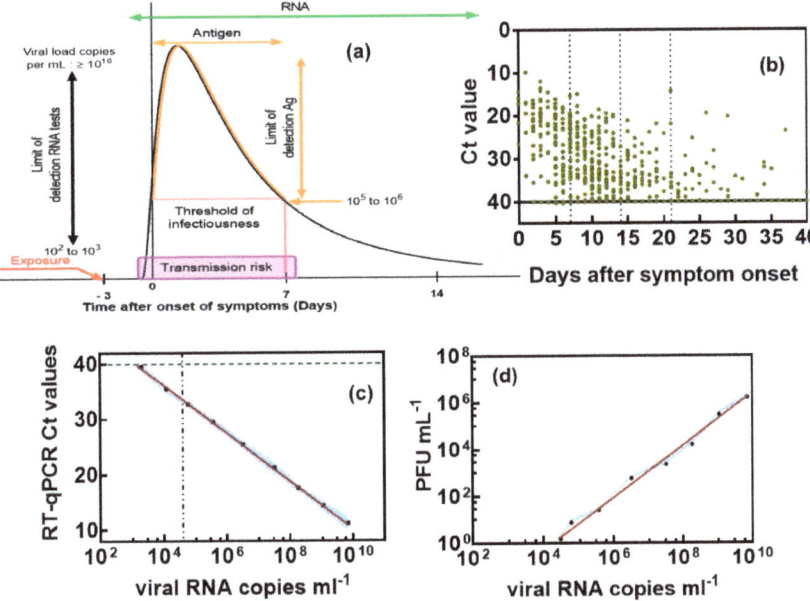

Figure 1. Clinical significance of Ct values and correlation with viral RNA copies as well as plaque-forming units (PFU): (**a**) Timeline of SARS-CoV-2 infectivity taking into account our own findings and those of others [12,14]. (**b**) Ct values as a function of time after symptom onset in nasopharyngeal swab specimens of COVID-19 patients. (**c**) Correlation of Ct counts with viral RNA copies. (**d**) Correlation of viral RNA copies mL^{-1} with plaque-forming units (PFU) of SARS-CoV-2 as a measure of infectivity. Vero E6 cells were infected with 10-fold dilutions of a SARS-CoV-2 isolate clade 20A.EU2 (EU variant). Calculation of estimated virus concentration was carried out by the Spearman and Karber method and expressed as TCID50/mL (1 pfu mL^{-1} = TCID50/mL $\times$ 0.7). The results are expressed as the mean $\pm$ SEM of at least three independent measurements for each group.

SARS-CoV-2 causes mild or asymptomatic disease in most cases; however, severe to critical illness occurs in a small proportion of infected individuals, with the highest rate seen in people older than 70 years. Compared to other viruses, SARS-CoV-2 has a medium reproduction rate of $R_0 = 2.5$ compared with $R_0 = 2.0$–3.0 for SARS-CoV and the 1918 influenza pandemic, $R_0 = 0.9$ for MERS-CoV and $R_0 = 1.5$ for the 2009 influenza pandemic [19]. It is generally true that for a rapid transmitted disease, such as SARS-CoV-2, the most efficient way to curb its spread is early detection to isolate patients. The gold standard for COVID-19 diagnosis is nucleotide-based testing (qRT-PCR) of viral RNA in nasopharyngeal swabs, collected from the upper respiratory tracts of suspected individuals. Next to viral ssRNA, most FDA-approved commercial antigen kits target the nucleocapsid (Figure 2).

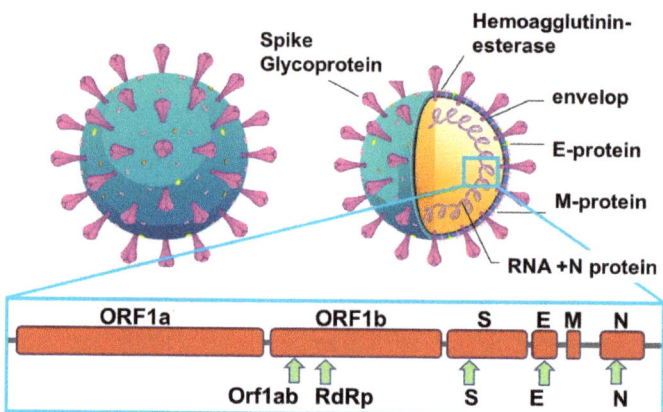

Figure 2. Structural proteins of SARS-CoV-2 for sensing: Viral replication requires other auxiliary genes, including open reading frame 1a (ORF1a), ORF1b and RNA-dependent RNA polymerase (RdRp).

The structural proteins of SARS-CoV-2 are next to the spike glycoproteins (S1, S2), the envelop (E), the membrane (M) and the nucleocapsid (N) proteins. The M protein is the most abundant protein on the viral particles, with the E protein being the smallest major structural protein of viral particles. The S envelop protein consists of two functional subunits, S1 and S2; the S1 subunit binds to the host cell receptors, while the S2 subunit fuses with the viral and cell membranes. The S-protein remains the main target for neutralizing antibody treatment upon infection and the focus of vaccine and therapeutic design. It is also a major target for the development of diagnostic approaches but has not been widely integrated into commercial antigen kits, which are mainly based on targeting the nucleocapsid protein. The N-protein is indeed the main structural protein and responsible for the replication and transcription of the viral RNA, the packaging of the enveloped genome into viral particles and interaction with the cell cycle of host cells. It is also the most abundant protein produced and released during viral infections and can be detected in serum and urine within the first hours of infection, reaching a maximum at about 10 days after infection. In addition, only about 100 spike trimers are present on each SARS-CoV-2 virion, with an estimated total of 300 monomers, which can be targeted for sensing, while around 1000 copies of the nucleocapsid are expressed in each virion [17,20]. A comparison was recently implemented using monoclonal anti-spike antibodies [21] in an in-house-developed antigenic test for SARS-CoV-2 and a comparable test targeting the nucleocapsid protein [20] using, in particular, a novel monoclonal antibody with an affinity constant K_D = 0.7 nM. The antigen choice in most commercial assays, the nucleocapsid was confirmed with higher sensitivity than the spike-based assay. The spike-based assays were, however, significantly more specific than the nucleocapsid-based ones. As escape mutants have found to be manifested in these spikes as well as in the nucleocapsid proteins, a combination of both antigens on the same diagnostic device might be the way to go forward and strengthen the reliability of COVID-19 tests, an approach recently proposed by Cai et al. [22]. So, where are we standing in terms of alternatives to enzyme-linked immunosorbent assay (ELISA) and PCR using S- and N-protein targets?

This review can be seen as an addition to other ones [23,24], with recent results on clinical samples [25], underlining the high potential of portable SPR as a viral diagnostic device. A special focus will be on the potential of SPR to characterize affinity constants between bioreceptors and COVID-19 targets, an aspect often not described in more detail.

However, localized surface plasmon resonance (LSPR) sensors will not be discussed, and voluble information can be found in the paper by Takemura [23]. The review will focus mainly on the detection of SARS-CoV-2 viral particles by SPR. While genes remain one of the most widely used viral biomarkers, and more sensitive and novel methods for the detection of viral genes have been implemented [26–29], such as CRISPR-associated protein 9 combined with SPR [28], we believed that molecular testing focusing on the presence of SARS-CoV-2 proteins, such as S- and N-proteins, to identify those individuals who are infected at the time of testing is more effective in directly correlating with infectivity if performed in a quantitative or at least semi-quantitative manner. In the discussion, which follows, viral-particles-based SPR sensing will be focused upon.

2. Surface Plasmon Resonance as a Tool for Binding Kinetics Analysis

The key to biological ligand development is understanding the binding interaction strength between the bioreceptor and the target (analyte) of interest. Classical biochemical approaches, such as Western blots, and co-immunoprecipitation approaches, only tell whether binding is occurring among biomolecules. ELISA provides more detailed information, such as binding affinity, but not without complicated and time-consuming enzyme-based amplification and labeling steps. The advantage of SPR, commercially available for more than 30 years [30], is that it uncovers accurately binding interactions in a label-free manner. In the classical gold-prism-based SPR approach, this information is obtained by flowing the analyte over the SPR prism modified with bioreceptors. The accumulation of analytes onto the sensor's surface due to bioreceptor–analyte interactions results in an increase in the refractive index near to the sensor surface, leading to changes in SPR conditions in real time and providing information about the binding efficiency in minutes. The approach requires minimal amounts of sample for binding kinetics experiment and provides information on the rates of association and dissociation events without the use of fluorescent, magnetic or radioactive labels. A handful of different bioreceptors can be integrated on SPR sensors using different surface chemistry approaches [31], ranging from the use of classical antibodies and engineered antibodies [25] to DNA [32], aptamers [33], sugars [34], etc. The cost and complexity of SPR analysis have been largely decreased in recent years with the advent of access to affordable and portable SPR technologies [25,35,36]. SPR methods remained, however, up to recent achievements, useless for the detection of single viral particles and low viral particle concentration in general. As their prompt detection and quantification remain extremely important for precise disease diagnostics, as exemplified for COVID-19, different efforts in this direction have been described recently and will be discussed in more detail in the following.

SARS-CoV-2 viral particles have a reported isoelectric point pI of 10.07 and are positively charged at physiological pH [37]. Non-specific interaction with the negatively charged backbones of aptamers might occur, requiring the design of highly specific bioreceptors. A handful of SARS-CoV-2 aptamers targeting the spike protein [38–40] as well as the N-protein [41] have indeed been reported. In this case, and others, SPR proved to be an efficient tool for understanding the affinity between the receptor binding domains (RBD) and the full S1 protein of SARS-CoV-2 and the surface bioreceptor, preferentially immobilized on the surface of the SPR chip to make the binding kinetics analysis comparable to future plasmonic sensing. In the case of the 20-base aptamer "CFA0688T" (Base Pair Bio) with one loop modified on the $5'$ end with a thiol-TTT-TTT to give the aptamer some flexibility for its anchoring onto gold interfaces, the binding affinity to the recombinant SARS-CoV-2 S1 spike protein was determined as $K_D = 3.4 \pm 0.2$ nM ($R^2 = 0.9985$) (Figure 3a). The attachment of the SARS-CoV-2 aptamer to gold SPR chips was based on maleimide-thiol chemistry by first coupling 3-mercaptopropionic acid to the gold chip followed by EDC/NHS linking of maleimide-PEG$_6$-amine (Figure 3a).

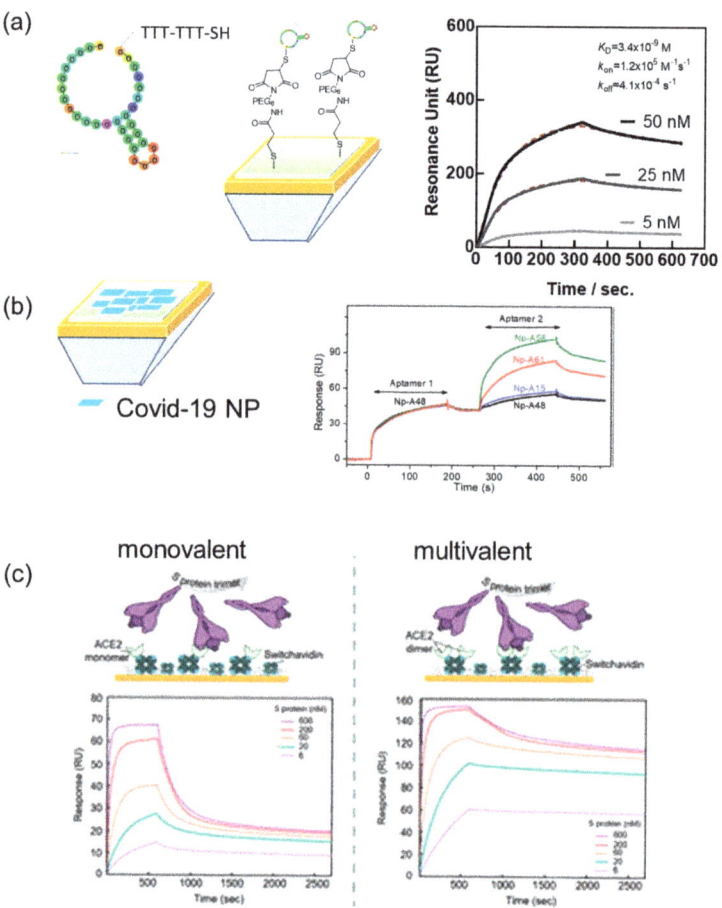

Figure 3. SPR as a valuable tool for the determination of affinity between SARS-CoV-2 bioreceptors and viral proteins: (**a**) SPR sensogram of the binding kinetics for S1 spike protein to 20-base aptamer "CFA0688T" from BasePairBio together with surface chemistry architecture. (**b**) SPR sensograms of the binding kinetics of N-protein specific aptamers to SARS-CoV-2 N-protein modified SPR chips (CM5 chip using EDC/NHS chemistry) with a sequence of different aptamers flown over the sensor chip (Reprinted with permission from Ref. [41]), 2020, RSC, (**c**) Schematic of SPR assay on monolayer and dimer ACE-2 modified SPR chips together with binding kinetics (Reprinted with permission from Ref. [42], 2021, ACS).

Zhang et al., reported a 58-base N-protein specific aptamer (A48) with a K_D of 0.49 nM, a $k_{on} = 8.80 \times 10^5$ M^{-1} s^{-1} and $k_{off} = 3.48 \times 10^{-4}$ s^{-1}, as determined by SPR. However, in this experiment, the N-protein was attached to the surface using a typical EDC/NHS protocol and the aptamers flown over the surface (Figure 3b). By adopting this approach, the possibility of sandwich-type binding between different aptamers and the N-protein can be evaluated. In the first run, aptamer A48 was flown over the channel resulting in a shift of 47 RU. In the following run, a second aptamer specific to the N-protein was flown over the same channel. If this aptamer binds to different epitopes of the protein, the response signal should feature a second plateau, which was observed for A58, A61 but not for A15 and A48 as controls.

Similarly, SPR was used for the deconvolution of the avidity-induced affinity enhancement for SARS-CoV-2 spike protein and the human receptor angiotensin-converting enzyme 2 (ACE-2) [42]. Indeed, similar to other coronaviruses, the glycosylated spike proteins of the SARS-CoV-2 envelop bind to host ACE-2 receptors to mediate the fusion of the viral particles and host cell membrane. It has been shown that the chimeric structure of the SARS-CoV-2 RBD possesses higher binding affinity toward the ACE-2 compared to SARS-CoV [43]. Geschinder and co-workers [42] pointed out that the commonly considered 1:1 binding interaction between an isolated RBD of the spike protein and a single ACE-2 monomer is oversimplified and does not account for avidity effects. By designing a sensor surface favoring monovalent interaction events between the full-length S-protein and ACE-2 as well as a surface that favors the generation of multivalent effects, a K_D of 60 nM was determined in the first case, while in the multivalent case, the signal accounts for a 125 nM affinity interaction (62%) but also a 4 nM affinity (28%). In the following, monomeric and multimeric ACE-2 species were linked to switch-avidin modified SPR chips, allowing resolving multiple binding events on each surface. On the dimeric ACE-2 surface, a high affinity of 283 pM was observed, mainly due to the lower k_{off} rate (Figure 3c).

Next to aptamers and ACE-2, the most widely investigated bioreceptors for SARS-CoV-2 remain the antibodies and engineered antibodies. Nanobodies have, in this respect, found a wider interest, and SPR was largely used to obtain their affinity characteristics to RBD and full-length S1 protein of SARS-CoV-2. We selected VHH-72 (PDB ID 6WAQ) [44], an anti SARS-CoV-1 anti-spike nanobody, which cross-neutralizes SARS-CoV-2, for SPR-based investigations and sensing. Despite the nanomolar affinity of VHH-72 for the SARS-CoV-2 RBD [44], the rapid dissociation is believed to negatively affect the SPR-based sensing. In addition, a common drawback of biosensors relates to the immobilization of proteins such as VHH-72 onto the transducer using EDC/NHS. Random attachment of VHH-72 is most likely to decrease the binding efficiency of a bulky target, such as the SARS-CoV-2 viral particle. Immunoglobulin or Fab fragments are the favorite binder candidates to surfaces, allowing the orientation of the nanobody's recognition epitope toward the solution and thus the viral target. The bivalence of VHH-72-Fc, due to the Fc domain of human IgG1 genetically linked by a HHHHHHRENLYFQG linker to the VHH domain, results in nanomolar affinity constant $K_D = 1.5 \times 10^{-9}$ M with a k_{on} of 1.2×10^5 M^{-1} s^{-1} and an improved k_{off} equal to 1.8×10^{-4} s^{-1} (Figure 4a).

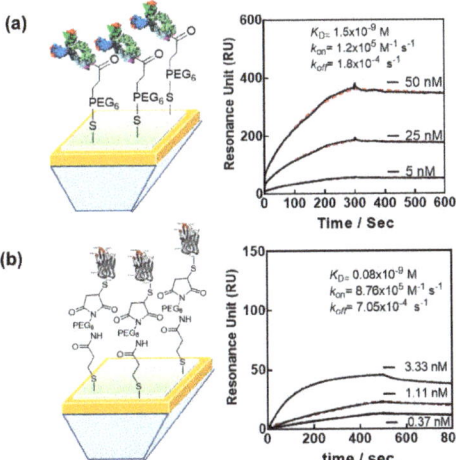

Figure 4. Affinity of different engineered SARS-CoV-2 antibodies: (a) Oriented linkage of nanobody VHH-72-Fc together with sensogram (Reprinted with permission from Ref. [25], 2022, RSC). (b) Binding affinities of nanoCLAMP P2712L (6His-P2710-linker-P2609-linker-Cys) to Wuhan-RBD. Gold chips were modified with a maleimide linker. Running buffer: 20 mM MOPS, 150 mM NaCl, 1 mM CaCl$_2$ and 1% BSA as blocking agent (pH 6.5). Black lines depict binding data, and red lines display the 1:1 binding model fit.

More recently, novel SARS-CoV-2 RBD-specific antibody mimetics called nanoCLAMPs (nano-CLostridial Antibody Mimetic Proteins) have been investigated with SPR [45]. nanoCLAMPs, derived from an immunoglobulin-like carbohydrate binding module from a Clostridium hyaluronidase, are 4 nm × 2.5 nm antibody mimetics with distinctive advantages over other antibody mimetics as well as nanobodies. They can be screened from a naïve phage display library for high specificity target affinity in as little as 6 weeks. Their production from the cytosol of E. coli is cheap, with yields over 200 g/L. The high melting point >75 °C makes them stable at room temperature and thus ideal for sensor development, as the modified interfaces might be stored at room temperature over an extended period of time without any degradation of their sensing performance. The absence of other cysteine units in nanoCLAMPs makes cysteine-based surface attachment particularly easy, as reducing agents, such DTT, do not alter the protein binding structure. An affinity maturation nanoCLAMP with cysteine end, nanoCLAMP P2712 (6His-P2710-linker-P2609-linker-Cys), was lately tested and showed a K_D of 80 pM for the Wuhan RBD (Figure 4b). The ligand was covalently conjugated to gold chips modified with maleimide units via its single C-terminal Cys and, in addition, could be easily refolded on the surface following chemical denaturation with 6 M GuHCl/0.1 N NaOH.

3. Plasmonic Sensors of SARS-CoV-2

The development of COVID-19-specific and high-affinity biomarkers is not only useful for the design of therapeutics but has become an essential part of plasmonic SARS-CoV-2 sensors [23,46–48]. One of the first examples of SPR, notably intensity-modulated SPR-based virus sensing, is that reported by Chang et al. [49]. An antibody-based H7N9 virus sensing was proposed with a detection limit of 144 copies mL^{-1}, a 20-fold increase in sensitivity compared with a homemade target-capture ELISA using the identical antibody. These conventional SPR testing machines were rather bulky and not adapted for implementation in clinical settings. Therefore, the SPR virus detection schemes performed in research laboratories were rarely considered as viable methods and accessible to clinical and point-of care applications. A low-cost nanoplasmonic sensor, allowing for one-step rapid detection and quantification of SARS-CoV-2 pseudoviral, was proposed by Huang et al. [50]. The concept was based on a gold nanocup array modified with antibodies; the attachment of SARS-CoV-2 to it results in a change in the plasmon resonance wavelength and intensity. Further interaction with gold nanoparticles modified with the ACE-2 protein resulted in a sensitive sandwich assay with sensing capability in the range of 10^2–10^7 viral particles mL^{-1} and a detection limit of 370 pseudoviral particles mL^{-1} (Table 1) within 15 min (Figure 5a). Graphene-coated SPR was proposed by Akib et al. for COVID sensing [51] with the main focus on the demonstration of the advantage of graphene SPR rather than on real sensing of virus samples.

As stated in a recent review by Jean-Francois Masson, plasmonic sensors are ideal for small and portable diagnostic devices [52]. The field has progressed lately from the use of prism-based approaches to the use of plasmonic nanomaterials, optical fibers and smartphones as optical components in the diagnostics system [53–56]. Indeed, plasmonic devices can be downscaled with limited loss in performance, as the optical measurements rely rather on wavelength or plasmonic resonance angle shift than on intensity. Signal to noise ratios remain consequently unchanged as long as the detector sensitivity is not compromised. The use of inexpensive light-emitting diode (LED) sources rather than lasers together with small USB spectrometers [57] or even smartphones [58] for read out makes the instrumentation portable and of low cost. The sensor chip can, in addition, be downscaled with no loss in analytical sensitivity, as the propagation length of plasmons is in the tens of micrometers range. The use of refractive index matching fluids, which are untidy and can interfere with the optical read out, can be avoided when disposable gold-coated prims are employed [35]. It is around sample handling where the costs of SPR and its complexity remain to be improved. The fluid handling in a portable device should be under low pressure or even without pumps required, such as passive transport of the analyte to the sensing chip [59]. Reproducible and bioreceptor-oriented surface chemistries remain, in addition, an ultimate step to be optimized for each analyte, even for portable SPR devices. The integration of deep- and machine-learning approaches to improve the detection characteristics of SPR is becoming an important and integral part for faster and sustainable sensing [25,60–62]. Some portable plasmonic devices had been reported, such as the smart-phone-based SPRI by Guner at al. [56], displaying refractive index changes as low as 4.12×10^{-5} RIU, comparable to the performance of commercial instruments as well as miniaturized platforms by PhotonicSys SPR H5 [36], Affinité Instrument [63,64] or the phase-sensitive compact IPOS-Lab SPR by Phaselab Instruments [65]. In the case of Affinité Instrument, the minimum in the spectral SPR signal is followed using a proprietary algorithm that provides a final instrumental resolution of 0.004 nm with a noise level < 5 RIU.

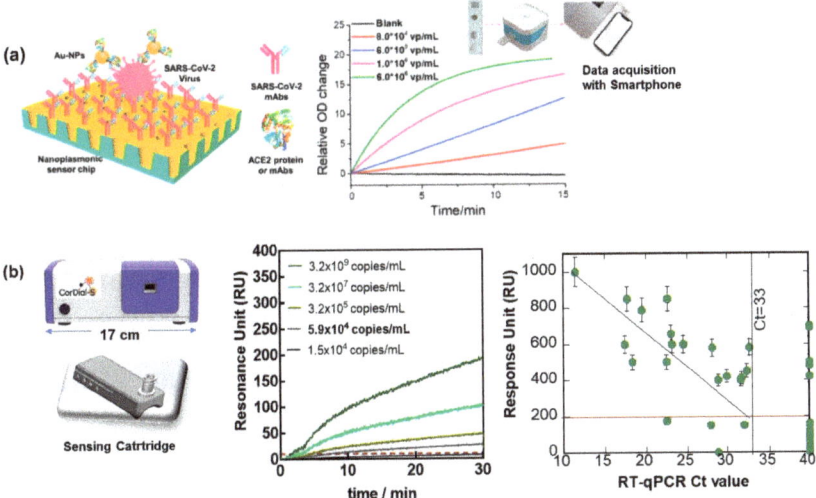

Figure 5. Portable SPR concepts applied to SARS-CoV-2 sensing: (**a**) Principle of nanoplasmonic resonance sensor for the detection of SARS-CoV-2 viral particles in a sandwich assay together with a photo of the developed sensor chip cartridge to be inserted into a handheld device with smartphone for data read out and binding curve to different SARS-CoV-2 pseudoviral particles concentrations (Reprinted with permission of Ref. [50], 2021, Elsevier).(**b**) (left) Image of a desk-top SPR POC testing device with cartridge-based sensing ability. (middle) SPR sensograms upon flowing cultured SARS-CoV-2 viral particles over cartridge-based SPR chip modified with VHH-72-Fc (Figure 4b), running buffer HBS-P + 1× containing 0.01 M HEPES, 0.15 M NaCl and 0.05% v/v Surfactant P20 as well as a correlation between RT-qPCR positive (50) and negative (69) nasopharyngeal samples and SPR data. Cut-off between positive and negative was 186 RIU (red line).

The use of portable SPR for diagnostics was also the focus point for studies during the COVID-19 pandemic. How to break the defect of conventional and portable SPR for their implementation in clinical settings was recently exemplified by us, using the sensing of the presence of the S1 protein of SARS-CoV-2 as an example [25]. To demonstrate how a portable SPR technology can be implemented for the sensing of SARS-CoV-2 viral particles via the S1 spike protein, we lately focused on three scientific and technological elements important for bringing SPR to the POC testing level: the oriented attachment of an engineered antibody of high affinity for the envelop S1 protein of SARS-CoV-2 and the use of a sensing cartridge, one of the first instrument considerations for achieving state-of-the-art point-of-care sensing (Figure 4b). The implementation of machine learning for predicting the cut-off value between positive and negative nasopharyngeal swab samples proved to also be essential for improving the performance of the sensor. When exposed to cultured SARS-CoV-2 viral particles (clade 20A.EU2, EU variant) of different concentrations, a sample of 5.9×10^4 viral particles mL^{-1} could still be distinguished from the noise, being RU = 10 (Figure 5b), and correlated with an RT-qPCR value of around Ct = 32. To push the analysis further, the number of viral particles required to kill 50% of Vero E6 cells allowed the determination of the infectious titer and was found to be 10 PFU mL^{-1} for 5.9×10^4 viral particles mL^{-1}.

The clinical performance of the cartridge-based sensor was, in addition, evaluated on 50 nasopharyngeal swab samples (25 positive and 25 negative samples, as identified by RT-qPCR collected from patients at a clinical testing facility). Using a cut-off value of 186 RU (Figure 5b), from the 50 nasal swab samples that had been confirmed by RT-qPCR to be positive, 4 were identified as COVID-19 positive. With 21 samples correctly identified out of 25, in accordance with RT-qPCR, an 84% positive percentage agreement (PPA) was determined. Out of 25 nasal samples confirmed by RT-qPCR as negative, 6 were identified as negative by SPR, revealing a 76% negative percentage agreement (NPA). Using a machine-learning algorithm with 250 ms sampling time and 1 min acquisition time instead of 15 min, it was still possible to match the same results. Interestingly, the results of the cartridge-based sensor are comparable to those of SPR using microfluid channels [25]. Such work opens up the possibility of point-of-care detection of SARS-CoV-2 infection due to the unique sensitivity and lateral flow assay-comparable response time and could add strongly to virus diagnosis scenarios.

How the performance of this and other COVID-19 SPR sensors compares to other alternative portable sensing approaches can be seen from Table 1. Indeed, RT-PCR remains the most sensitive approach for viral diagnostics. Comparing an optical [25] and electrochemical sensor [18] using the same surface ligand resulted in comparable sensitivities. Both of them outperformed the lateral-flow-based assays.

Table 1. Comparison of different SARS-CoV-2 detection principles.

Method	Ligand Target	LoD Viral Particles mL^{-1}	Ref.
RT-PCR	Nucleic acid against ORF/N	<10	[66]
RT-LAMP	Nucleic acid against N	50	[67]
GFET	antibody against S1	242	[68]
Nanoplasmonic	Antibody against S1/Au-NP with ACE2	370	[50]
paper-based EC sensor	Nucleic acid	6.9×10^3	[69]
Portable EC sensor	Nanobody against S1	1.2×10^4	[18]
SPR	Nanobody against S1	5.9×10^4	[25]
Lateral flow assays	N gene	3.0×10^6	[6]

EC = electrochemical; GFET = graphene-based field effect transistor; RT-LAMP: Reverse transcription loop-mediated isothermal amplification.

4. Conclusions and Perspectives

Currently, various commercial POCT devices have been developed for the purpose of detecting early pandemic outbreaks. Innovative advances in microfluidics, microelectronmechanical systems technology, nanotechnology and 3D printing, as well as data analytics and development of efficient surface ligands have significantly facilitated the development of POCT diagnosis in the last two years. POCT is still in its infancy on a global scale, with technological advancements needing to be addressed in the future. This is also valid for an SPR-based sensor. While still mostly research-based instrumentations, portable surface plasmon resonance devices have proven to be of great value for the current SARS-CoV-2 pandemic. We hope to have shown here that some of the disadvantages of conventional SPR testing, such as bulky instrumentation and its difficult implementation in clinical settings, have been partially overcome with such miniaturized approaches. Their miniaturized nature combined with adequate surface architecture allow for their implementation in biosafety-level-3 conditions to screen novel bioreceptors for their affinity to different virus epitopes and results in a handful of sensitive SARS-CoV-2 diagnostic platforms. With reliable SPR tests down to 10 PFU/mL, they can be seen as alternative to lateral flow antigenic assays for which most reliable tests detect 50 PFU/mL equivalent to about 3×10^6 RNA copies/mL. The possibility of multichannel and multianalyte analysis might offer SPR additional advantages in clinical settings. The clinical performance was tested more closely in at least one approach under an EU-funded project, CorDial-S. The evaluation of 119 nasopharyngeal swab samples achieved an 88% positive percentage agreement (PPA) and a 92% negative percentage agreement (NPA). The sensors could only be used one time, as the regeneration of the surface resulted in decreased performance, i.e., an 86% positive percentage agreement (PPA) and an 82% negative percentage agreement (NPA). Interestingly, the regeneration of the surface mainly had a large effect on the negative samples, with false positive responses obtained. Out of 50 negative samples screened on reused interfaces, 41 were assigned by RT-PCR and SPR as negative.

With these results at hand, what are the SPR perspectives in viral detection? The liquid sample volumes as well as power consumption of SPR-based biosensors remain the main bottlenecks for biomedical applications. To circumvent these drawbacks, improved and compact microfluid devices, as power-free pump systems, have to be considered for the next generation of integrated SPR-based biosensors. The use of sensing cartridges is one attempt taken by Affinité Instruments together with us to reduce the implementation of costly pumps. These disposable SPR sensors are low-cost and easy-to-use sensing devices intended for rapid single-point measurements. The integration of nanomaterials into SPR-based sensors needs to be pursued in this field if ultra-sensitivity becomes an important parameter. The integration of magnetic fields into SPR and the use of magnetic particles might be a way toward improved viral sensing. A magnetically enhanced SPR (M-SPR) was investigated lately (unpublished data) and showed to result in a detection limit as low as 1.5×10^3 viral particles mL^{-1}, two orders lower than the detection limit of conventional SPR, being 5.9×10^4 viral particles mL^{-1}. This and other concepts will allow driving the SPR field in the future.

It can be inferred that the plasmonic approach might also be adapted for the post-COVID crisis, notably for providing diagnostic parameters for distinguishing long-COVID patients from others. It is now recognized that many patients infected with SARS-CoV-2- can develop post-acute COVID syndromes a few months after the initial infection. This health stage, called long-COVID, occurs in 30–50% of COVID-19 patients and is characterized by multisystem symptoms, persistent fatigue and cogitative impairment more present with increasing age and female sex. In spite of the early impression that long COVID can only develop in patients who were hospitalized and intubated, increasing evidence indicates that long COVID can develop regardless of the severity of the original symptoms [70].

Author Contributions: Conceptualization, S.S.; writing—original draft preparation, R.B.; writing—review and editing, H.S. and Q.P.; images. All authors have read and agreed to the published version of the manuscript.

Funding: This research was funded by the Horizon 2020 framework programme of the European Union under grant agreement No 101016038 (CorDial-S). Financial support by ANR CorDial-FLU (ANR-21-HDF1-0003) and CPER "Photonics for Society" is also acknowledged.

Institutional Review Board Statement: The presented clinical data were conducted in accordance with the Declaration of Helsinki, and approved by the CHU Lille Ethics Committee on 7 April (CNRIPH: 21.02.11.57302; Promoter: CHU Lille; No ID RCB: 2021-A00387-34; ClinicalTrials.gov ID: NCT04780334).

Informed Consent Statement: Informed consent was obtained from all subjects involved in the study.

Acknowledgments: The authors wish to thank Ilka Engelmann, David Devos, Emmanuel Faure, Ann -Sophie Rolland, Yanick Njosse, Khadija Alioui and all the staff of CHU Lille for support in COVID-19-related projects. The constant support of Affinité Instruments is acknowledged. We want to thank Alain Roussel for inspiring us with nanobody technology and Richard Suderman form Nectagen for trusting us with the proper use of nanoCLAMP bioreceptors for sensing.

Conflicts of Interest: The authors declare no conflict of interest.

References

1. Kwon, S.; Joshi, A.D.; Lo, C.-H.; Drew, D.A.; Nguyen, L.H.; Guo, C.-G.; Ma, W.; Mehta, R.S.; Shebl, F.M.; Warner, E.T.; et al. Association of social distancing and face mask use with risk of COVID-19. *Nat. Commun.* **2021**, *12*, 3737. [CrossRef] [PubMed]
2. Chu, D.K.; Akl, E.A.; Duda, S.; Solo, K.; Yaacoub, S.; Schünemann, H.J. Physical distancing, face masks, and eye protection to prevent person-to-person transmission of SARS-CoV-2 and COVID-19: A systematic review and meta-analysis. *Lancet* **2020**, *395*, 1973–1987. [CrossRef]
3. Peeling, R.W.; Heymann, D.L.; Teo, Y.-Y.; Garcia, P.J. Diagnostics for COVID-19: Moving from pandemic response to control. *Lancet* **2022**, *399*, 757–768. [CrossRef]
4. Available online: https://ec.europa.eu/health/system/files/2022-05/covid-19_rat_common-list_en.pdf (accessed on 8 July 2022).
5. Vandenberg, O.; Martiny, D.; Rochas, O.; van Belkum, A.; Kozlakidis, Z. Considerations for diagnostic COVID-19 tests. *Nat. Rev. Microbiol.* **2021**, *19*, 171–183. [CrossRef] [PubMed]
6. Pickering, S.; Batra, R.; Merrick, B.; Snell, L.B.; Nebbia, G.; Douthwaite, S.; Reid, F.; Patel, A.; Ik, M.T.K.; Patel, B.; et al. Comparative performance of SARS-CoV-2 lateral flow antigen tests and association with detection of infectious virus in clinical specimens: A single-centre laboratory evaluation study. *Lancet Microbe* **2021**, *2*, e461–e471. [CrossRef]
7. Pokhrel, P.; Hu, C.; Mao, H. Detecting the Coronavirus (COVID-19). *ACS Sens.* **2020**, *5*, 2283–2296. [CrossRef]
8. Marks, M.; Millat-Martinez, P.; Ouchi, D.; Roberts, C.H.; Alemany, A.; Corbacho-Monné, M.; Ubals, M.; Tobias, A.; Tebé, C.; Ballana, E.; et al. Transmission of COVID-19 in 282 clusters in Catalonia, Spain: A cohort study. *Lancet Infect. Dis.* **2021**, *21*, 629–636. [CrossRef]
9. Kim, S.E.; Jeong, H.; Yu, Y.; Shin, S.U.; Kim, S.I.; Oh, T.H.; Kim, U.J.; Kang, S.-J.; Jang, H.-C.; Jung, S.-I.; et al. Viral kinetics of SARS-CoV-2 in asymptomatic carriers and presymptomatic patients. *Int. J. Infect. Dis.* **2020**, *95*, 441–443. [CrossRef]
10. Walsh, K.A.; Jordan, K.; Clyne, B.; Rohde, D.; Drummond, L.; Bryne, P.; Ahern, S.; Carty, P.G.; O'Brien, K.K.; O'Murchu, E.; et al. SARS-CoV-2 detection, viral load and infectivity over the course of an infection. *J. Infect.* **2020**, *81*, 357–371. [CrossRef]
11. Jefferson, T.; Spencer, E.A.; Brassey, J.; Heneghan, C. Viral cultures for COVID-19 infectivity assessment—A systematic review (Update 4. *medRxiv* **2020**. [CrossRef]
12. Byrne, A.W.; McEveoy, D.; Collins, A.B.; Hunt, K.; Casey, M.; Barber, A.; Butler, F.; Griggin, J.; Lane, E.A.; McAloon, C.; et al. Inferred duraiton of infectious periode of SARS-CoV-2: Rapid scoping review and analysis of avalaible evidence for asymptpomatic and symptomatic COVID-19 cases. *BMJ Open* **2020**, *10*, e039856. [CrossRef] [PubMed]
13. Engelmann, I.; Alidjinou, E.K.; Ogiez, J.; Pagneux, Q.; Miloudi, S.; Benhalima, I.; Ouafi, M.; Sane, F.; Hober, D.; Roussel, A.; et al. Preanalytical Issues and Cycle Threshold Values in SARS-CoV-2 Real-Time RT-PCR Testing: Should Test Results Include These? *ACS Omega* **2021**, *6*, 6528–6536. [CrossRef]
14. Available online: https://assets.publishing.service.gov.uk/government/uploads/system/uploads/attachment_data/file/926410/Understanding_Cycle_Threshold_Ct_in_SARS-CoV-2_RT-PCR_.pdf.UCTCiS-C-R-P (accessed on 8 July 2022).
15. Guglielmi, G. Rapid coronavirus tests: A guide for the perplexed. *Nature* **2021**, *590*, 202–205. [CrossRef]
16. Alidjinou, E.K.; Poissy, J.; Ouafi, M.; Caplan, M.; Benhalima, I.; Goutay, J.; Tinez, C.; Faure, K.; Chopin, M.-C.; Yelnik, C.; et al. Spatial and Temporal Virus Load Dynamics of SARS-CoV-2: A Single-Center Cohort Study. *Diagnostics* **2021**, *11*, 3. [CrossRef] [PubMed]
17. Bar-On, Y.M.; Flamholz, A.; Phillips, R.; Milo, R. SARS-CoV-2 (COVID-19) by the numbers. *eLife* **2020**, *9*, e57309. [CrossRef] [PubMed]
18. Pagneux, Q.; Roussel, A.; Saada, H.; Cambillau, C.; Amigues, B.; Delauzun, V.; Engelmann, I.; Alidjinou, E.K.; Ogiez, J.; Rolland, A.S.; et al. SARS-CoV-2 detection using a nanobody-functionalized voltammetric device. *Commun. Med.* **2022**, *2*, 56. [CrossRef] [PubMed]
19. Petersen, E.; Koopmans, M.; Go, U.; Hamer, D.H.; Petrosillo, N.; Castelli, F.; Storgaard, M.; Al Khalili, S.; Simonsen, L. Comparing SARS-CoV-2 with SARS-CoV and influenza pandemics. *Lancet Infect Dis.* **2020**, *20*, e238–e244. [CrossRef]
20. Barlev-Gross, M.; Shay Weiss, S.; Ben-Shmuel, A.; Sittner, A.; Eden, K.; Mazuz, N.; Glinert, I.; Bar-David, E.; Puni, R.; Amit, S.; et al. Spike vs nucleocapsid SARS-CoV-2 antigen detection: Application in nasopharyngeal swab specimens. *Anal. Bioanal. Chem.* **2021**, *413*, 3501–3510. [CrossRef]
21. Noy-Poarat, T.; Makdasi, E.; Alcalay, R.; Mechaly, A.; Levy, Y.; Bercovich-Kinori, A.; Zauberman, A.; Tamir, H.; Yahalom-Ronen, Y.; Israeli, M.; et al. A panel of human neutralizing mAbs targeting SARS-CoV-2 spike at multiple epitopes. *Nat. Commmun.* **2020**, *11*, 4303. [CrossRef]
22. Cai, Q.; Mu, J.; Lei, Y.; Ge, J.; Aryee, A.A.; Zhang, X.; Li, Z. Simultaneous detection of the spike and nucleocapsid proteins from SARS-CoV-2 based on ultrasensitive single molecule assays. *Anal. Bioanal. Chem.* **2021**, *413*, 4645. [CrossRef]
23. Takemura, K. Surface Plasmon Resonance (SPR)- and Localized SPR (LSPR)-Based Virus Sensing Systems: Optical Vibration of Nano- and Micro-Metallic Materials for the Development of Next-Generation Virus Detection Technology. *Biosensors* **2021**, *11*, 250. [CrossRef] [PubMed]
24. Zhang, Y.; Ding, D. Portable and visual assays for the detection of SARS-CoV-2. *View* **2022**, *3*, 20200138. [CrossRef]
25. Saada, H.; Pagneux, Q.; Wei, J.; Live, L.; Roussel, A.; Dogliani, A.; Die Morini, L.; Engelmann, I.; Alidjinou, E.K.; Rolland, A.S.; et al. Sensing of COVID-19 spike protein in nasopharyngeal samples using a portable surface plasmon resonance diagnostic system. *Sens. Diagn.* **2022**. [CrossRef]

26. Moitra, P.; Alafeef, M.; Dighe, K.; Frieman, M.B.; Pan, D. Selective Naked-Eye Detection of SARS-CoV-2 Mediated by N Gene Targeted Antisense Oligonucleotide Capped Plasmonic Nanoparticles. *ACS Nano* **2020**, *14*, 7617–7627. [CrossRef]
27. Karami, A.; Hasani, M.; Jalilian, F.A.; Ezati, R. Conventional PCR assisted single-component assembly of spherical nucleic acids for simple colorimetric detection of SARS-CoV-2. *Sens. Actuators B* **2021**, *328*, 128971. [CrossRef]
28. Zheng, F.; Chen, Z.; Li, J.; Wu, R.; Zhang, B.; Nie, G.; Xie, Z.; Zhang, H. A Highly Sensitive CRISPR-Empowered Surface Plasmon Resonance Sensor for Diagnosis of Inherited Diseases with Femtomolar-Level Real-Time Quantification. *Adv. Sci.* **2022**, *9*, e2105231. [CrossRef]
29. Broughton, J.P.; Deng, X.; Yu, G.; Fasching, C.L.; Servellita, V.; Singh, J.; Miao, X.; Streithorst, J.A.; Granados, A.; Sotomayor-Gonzalez, A.; et al. CRISPR–Cas12-based detection of SARS-CoV-2. *Nat. Biotechnol.* **2020**, *38*, 870–874. [CrossRef]
30. Available online: https://www.who.int/emergencies/diseases/novel-coronavirus-2019 (accessed on 8 July 2022).
31. Wijaya, E.; Lenaerts, C.; Maricot, S.; Hastanin, J.; Habraken, S.; Vilcot, J.-P.; Boukherroub, R.; Szunerits, S. Surface plasmon resonance-based biosensors: From the development of different SPR structures to novel surface functionalization strategies. *Curr. Opin. Solid State Mater. Sci.* **2011**, *15*, 208–224. [CrossRef]
32. Zagorodko, O.; Spadavecchia, J.; Serrano, A.Y.; Larroulet, I.; Pesquera, A.; Zurutuza, A.; Boukherroub, R.; Szunerits, S. Highly Sensitive Detection of DNA Hybridization on Commercialized Graphene-Coated Surface Plasmon Resonance Interfaces. *Anal. Chem.* **2014**, *86*, 11211–11216. [CrossRef]
33. Chang, C.-C. Recent Advancements in Aptamer-Based Surface Plasmon Resonance Biosensing Strategies. *Biosensors* **2021**, *11*, 223. [CrossRef]
34. Subramanian, P.; Barka-Bouaifel, F.; Bouckaert, J.; Yamakawa, N.; Boukherroub, R.; Szunerits, S. Graphene-Coated Surface Plasmon Resonance In-terfaces for Studying the Interactions between Bacteria and Surfaces. *ACS Appl. Mater. Interfaces* **2014**, *6*, 5422–5431. [CrossRef] [PubMed]
35. Zhao, S.S.; Bukar, N.; Toulouse, J.L.; Pelechacz, D.; Robitaille, R.; Pelletier, J.N.; Masson, J.-F. Miniature multi-channel SPR instrument for methotrexate monitoring in clinical samples. *Biosens. Bioelectron.* **2015**, *64*, 664–670. [CrossRef] [PubMed]
36. Harpaz, D.; Koh, B.; Marks, R.S.; Seet, R.C.S.; Abdulhalim, I.; Tok, A.I.Y. Point-of-Care Surface Plasmon Resonance Biosensor for Stroke Biomarkers NT-proBNP and S100β Using a Functionalized Gold Chip with Specific Antibody. *Sensors* **2019**, *19*, 2533. [CrossRef] [PubMed]
37. Scheller, C.; Krebs, F.; Minkner, R.; Astner, I.; Gil-Moles, M.; Wätzig, H. Physicochemical properties of SARS-CoV-2 for drug targeting, virus inactivation and attenuation, vaccine formulation and quality control. *Electrophoresis* **2020**, *41*, 1137–1151. [CrossRef] [PubMed]
38. Szunerits, S.; Pagneux, Q.; Swaidan, A.; Mishyn, V.; Roussel, A.; Cambillau, C.; Devos, D.; Engelmann, I.; Alidjinou, E.K.; Happy, H.; et al. The role of the surface ligand on the performance of electrochemical SARS-CoV-2 antigen biosensors. *Anal. Bioanal. Chem.* **2021**, *414*, 103–113. [CrossRef]
39. Daniels, J.; Wadekar, S.; DeCubellis, K.; Jackson, G.W.; Chiu, A.S.; Pagneux, Q.; Saada, H.; Engelmann, I.; Judith Ogiez, J.; Loze-Warot, D.; et al. A mask-based diagnostic platform for point-of-care screening of COVID-19. *Biosens. Bioelectron.* **2021**, *192*, 113486. [CrossRef]
40. Torabi, R.; Ranjbar, R.; Halaji, M.; Heiat, M. Aptamers, the bivalent agents as probes and therapies for coronavirus infections: A systematic review. *Mol. Cell. Probes* **2020**, *53*, 101636. [CrossRef]
41. Zhang, L.; Fang, X.; Liu, X.; Ou, H.; Zhang, H.; Wang, J.; Li, Q.; Cheng, H.; Zhang, W.; Luo, Z. Discovery of sandwich type COVID-19 nucleocapsid protein DNA aptamers. *Chem. Commun.* **2020**, *56*, 10235. [CrossRef]
42. Gutgsell, A.R.; Gunnarsson, A.; Forssén, P.; Gordon, E.; Fornstedt, T.; Geschwindner, S. Biosensor-Enabled deconvolution of the avidity-induced affinity enhancement. *Anal. Chem.* **2021**, *94*, 1187–1194. [CrossRef]
43. Shang, J.; Ye, G.; Shi, K.; Wan, Y.; Luo, C.; Aihara, H.; Geng, Q.; Auerbach, A.; Li, F. Structural basis of receptor recognition by SARS-CoV-2. *Nature* **2020**, *581*, 221–224. [CrossRef]
44. Wrapp, D.; De Vlieger, D.; Corbett, K.S.; Torres, G.M.; Wang, N.; Van Breedam, W.; Roose, K.; Schie, L.; Team, V.-C.C.-R.; Hoffmann, M.; et al. Structural Basis for Potent Neutralization of Betacoronaviruses by Single-Domain Camelid Antibodies. *Cell* **2020**, *181*, 1004–1015. [CrossRef] [PubMed]
45. Suderman, R.; Rice, D.A.; Gibson, S.D.; Strick, E.J.; Chao, D.M. Development of polyol-responsive antibody mimetics for single-step protein purification. *Protein Expr. Purif.* **2017**, *134*, 114–124. [CrossRef] [PubMed]
46. Parihar, A.; Ranjan, P.; Sanghi, S.K.; Srivastava, A.K.; Khan, R. Point-of-Care Biosensor-Based Diagnosis of COVID-19 Holds Promise to Combat Current and Future Pandemics. *ACS Appl. Bio Mater.* **2020**, *3*, 7326–7343. [CrossRef] [PubMed]
47. Shrivastav, A.M.; Cvelbar, U.; Abdulhalim, I. A comprehensive review on plasmonic-based biosensors used in viral diagnostics. *Commun. Biol.* **2021**, *4*, 70. [CrossRef] [PubMed]
48. Cognetti, J.S.; Miller, B.L. Monitoring Serum Spike Protein with Disposable Photonic Biosensors Following SARS-CoV-2 Vaccination. *Sensors* **2021**, *21*, 5857. [CrossRef]
49. Chang, Y.-F.; Wang, W.-H.; Hong, Y.-H.; Yuan, R.-Y.; Chen, K.-H.; Huang, Y.-W.; Lu, P.-L.; Chen, Y.-H.; Chen, Y.-M.A.; Su, L.-C.; et al. Simple Strategy for Rapid and Sensitive Detection of Avian Influenza A H7N9 Virus Based on Intensity-Modulated SPR Biosensor and New Generated Antibody. *Anal. Chem.* **2018**, *90*, 1861–1869. [CrossRef]

50. Huang, L.; Ding, L.; Zhou, J.; Chen, S.; Chen, F.; Zhao, C.; Xu, J.; Hu, W.; Ji, J.; Xu, H.; et al. One-step rapid quantification of SARS-CoV-2 virus particles via low-cost nanoplasmonic sensors in generic microplate reader and point-of-care device. *Biosens. Bioelectron.* **2021**, *171*, 112685. [CrossRef]
51. Akib, T.B.A.; Mou, S.F.; Rahman, M.M.; Rana, M.M.; Islam, M.R.; Mehedi, I.M.; Mahmud, M.P.; Kouzani, A.Z. Design and Numerical Analysis of a Graphene-Coated SPR Biosensor for Rapid Detection of the Novel Coronavirus. *Sensors* **2021**, *21*, 3491. [CrossRef]
52. Masson, J.F. Portable and field-deployed surface plasmon resonance and plasmonic sensors. *Analyst* **2020**, *145*, 3376–3800. [CrossRef]
53. Zeni, L.; Perri, C.; Cennamo, N.; Arcadio, F.; D'Agostino, G.; Salmona, M.; Beeg, M.; Gobbi, M. A portable opticla-fiber based surface plasmon resonance biosensor for the deteciton of therapeutic antibodies in human serum. *Sci. Rep.* **2020**, *10*, 11154. [CrossRef]
54. Huang, Y.; Zhang, L.; Zhang, H.; Li, Y.; Liu, L.; Chen, Y.; Qiu, X.; Yu, D. Development of a portable SPR sensor for nucleic acid detection. *Micromachines* **2020**, *11*, 526. [CrossRef] [PubMed]
55. Rifat, A.A.; Ahmed, R.; Yerisen, A.K.; Butt, H.; Sabouri, A.; Mahdiraji, G.A.; Yun, S.H.; Adikan, F.R.M. Phonit crystal bibre based plasmonic sensors. *Sens. Actuators B* **2017**, *243*, 311–325. [CrossRef]
56. Guner, H.; Ozguer, E.; Kokturk, G.; Celik, L.; Esen, F.; Topal, A.E.; Ayas, S.; Uludag, Y.; Elbuken, C.; Dana, A. A smartphone based surface plasmon resonance imaging (SPRi) platform for on-site biodetection. *Sens. Actuators B* **2017**, *239*, 571–577. [CrossRef]
57. Johnston, K.S.; Booksh, K.S.; Chinowsky, T.M.; Yee, S.S. Performance comparision between high and low resolution spectrophotometers used in a chite light surface plasmon resonance sensor. *Sens. Actuators B* **1999**, *54*, 80–88. [CrossRef]
58. Liu, Y.; Liu, Q.; Chen, S.; Cheng, F.; Wang, H.; Peng, W. Surface Plasmon Resonance Biosensor Based on Smart Phone Platforms. *Sci. Rep.* **2015**, *5*, 12864. [CrossRef]
59. Horiuchi, T.; Miura, T.; Iwasaki, Y.; Seyama, M.; Inoue, S.; Takahashi, J.; Haga, T.; Tamechika, E. Passive Fluidic Chip Composed of Integrated Vertical Capillary Tubes Developed for on-site SPR immunoassay analysis targeting real samples. *Sensors* **2012**, *12*, 13964–13984. [CrossRef]
60. Moon, G.; Son, T.; Lee, H.; Kim, D. Deep Learning Approah for enhanced Deteciton of surface plasmon scattering. *Anal. Chem.* **2019**, *91*, 9538–9545. [CrossRef]
61. Wang, X.; Zeng, Y.; Zhou, J.; Chen, J.; Miyan, R.; Zhang, H.; Qu, J.; Ho, H.-P.; Gao, B.Z.; Shao, Y. Ultrafast Surface Plasmon resonance imaging sensor via the high-precise four-parameter-based spectral curve readjusting method. *Anal. Chem.* **2021**, *93*, 828–833. [CrossRef]
62. Arzola-Flores, J.A.; Gonzalez, A.L. Machine Learning for predicitng the surface plamson resonane of perfect and concave gold nanocubes. *J. Phys. Chem. C* **2020**, *124*, 25447–25454. [CrossRef]
63. Brulé, T.; Granger, G.; Bukar, N.; Deschênes-Rancourt, C.; Havard, T.; Schmitzer, A.R.; Martel, R.; Masson, J.-F. A field-deployed surface plasmon resonance (SPR) sensor for RDX quantification in environmental water. *Analyst* **2017**, *142*, 2161–2168. [CrossRef]
64. Hojjat Jodaylami, M.; Djaïleb, A.; Ricard, P.; Lavallée, É.; Cellier-Goetghebeur, S.; Parker, M.-F.; Coutu, J.; Stuible, M.; Gervais, C.; Durocher, Y.; et al. Cross-validation of ELISA and a portable surface plasmon resonance instrument for IgG antibodies serology with SARS-CoV-2 positive individuals. *Sci. Rep.* **2021**, *11*, 21601. [CrossRef] [PubMed]
65. Available online: https://www.phaselabinstrument.com/?gclid=CjwKCAjwtcCVBhA0EiwAT1fY75lurA6W-cJfqdC0FNx7zsqqOlxeooXrgD3OK_z1F2GsCIDiwxInaBoCSqsQAvD_BwE#solutions_section (accessed on 8 July 2022).
66. Chu, D.K.W.; Pan, Y.; Cheng, S.M.S.; Hui, K.P.Y.; Krsihan, P.; Liu, Y.; Ng, D.Y.M.; Wan, C.K.C.; Yang, P.; Wang, Q.; et al. Molecular Diagnosis of a Novel Coronavirus (2019-nCoV) Causing an Outbreak of Pneumonia. *Clin. Chem.* **2020**, *66*, 549–555. [CrossRef] [PubMed]
67. Rabe, B.A.; Cepko, C. SARS-CoV-2 detection using isothermal amplification and a rapid, inexpensive protocol for sample inactivation and purification. *Proc. Natl. Acad. Sci. USA* **2020**, *117*, 24450–24458. [CrossRef]
68. Seo, G.; Lee, G.; Kim, M.J.; Baek, S.-H.; Choi, M.; Ku, K.B.; Lee, C.-S.; Jun, S.; Park, D.; Kim, H.G.; et al. Rapid Detection of COVID-19 Causative Virus (SARS-CoV-2) in Human Nasopharyngeal Swab Specimens Using Field-Effect Transistor-Based Biosensor. *ACS Nano* **2020**, *14*, 5135–5142. [CrossRef]
69. Alafeef, M.; Dighe, K.; Moitra, P.; Pan, D. Rapid, Ultrasensitive, and Quantitative Detection of SARS-CoV-2 Using Antisense Oligonucleotides Directed Electrochemical Biosensor Chip. *ACS Nano* **2020**, *14*, 17028–17045. [CrossRef] [PubMed]
70. Theoharides, T.C. Could SARS-CoV-2 Spike Protein Be Responsible for Long-COVID Syndrome? *Mol. Neurobiol.* **2022**, *59*, 1850–1861. [CrossRef] [PubMed]

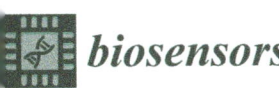

Article

Asymmetric Mach–Zehnder Interferometric Biosensing for Quantitative and Sensitive Multiplex Detection of Anti-SARS-CoV-2 Antibodies in Human Plasma

Geert Besselink [1,*], Anke Schütz-Trilling [1], Janneke Veerbeek [1], Michelle Verbruggen [1], Adriaan van der Meer [1], Rens Schonenberg [1], Henk Dam [1], Kevin Evers [1], Ernst Lindhout [2], Anja Garritsen [3], Aart van Amerongen [4], Wout Knoben [1] and Luc Scheres [1]

[1] Surfix Diagnostics, Plus Ultra Building, Bronland 12 B-1, 6708 WH Wageningen, The Netherlands; anke.trilling@surfixdx.com (A.S.-T.); janneke.veerbeek@surfixdx.com (J.V.); michelle.verbruggen@surfixdx.com (M.V.); adriaan.vandermeer@surfixdx.com (A.v.d.M.); rens.schonenberg@surfixdx.com (R.S.); henk.dam@surfixdx.com (H.D.); kevin.evers@surfixdx.com (K.E.); wout.knoben@surfixdx.com (W.K.); luc.scheres@surfixdx.com (L.S.)
[2] Future Diagnostics Solutions, Nieuweweg 279, 6603 BN Wijchen, The Netherlands; lindhout.e@future-diagnostics.nl
[3] Innatoss Laboratories B.V., Kloosterstraat 9, 5349 AB Oss, The Netherlands; anja.garritsen@innatoss.com
[4] Wageningen Food & Biobased Research, Bornse Weilanden 9, 6708 WG Wageningen, The Netherlands; aart.vanamerongen@wur.nl
* Correspondence: geert.besselink@surfixdx.com

Abstract: The Severe Acute Respiratory Syndrome Coronavirus 2 (SARS-CoV-2) pandemic has once more emphasized the urgent need for accurate and fast point-of-care (POC) diagnostics for outbreak control and prevention. The main challenge in the development of POC in vitro diagnostics (IVD) is to combine a short time to result with a high sensitivity, and to keep the testing cost-effective. In this respect, sensors based on photonic integrated circuits (PICs) may offer advantages as they have features such as a high analytical sensitivity, capability for multiplexing, ease of miniaturization, and the potential for high-volume manufacturing. One special type of PIC sensor is the asymmetric Mach–Zehnder Interferometer (aMZI), which is characterized by a high and tunable analytical sensitivity. The current work describes the application of an aMZI-based biosensor platform for sensitive and multiplex detection of anti-SARS-CoV-2 antibodies in human plasma samples using the spike protein (SP), the receptor-binding domain (RBD), and the nucleocapsid protein (NP) as target antigens. The results are in good agreement with several CE-IVD marked reference methods and demonstrate the potential of the aMZI biosensor technology for further development into a photonic IVD platform.

Keywords: biosensor; photonics; SARS-CoV-2; antibodies; diagnostics; serology

Citation: Besselink, G.; Schütz-Trilling, A.; Veerbeek, J.; Verbruggen, M.; van der Meer, A.; Schonenberg, R.; Dam, H.; Evers, K.; Lindhout, E.; Garritsen, A.; et al. Asymmetric Mach–Zehnder Interferometric Biosensing for Quantitative and Sensitive Multiplex Detection of Anti-SARS-CoV-2 Antibodies in Human Plasma. *Biosensors* 2022, 12, 553. https://doi.org/10.3390/bios12080553

Received: 29 June 2022
Accepted: 20 July 2022
Published: 22 July 2022

Publisher's Note: MDPI stays neutral with regard to jurisdictional claims in published maps and institutional affiliations.

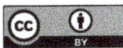

Copyright: © 2022 by the authors. Licensee MDPI, Basel, Switzerland. This article is an open access article distributed under the terms and conditions of the Creative Commons Attribution (CC BY) license (https://creativecommons.org/licenses/by/4.0/).

1. Introduction

Biosensors are valuable tools in a wide range of application areas such as medical diagnostics, agri-food, and environmental monitoring [1,2]. Application of biosensors in point-of-care (POC) in vitro diagnostics (IVD) is promising as they may fulfill the need for sensitive, robust, and cost-effective POC testing platforms for disease diagnosis outside of the lab. Early diagnosis and effective treatment enabled by POC diagnostics support a more efficient and patient-centered healthcare system. Moreover, the availability of affordable POC diagnostics is of crucial importance for developing countries, where resources and access to healthcare facilities are limited [3]. The Severe Acute Respiratory Syndrome Coronavirus 2 (SARS-CoV-2) pandemic has once more emphasized the value of and the urgent need for accurate and fast POC diagnostics for outbreak control and prevention [4–6].

Infection with SARS-CoV-2 induces an immune response in the host that normally results in the generation of different isotype antibodies (IgM, IgG, and IgA) against specific viral antigens such as the spike protein (SP), the receptor-binding domain (RBD), and the nucleocapsid protein (NP) [7]. Seroconversion for IgG typically takes about two to three weeks after symptoms onset while IgG antibody waning typically sets in after two to three months [8,9]. Serological testing is useful for confirming if individual cases have been infected in the past, for assessing seroprevalence and overall exposure of the host population [10], and for assessing vaccination response and efficiency.

Various IVD tests for SARS-CoV-2 specific antibodies are being used in the laboratory. Up till now, worldwide, 356 IVD registered serology tests are available, of which 219 are CE-IVD marked and 73 have obtained the FDA Emergency Use Authorization (EUA) [11]. Most of these tests involve enzyme-linked immunosorbent assay (ELISA), chemiluminescent immunoassay (CLIA), and lateral flow assay (LFA) test formats. Each test format has its own advantages and disadvantages: ELISA is a well-known and proven quantitative test, but the method is laborious and time-consuming and has to be performed by skilled personnel. CLIA is a highly automated and high-throughput quantitative method, but mostly depends on bulky and expensive measurement platforms. LFA is fast, simple, and relatively inexpensive, which explains why testing with lateral flow test strips has become rather customary for POC applications. However, LFA is not a quantitative test and may have a lower performance, especially with regard to sensitivity [12].

To bridge the gap between POC testing with LFA and remote (clinical lab) testing with ELISA or CLIA, several alternative POC testing formats are being developed such as lab-on-a-chip (LOC) and lab-on-a-disc (LOAD) [4,13–15]. Integration of microfluidics in the POC device might be beneficial as it offers possibilities for improving compactness and limiting reagent consumption and might also help in further reducing the amount of required patient sample [16]. To improve POC biomarker detection, different types of sensitive and real-time measuring biosensors have been suggested for implementation in POC devices [5,17–19] such as electrochemical sensors and optical sensors based on surface plasmon resonance (SPR), surface-enhanced Raman scattering (SERS), fluorescence, and chemiluminescence. Photonic biosensing technologies that have been explored for the possible use in SARS-CoV-2 serology include SPR [20–24], biolayer interferometry (BLI) [25], and microring resonators (MRRs) [26,27]. The last mentioned is a member of a special group of sensors called the photonic integrated circuit (PIC) biosensors.

PIC biosensors offer advantageous features such as a high analytical sensitivity, the capability for multiplexing and miniaturization, and the suitability for integration in optofluidic devices [28,29]. Additionally, these sensors offer advantages such as the prospect of label-free detection, the possibility of real-time measurement, immunity to electromagnetic interference, and the high potential for integration with other (micro) components. In addition, the photonic chips are manufactured by standard complementary metal-oxide semiconductor (CMOS)-compatible fabrication techniques. This is important to reduce the cost price of the chips as CMOS technology is ideally suited for high-volume manufacturing. Many types of PIC sensors have been described in the literature such as MRRs, grating coupler devices, photonic crystals, and interferometric waveguide sensors [19].

Surfix Diagnostics has developed a photonic biosensor platform based on the asymmetric Mach–Zehnder Interferometer (aMZI), which is intended for generic, label-free, and sensitive multiplex detection of a wide variety of targets, such as proteins, DNA, RNA, viruses, bacteria, etc. A major advantage of the aMZI design is that the sensor sensitivity can be tailored by increasing the geometrical pathlength of the sensing arm and/or by decreasing the asymmetry of the aMZI (the difference in pathlength between the two interferometer arms) [30,31]. When combining the high intrinsic sensitivity of the aMZI sensor with Surfix's proprietary material-selective surface modification, the analytical sensitivity can be even further enhanced [32]. In previous studies, aMZI-based biosensors have been used for the detection of food contaminants [33,34], ocean pollutants [35], streptavidin [36], and protein biomarkers for cancer [30]. While these studies show the potential and broad applicability of the technology, the amount of data presented was limited.

This paper describes the detection of different anti-SARS-CoV-2 specific antibodies (anti-SP, anti-RBD, and anti-NP) in a dilution series of an NIBSC-verified plasma calibrant in order to assess the analytical sensitivity and dynamic range of the photonic biosensor platform. Moreover, the diagnostic performance of the platform was evaluated by the detection of anti-SARS-CoV-2 specific antibodies in plasmas from a NIBSC verification panel. All results were compared to testing results obtained with several CE-IVD marked serology tests. Calibrant dilution tests showed a good limit of detection (LODs down to 0.3 IU/mL of calibrant) and dynamic ranges that were in accordance with most of the reference methods. The data obtained with the verification panel showed good scores for the Surfix photonic biosensor for distinguishing anti-SARS-CoV-2 antibody positive and anti-SARS-CoV-2 antibody negative plasmas.

In this explorative validation study, the performance of the Surfix photonic biosensor platform was successfully tested in a comparison with different CE-IVD marked reference methods, which demonstrates the potential of the method. Currently, efforts are directed at increasing the manufacturability of the system and developing it into an IVD platform for POC testing.

2. Materials and Methods

2.1. Materials

N-Hydroxysuccinimide (NHS), (1-ethyl-3-(3-dimethylaminopropyl)carbodiimide hydrochloride (EDC), trehalose, bovine serum albumin (BSA; heat shock fraction, $\geq$98%), sodium dodecyl sulfate solution (SDS, 10% in H_2O), Tween 20, sodium chloride (NaCl), sodium hydroxide (NaOH), hydrochloric acid solution (1 M), phosphate-buffered saline (PBS) tablets (0.01 M phosphate buffer, 0.0027 M potassium chloride and 0.137 M sodium chloride, pH 7.4), sodium phosphate (dibasic dihydrate and monobasic monohydrate, respectively), bicine ($\geq$99%), sodium carbonate, and sodium bicarbonate were purchased from Sigma-Aldrich (St. Louis, MO, USA). Methanol ($\geq$99.5%) was obtained from VWR. 2-(N-morpholino)ethanesulfonic acid (MES hydrate, $\geq$99.5%) was obtained from Fluka. SARS-CoV-2 (2019-nCoV) Spike S1 + S2 ECD-His (referred to as SP; 40589-V08H4, host: HEK293 cells), SARS-CoV-2 Nucleocapsid-His SARS-CoV-2 (2019-nCoV) Nucleocapsid-His (referred to as NP; 40588-V07E, supplied in PBS, host: *E. coli*), and SARS-CoV-2 (2019-nCov) Spike RBD-His (referred to as RBD; 40592-V08H, supplied in PBS, host: HEK293 cells) recombinant proteins were obtained from Sino Biological Europe GmbH (Eschborn, Germany). Affinity-purified polyclonal rabbit anti-human IgG (Fcγ fragment-specific, 309-005-008) was obtained from Jackson ImmunoResearch (Cambridgeshire, UK). Affinity-purified polyclonal rabbit anti-nucleocapsid IgG (GTX135361) was obtained from GeneTex, Inc. (Irvine, CA, USA). Affinity-purified polyclonal goat anti-rabbit IgG (heavy&light chain-specific, Atto 488 labeled, ABIN964982) was purchased from antibodies-online GmbH (Aachen, Germany). Anti-SARS-CoV-2 antibody negative plasma panel (DSPA 4.9.11.1) was obtained from in.vent Diagnostica GmbH (Hennigsdorf, Germany). CE-marked material anti-SARS-CoV-2 verification panel for serology assays (20/B770-02) and Anti-SARS-CoV-2 antibody diagnostic calibrant reagent (20/162) were obtained from the National Institute for Biological Standards and Control (NIBSC, Potters Bar, UK). Ultrapure water (18.2 MΩ.cm at 25 °C) was prepared using the Puranity TU3 UV/UF+ system (VWR International).

2.2. Chip Design and Operation

The heart of the system is the photonic chip, which contains an array of planar waveguide-based aMZI biosensors (Figure 1). The chips were fabricated by LioniX International (Enschede, The Netherlands). The photonic chips have dimensions of 10 mm × 5 mm and are based on a single stripe TriPleX™ geometry [37] containing a stoichiometric Si_3N_4 core (a height of 100 nm and a width of 1000 nm), on top of a 6 μm thermal SiO_2 substrate, and 4 μm top cladding. The on-chip circuitry consists of a spot-size convertor (allowing for a very efficient fiber-to-chip light coupling) and a 1 × 8 splitter (based on subsequent Y-branches) in order to achieve an even distribution of the input light over the 8 individual aMZI sensor elements (6 aMZI biosensors and 2 auxiliary aMZI's), with each aMZI sensor being connected to an individual output waveguide.

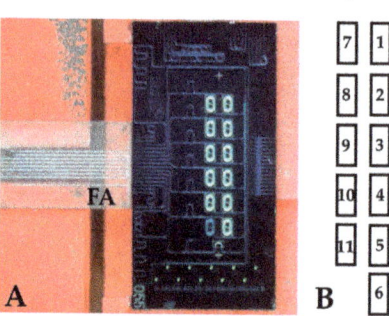 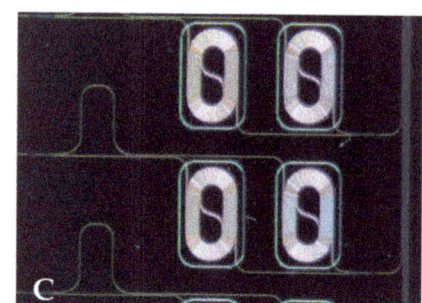

Figure 1. (**A**) Photomicrograph of the asymmetric Mach–Zehnder (aMZI) chip (dimensions: 5 × 10 mm) with an aligned Fiber Array (FA). (**B**) Assignment scheme for the five balanced and the one unbalanced aMZI biosensors regarding the spotting of viral antigens: 1, 4: spike protein (SP); 2: receptor binding domain (RBD); 3, 5: nucleocapsid protein (NP); 6–11: bovine serum albumin (BSA). (**C**) Zoom-in on two balanced aMZI sensors with a view of the waveguide spirals and sensing windows.

In-coupling and out-coupling of light was realized by butt-end coupling of fibers to the chip facet by means of an optimized fiber array (Figure 1A). The operating wavelength is about 850 nm, allowing the use of cost-effective and high-quality light sources (vertical-cavity surface-emitting lasers (VCSELs)) and detectors (photodiodes). A large part of the mode field of the light is confined to the waveguide core but a significant part propagates outside the waveguide. This component is called the evanescent field, which decays exponentially as a function of the distance to the waveguide surface (penetration depth ≈ 200 nm). At places where the sensor needs to interact with the sample, the SiO_2 top cladding had been etched away locally (yielding the so-called sensing window) for exposing the Si_3N_4 waveguide to the sample or buffer solution. The specific binding of antibodies or other (bio)molecules onto the waveguide surface causes a local increase of the effective index of the propagating mode of the aMZI arm and, concomitantly, an increase of the optical pathlength. This leads to a phase shift in the sinusoidal optical power transfer function of the aMZI that can be measured as a shift in the transmission spectrum [30,33]. The transmission spectrum is continuously determined by measuring the optical power output of the aMZI as a function of the operating wavelength of the incoming light during wavelength scanning (Figure 2), which enables monitoring of the shift (in picometer) of the transmission spectrum. Wavelength scanning is performed by electrical modulation of the VCSEL at a frequency of 10 Hz (see Section 2.3).

Each aMZI biosensor contains two spiral-shaped sensor arms (a signal arm and a reference arm) with a geometrical pathlength of the waveguide within the sensing window of 12.5 mm (Figure 1C). The bulk sensitivity of each sensor is about 2000 nm per refractive index unit (RIU). Each chip contains five balanced biosensors and one unbalanced aMZI biosensor (Figure 1A,B). The term balanced means that both the signal arm and the reference arm are in direct contact with the sample or buffer solutions at the place of the sensing window (Figure 1C). Use of a reference arm that contacts the fluid has advantages as it allows for compensation for differences in bulk refractive index (as may exist, for example, between sample and run buffer) and is relatively insensitive to changes in temperature. The unbalanced aMZI (Figure 1B: sensor 6) has a signal arm that is in contact with the sample or buffer solutions and a reference arm that is covered with a SiO_2 layer. This unbalanced aMZI was used to measure bulk refractive index changes in the liquid in order to monitor the injection and washing away of plasma sample.

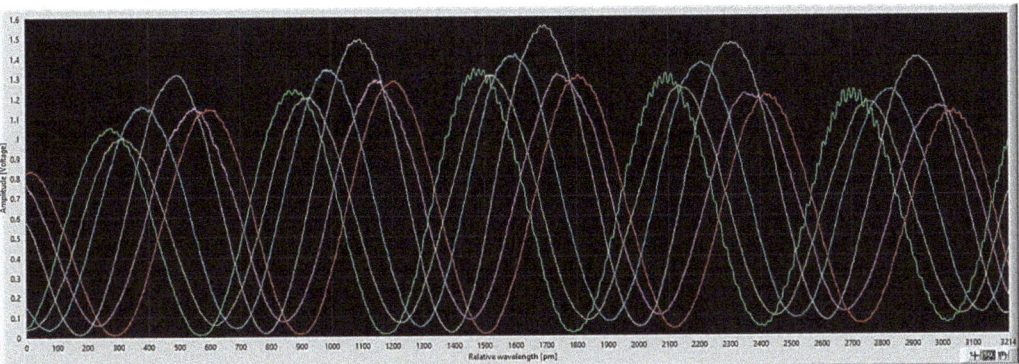

Figure 2. Example of a transmission spectrum overlay determined for the 6 different aMZI biosensors (x-axis: wavelength scan position (in picometer), y-axis: optical power output (in Volt)).

2.3. Measurement Platform

The measurement platform consists of a liquid handling unit and an alignment stage (see below), and an optical signal read-out module (OSROM) [38]. The OSROM contains a tunable light source and 8 photodiode detectors, plus associated electronics and a built-in data acquisition (DAQ) unit (USB-6363, National Instruments, Austin, TX, USA). As a light source, a pigtailed VCSEL (type ULM850, TO46, 2.0 mW; obtained from Philips Technology GmbH, U-L-M Photonics, Ulm, Germany) with a nominal wavelength of 850 nm was used. The VCSEL is part of a thermally isolated compartment that is temperature controlled at about 40 °C (with a temperature stability of about 0.02 °C) by means of a Peltier element and a thermocouple. By varying the voltage/drive current over the VCSEL diode, a linear wavelength scan of the VCSEL light output is performed over a range of about 3 nm and at a frequency of 10 Hz, and simultaneously the optical power output of all 8 aMZI sensor elements is being monitored by means of the connected 8 photodiodes. The photodiode signals are amplified with low noise transimpedance amplifiers with adjustable gains. The obtained output is measured with the DAQ card enabling data transfer at 2 MB/s to the laptop.

The liquid handling unit contains components such as a peristaltic pump (P625/TS020P; Instech Laboratories, Inc., Plymouth Meeting, PA, USA), a syringe pump (NE-501; KF Technology, Rome, Italy), three automated stream selector valves (1 × 8, 1 × 6, and adapted load/inject valve; VICI AG, Schenkon, Switzerland) and associated polyether ether ketone (PEEK) tubing (inner diameter 0.01″, 0.02″ and 0.03″) with supply vials. All these components are brought together and connected to driving electronics and controlled by the software. Pumps and valves are operated via LabView based user-defined liquid handling scripts. Supply of liquid to the chip proceeds via a load/inject valve that is connected to a sample loop with an internal volume of 200 µL.

The photonic chip is placed on an alignment stage (Figure 3) to allow in-coupling and out-coupling of light, and to allow the flow of liquids over the chip. The alignment stage is custom designed and manufactured and has three main components: a frame that holds the chip, a clamp with a Teflon holder for the fluidic connection, and two piezoelectric linear stages with a control unit (12 mm travel, SLC; SmarAct GmbH, Oldenburg, Germany) to align the fiber array with respect to the chip (Figure 3).

2.4. Chip Functionalization

Functionalization of the chip surface was done by Surfix's proprietary material-selective coating technology. This results in a carboxylate-terminated layer on the Si_3N_4 waveguide surface while the surrounding SiO_2 surface is modified with a polyethylene glycol (PEG)-based antifouling layer. This way, bioreceptor immobilization and, consequently, analyte binding are confined exclusively to the waveguide surface, which leads to a higher analytical sensitivity and improved limit of detection [32].

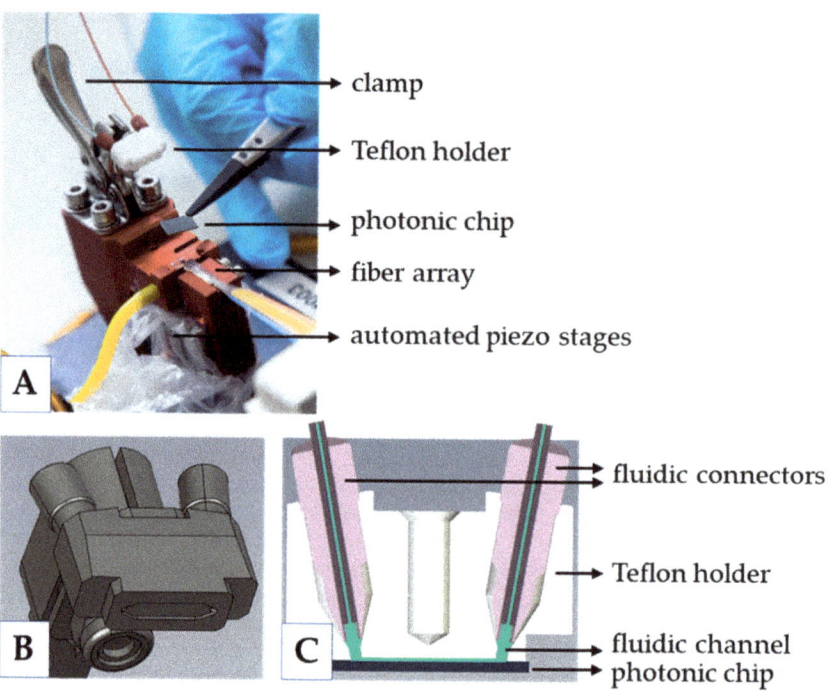

Figure 3. (A) Photograph of the alignment unit, where the chip is placed and brought in close contact with the fiber array. The flow cell is realized by clamping the Teflon holder on the chip. (B) Teflon holder close-up. (C) Cross-section of the Teflon holder on the chip, which defines the flow cell (liquid indicated in blue).

Shortly before spotting of protein, the coated aMZI chip was sonicated in ultrapure water for 10 min and this step was repeated in methanol after which the chip was dried quickly by means of nitrogen blowing. Subsequently, a chemical activation of the carboxylate coating was performed by application on top of the chip of a 60 μL sessile drop of a freshly prepared EDC/NHS solution (0.2 M EDC and 0.1 M NHS in 10 mM MES pH 5.5) for 15 min. Then, after a quick rinse with ultrapure water and drying by means of nitrogen blowing, spotting was performed by means of the sciFLEXARRAYER S3 piezoelectric arrayer spotter (Scienion, Berlin, Germany). Spotting was performed with 4 different proteins according to the assignment shown in the caption of Figure 1B. The viral antigens were spotted at a concentration of 100 μg/mL in spotting buffer (for SP: 10 mM MES pH 5.3, for RBD: 10 mM bicine pH 9.0, for NP: 10 mM bicarbonate pH 9.8, all with 3% trehalose), while bovine serum albumin (BSA) was spotted in the MES spotting buffer at a concentration of 500 μg/mL. The spotted chips were incubated for 15 min and afterwards blocked by incubation with blocking buffer (PBS + 7% BSA) for 30 min. Finally, the chips were washed with buffer (PBS + 0.05% v/v Tween 20) for 5 min under gentle shaking followed by washing for 5 min with storage buffer (PBS + 3% trehalose) also under gentle shaking. The chips were stored in storage buffer at 4 °C for a maximum of three days until further use.

2.5. Plasma Measurements

Using the liquid handling system, the spotted photonic chips were conditioned for a maximum of 30 min at a flow of 15 μL/min with run buffer (PBS + 1% BSA + 0.05%

v/v Tween 20). Then, sample was injected over the sensor surface for 10 min at a flow of 15 µL/min. For the NIBSC calibrant study, the calibrant (stock concentration 1000 IU/mL) was diluted with different amounts of anti-SARS-CoV-2 antibody negative plasma (pooled from three plasmas) resulting in calibrant concentrations of 0.25, 0.5, 1, 2, 5, 10, 20, 50, 100, 200, and 500 IU/mL. These different plasma mixtures were then diluted 10-fold with run buffer, resulting in 10% v/v plasma. The plasmas of the NIBSC verification panel were diluted 25-fold with run buffer, resulting in 4% v/v plasma. All samples from the NIBSC verification panel were measured in a blind manner, meaning that the operator did not know if the plasma was anti-SARS-CoV-2 positive or anti-SARS-CoV-2 negative. After plasma sample injection, the chips were washed with run buffer followed by an injection of secondary antibody (rabbit anti-human IgG, 24 µg/mL in run buffer) for 10 min at a flow of 15 µL/min. The resulting sensorgrams were recorded and from this, the total shifts in transmission spectrum (in picometer) that resulted from the incubation with human plasma sample and the incubation with secondary antibody, were determined. After each measurement, and before inserting a new aMZI chip, the liquid handling system was cleaned by flowing of 0.5% SDS solution for 6 min at a flow of 15 µL/min.

For comparison with the biosensor, plasma samples were also tested at Innatoss Laboratories (Oss, The Netherlands) with two commercial CE-IVD marked ELISAs: the Euroimmun SARS-CoV-2 IgG-S1 ELISA, which employs the S1-domain, and the Euroimmun SARS-CoV-2 IgG–NCP ELISA, modified to only contain diagnostically relevant epitopes of the NP antigen (Euroimmun, Lubeck, Germany). Furthermore, plasma samples were tested at Future Diagnostics (Wijchen, The Netherlands) with two commercial CE-IVD-marked CLIAs: the Abbott Architect SARS-CoV-2 IgG II assay, which uses the NP antigen (reference 06R8622, Abbott Laboratories Inc., Chicago, IL, USA), and the ADVIA Centaur SARS-CoV-2 IgG (sCOVG) assay, which uses the RBD domain (Siemens Centaur sCOVG assay, reference 11207376, Siemens Healthcare Diagnostics Inc., New York, NY, USA). All reference tests were performed in accordance with the manufacturer's instructions.

For representation in dose-response curves, all data obtained on the calibrant were fitted by non-linear regression using a 4-parameter logistic (4PL) model (GraphPad Prism 9). Blank measurements were done in replicate (n = 10) on the anti-SARS-CoV-2 antibody negative plasma (pooled from three plasmas), used for diluting the calibrant, yielding values for each antigen (SP, RBD, NP) for both assay steps (incubation with plasma and with secondary antibody) from which the means and standard deviations were calculated.

3. Results

3.1. Material-Selective Sensor Modification

To demonstrate the effectiveness of the material-selective functionalization (a carboxylate-terminated layer on Si_3N_4 and a polyethylene glycol (PEG)-based layer on SiO_2) for achieving selective immobilization of viral antigen to the Si_3N_4 waveguide surface, functionalized photonic chips were spotted with NP (viral antigen) and BSA (negative control protein). Next, the modified chips were incubated with rabbit anti-NP antibody followed by incubation with Atto 488 labeled goat anti-rabbit IgG. Finally, the chips were examined by means of fluorescence microscopy. As can be seen in Figure 4A, the resulting fluorescence was exclusively localized on the waveguide spiral indicating that modification of the sensor with NP antigen was confined to the carboxylate-terminated Si_3N_4 waveguide surface. In previous work, the added value of material-selective functionalization was demonstrated for improving the analytical sensitivity of a model system [32]. In addition, spiral arms modified with BSA (the negative control protein) did not show any fluorescence signal indicating a virtual absence of non-specific binding (Figure 4B).

3.2. Testing on Calibrant Dilution Series

To examine the dynamic range and analytical sensitivity of the six Surfix assays (direct and indirect detection of each of three antigens), a dilution series of anti-SARS-CoV-2 antibody plasma calibrant (NIBSC, 20/162) was measured. For comparison, the same dilution series was also measured by four CE-IVD-marked reference assays (two ELISA and two CLIA methods).

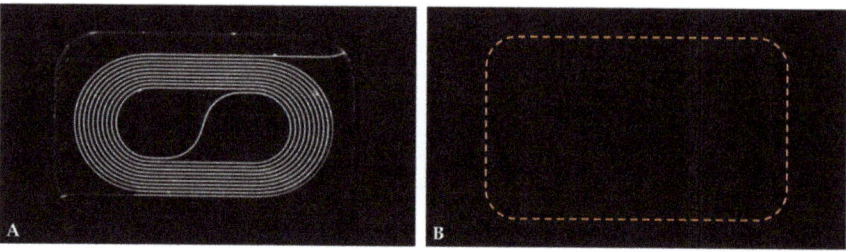

Figure 4. Fluorescence photomicrograph of (**A**) an NP-modified and (**B**) a BSA-modified spiral arm after incubation with polyclonal rabbit anti-NP antibody and subsequent incubation with Atto 488 labeled goat anti-rabbit IgG antibody. Note: the dotted orange line indicates the perimeter of the sensing window.

Figure 5A shows a schematic of the binding complex that is formed on the biosensor surface illustrating the direct and indirect assay option. Also shown are sensorgrams (Figure 5B) obtained with the Surfix method on a negative control sample (10 times diluted negative plasma in buffer) and a calibrant sample (10 times diluted calibrant stock in buffer). Incubation with negative plasma did not lead to a shift in signal indicating the absence of non-specific binding. Incubation with calibrant plasma induced a large shift of the signal, which indicated binding of a plasma component, most probably IgG. Subsequent incubation with anti-human IgG secondary antibody also resulted in a substantial binding, confirming the identity of the previously bound component.

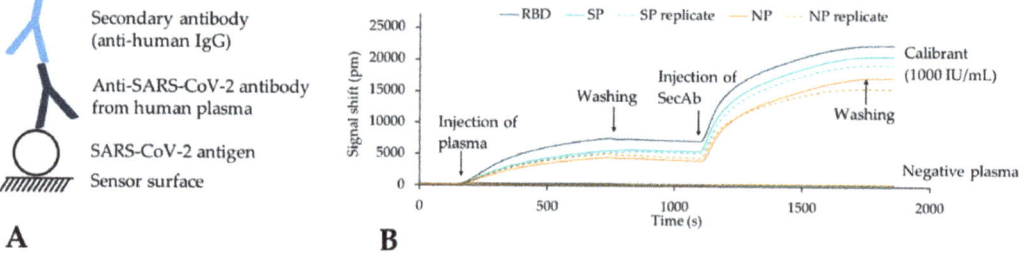

Figure 5. (**A**) Schematic representation of the binding complex that is formed during the assay. SARS-CoV-2 antigens (NP, RBD, and SP) are immobilized onto the sensor surface; during injection of plasma sample, SARS-CoV-2 specific antibodies (if present) bind to the antigens and, in turn, can be recognized and bound by secondary antibodies during the second incubation step. (**B**) Overlay of sensorgrams obtained for plasma calibrant (1000 IU/mL) and anti-SARS-CoV-2 antibody negative plasma.

The dose-response curves of all Surfix assays as obtained on the calibrant dilution series (12 concentrations) are shown in Figure 6. For both the direct and the indirect assay, a difference between the antigens was found with an increase of the signal in the order NP < SP < RBD. Furthermore, the indirect assay showed an amplification with a factor of about three as compared to the signal obtained with the direct assay.

Replicate measurements (n = 10) were done on the anti-SARS-CoV-2 antibody negative pooled plasma while employing a new chip for each measurement. For each assay, the mean and standard deviation (SD) of the replicate measurements on negative pooled plasma were calculated and used to derive the limit of detection (LOD). The LOD was defined as the calibrant concentration at which the signal was equal to the mean plus three times the SD of the blank measurement (Table 1).

The samples from the dilution series of the plasma calibrant were also tested with four CE-IVD-marked reference methods in order to validate the results from the photonic biosensor. Comparison of the dose-response curves generally shows a high resemblance between the Surfix indirect immunoassay and the reference tests (Figure 7).

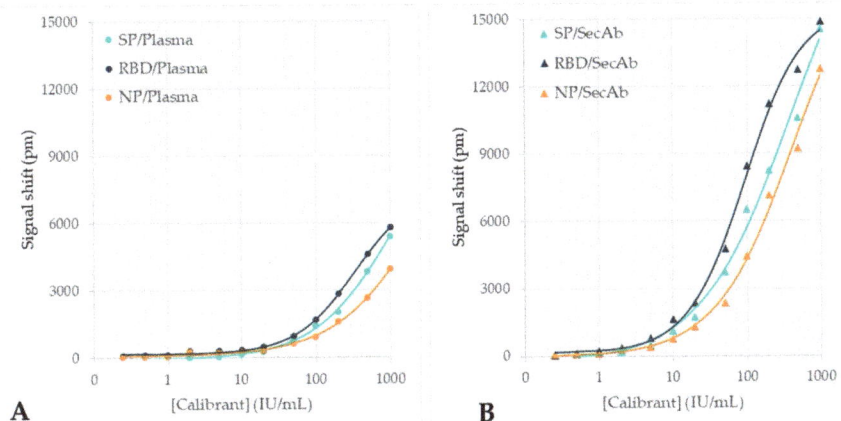

Figure 6. Dose-response curves obtained with the photonic biosensor when measuring the dilution series of plasma calibrant. Results are shown for (**A**) the incubation with diluted calibrant (direct assay) and (**B**) the incubation with anti-human IgG secondary antibody (indirect assay).

Table 1. Overview of the blank signals (mean ± standard deviation (SD), $n = 10$) as were found for each of the Surfix assays, and the calculated limits of detection (LODs).

Assay	Mean ± SD (pm)	LOD (IU/mL)
SP/Direct	−66 ± 21	1.4
SP/Indirect	22 ± 10	0.3
RBD/Direct	201 ± 40	9.7
RBD/Indirect	57 ± 25	0.5
NP/Direct	79 ± 34	4.8
NP/Indirect	111 ± 40	2.0

The LODs of the Surfix indirect immunoassay (Table 1) are indicated in Figure 7 (arrow symbols near the x-axis) in order to mark the large dynamic range of the photonic biosensor, which is more than 3 decades. These LODs are comparable to the detection capability of the reference assays used in the comparison study.

Subsequently, correlation plots were constructed in order to assess the linear relation between the results obtained on the calibrant dilution series with the Surfix method and the reference methods (Figure 8). Very strong, up to near-perfect linear correlations ($0.9 < R^2 < 1$) were found when comparing the data from the Surfix direct assay method and all reference methods; the same applies to the Surfix indirect assay method and three of the four (the ELISAs and Abbott CLIA) reference methods, indicating that the dynamic ranges are comparable. Only for the Siemens CLIA method, the correlation was non-linear in the comparison with the Surfix indirect assay method (Figure 8B), which may be related to the higher sensitivity of the Surfix method at lower concentrations (see also Figure 7B).

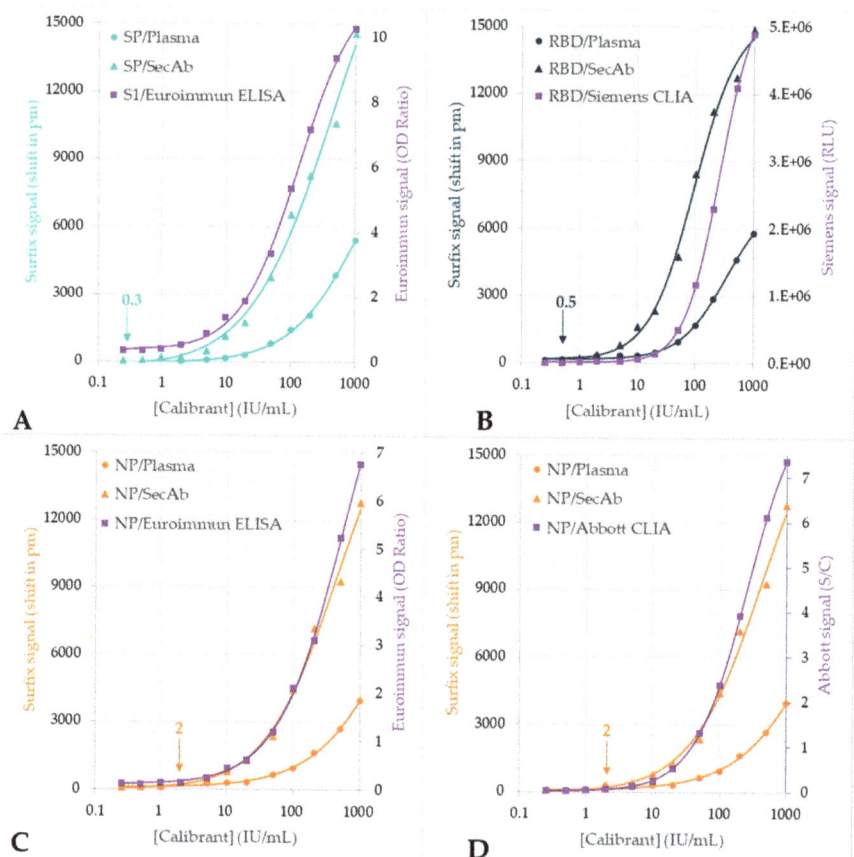

Figure 7. Dose-response curves for the plasma calibrant dilution series obtained with the photonic biosensor (n = 2) in a comparison with the outcome of the relevant reference test: (**A**) S1/reference test: Euroimmun SARS-CoV-2 IgG-S1 ELISA (IgG) (n = 3). (**B**) RBD/reference test: Siemens ADVIA Centaur SARS-CoV-2 IgG (sCOVG)) (n = 2). (**C**) NP/reference test: Euroimmun SARS-CoV-2 IgG-NCP ELISA (n = 3). (**D**) NP/reference test: Abbott Architect SARS-CoV-2 IgG (n = 2). Meaning of symbols: circles = plasma (direct assay), triangles = secondary antibody (indirect assay), squares: reference test. Note: the arrow near the x-axis indicates the LOD of each indirect Surfix assay.

3.3. Testing of the Plasma Verification Panel

In a second set of experiments, the diagnostic performance (sensitivity and specificity) of the six Surfix assays was examined by testing 23 anti-SARS-CoV-2 antibody positive and 14 anti-SARS-CoV-2 antibody negative plasma samples of the NIBSC anti-SARS-CoV-2 verification panel. Figure 9 shows a few examples of sensorgrams. Figure 9A is a representative example obtained with one of the negative plasmas (panel #27) exhibiting low but significant binding (signal shift of 100–300 pm) to the immobilized NP and RBD antigens and virtually no binding to the SP antigen (see also the inset). The two positive plasmas (panel #1 (Figure 9B) and #10 (Figure 9C)) both showed substantial binding but on a different overall level and with a different selectivity profile. Plasma #1 showed a clear order in the extent of antibody binding to the different antigens (i.e., NP > RBD > SP), whereas plasma #10 demonstrated a near equal binding outcome for RBD and NP, and a somewhat lower signal for SP. The average binding signal for the three antigens obtained during the incubation with plasma #10 (first incubation step) was approximately 5000 picometer, which corresponds to a calculated binding amount of protein of about 150 ng/cm². The way to calculate the adsorbed surface mass density of protein (ng/cm²) from the signal (shift in transmission spectrum in picometer) is explained elsewhere [36]. Assuming that the bound protein consists of head-on oriented IgG (Fc-up; both Fabs bound to the antigen on the surface), a value of 150 ng/cm² represents about half of a monolayer [39]. The ratio between the binding signal that results from the first (plasma) and the second incubation (secondary antibody) is about 1:4 and 1:2 for the sensorgrams in Figure 9B and C, respectively. This signal amplification is in reasonable agreement with the average threefold signal amplification that was found in the calibrant dilution experiments (see above).

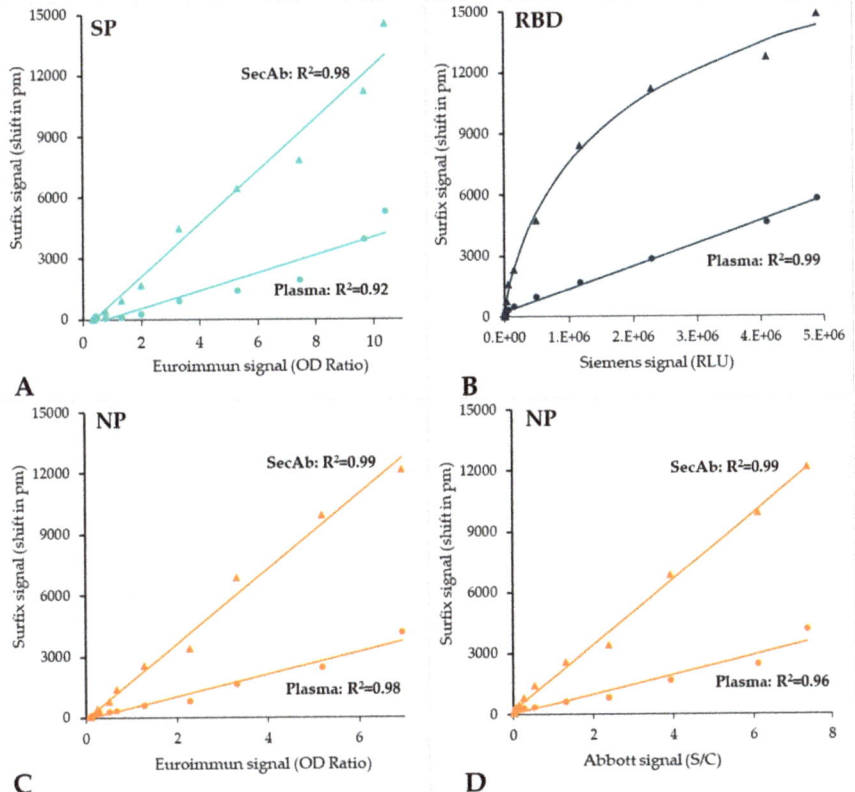

Figure 8. Correlation plots of the Surfix photonic biosensor results versus the results obtained with each of the reference methods: (**A**) Euroimmun SARS-CoV-2 IgG-S1 ELISA (IgG); (**B**) Siemens ADVIA Centaur® SARS-CoV-2 IgG (sCOVG) CLIA; (**C**) Euroimmun SARS-CoV-2 IgG-NCP ELISA; (**D**) Abbott Architect SARS-CoV-2 IgG CLIA. Meaning of symbols: circles = plasma (direct immunoassay), triangles = secondary antibody (indirect immunoassay).

A summary of the results obtained with the plasma panel is shown in Figure 10, which shows the binding signal distributions for the plasma incubation (direct assay) and the secondary antibody incubation (indirect assay) as found for the SP, RBD, and NP antigen. What stands out is the excellent performance of the SP assay regarding the distinction between negative and positive samples, which is related to the very low background level of the binding signal as was found for all negative samples. Compared to the SP assay, the RBD and NP assays showed a relatively high and more variable amount of non-specific binding in plasma. At least part of this unwanted background binding signal can be attributed to IgG antibodies since subsequent incubation with the anti-human IgG secondary antibody resulted in a further increased signal.

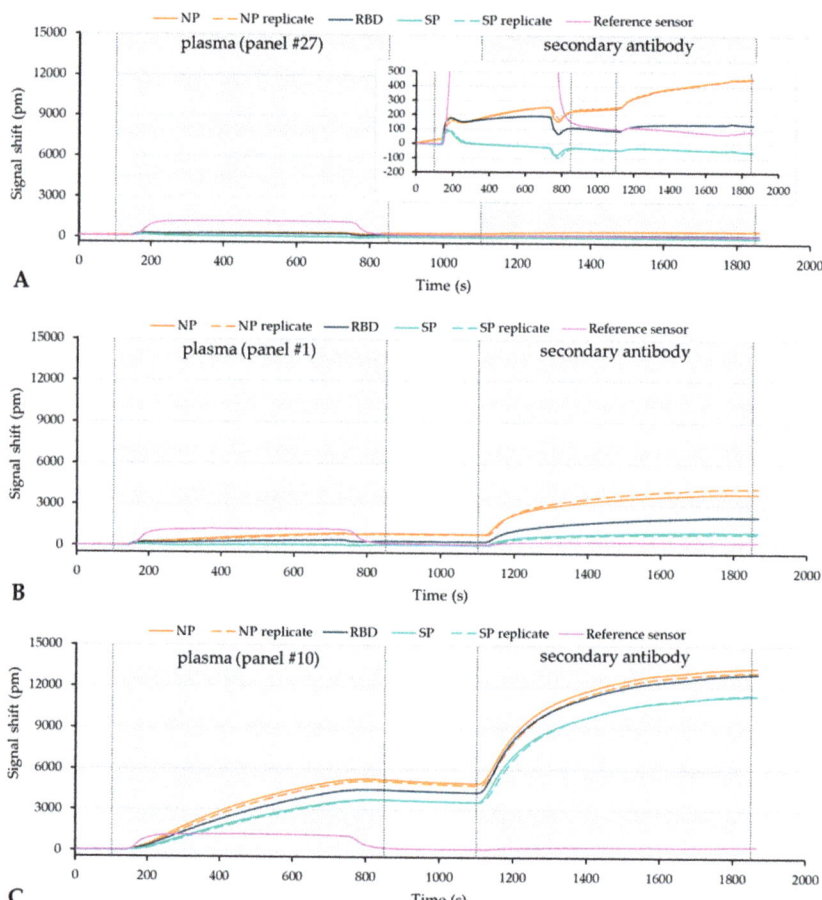

Figure 9. Sensorgrams showing the plasma incubation (direct assay) and the secondary antibody incubation (indirect assay) for (**A**) plasma #27, an anti-SARS-CoV-2 antibody negative plasma (the inset shows a zoom-in), and (**B**) plasma #1, and (**C**) plasma #10, both anti-SARS-CoV-2 antibody positive plasmas.

Cut-off values were determined as the mean plus three times the standard deviation of the binding signals obtained for all negative plasmas. Based on these cut-off values, diagnostic sensitivity and specificity were calculated for each assay (Figure 10). All assays showed a specificity of 100%. Furthermore, four out of the six assays showed a sensitivity of 100%; only the direct immunoassay with RBD and NP antigen revealed a lower sensitivity of 87%. Please note that these values should be treated with care as the number of samples was limited (23 positive and 14 negative plasmas), which is reflected in the calculated 95% confidence interval (CI) of 85.2–100% and 76.8–100% for the sensitivity and specificity, respectively.

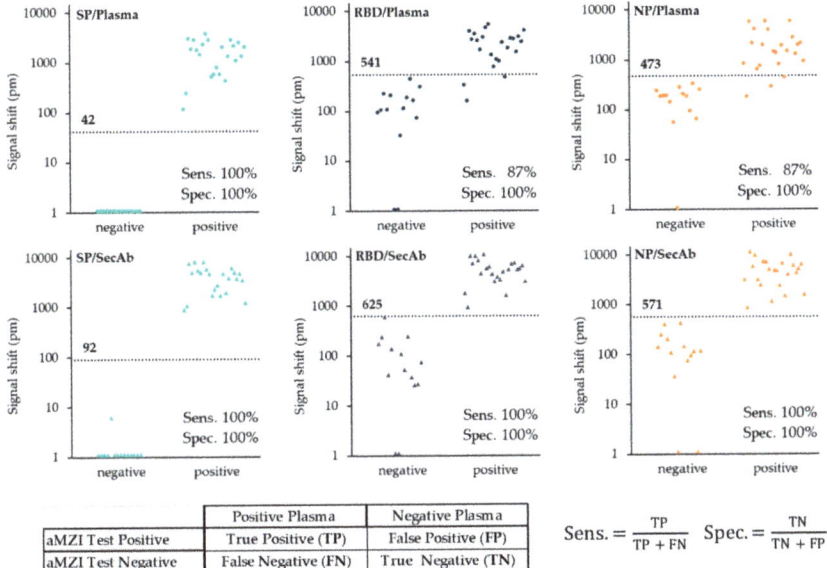

Figure 10. Binding signal distribution of 23 anti-SARS-CoV-2 antibody positive and 14 anti-SARS-CoV-2 antibody negative human plasma samples obtained for the plasma incubation (direct assay: top row) and the secondary antibody incubation (indirect assay: bottom row) shown for the SP (**left**), RBD (**middle**) and NP antigen (**right**). Note 1: for the SP assay, all but one of the negative plasma samples had a small negative binding signal (mean ± standard deviation: −32 ± 13 pm). In order to enable logarithmic presentation all negative values were assigned a value of 1 picometer. Note 2: the small table and the equations at the bottom explains how the sensitivity and specificity was calculated.

4. Discussion

The outcome of this explorative study shows very promising results for the Surfix photonic biosensor platform especially regarding its analytical performance in terms of analytical sensitivity and dynamic range. Furthermore, the measurement results are in accordance with the results obtained by different CE-IVD marked ELISA and CLIA reference methods. The aMZI-based approach is a label-free mass sensing method that very efficiently measures changes in surface mass amounts that come about by the binding of molecules to the sensor surface [40]. Despite the fact that no exogenous labeling (such as chemiluminescence or enzyme labeling) is needed for detection, the added value of the use of a secondary antibody has been clearly demonstrated in the current work by the much improved detection levels of the indirect assay (Table 1). That said, very sensitive detection may not be very relevant for SARS-CoV-2 serology testing but might be relevant for other applications where small analytes or lower clinically relevant concentrations of biomarkers are involved.

The upper limit of the dynamic range of the Surfix assays could not be accurately determined, since no signal saturation was observed at the highest calibrant concentration used (1000 IU/mL, Figure 6). Especially the direct assays are expected to have a very high upper limit. It may therefore be worthwhile to explore the performance of the Surfix assays at higher concentrations of calibrant, since this might be relevant for applications where high antibody titers are expected, for example, in studies concerning vaccine effectiveness. For such applications, the upper limit of currently available assays may be too limited.

Prevention of non-specific binding in the case of plasma sample is challenging because of its high and complex biochemical content. Especially in the case of a direct binding approach, non-specific binding of plasma constituents onto the biosensor surface (fouling) is unwanted, as discrimination between non-specific and specific binding events will be limited [41]. Due to the ease of multiplexing on the photonic biosensor platform, negative control or reference sensors can be easily implemented to compensate for this non-specific binding. Use of an internal reference arm in the balanced aMZI configuration (self-referencing) has an extra advantage as it allows for the direct compensation of the effect from changes in bulk refractive index as can be seen in Figure 9A where the one unbalanced reference sensor exhibits a step-in signal upon introduction of the plasma sample while the other (balanced) sensors show no response. Also shown in Figure 9A is that the SP/BSA balanced aMZI sensor reveals no sign of non-specific binding, but instead, it even shows a slight decrease of signal during incubation with negative control plasma. This is probably explained by a lower degree of non-specific binding that takes place to SP as compared to BSA. In contrast to SP, sensors modified with the RBD and NP antigen did show low but significant non-specific binding when testing the negative controls of the plasma panel (Figure 9A). As a consequence, a poorer discrimination between the anti-SARS-CoV-2 antibody negative and anti-SARS-CoV-2 antibody positive plasma samples was found for the RBD and NP as compared to the SP antigen (Figure 10). The higher level of non-specific binding is very likely attributed to a higher cross-reactivity and/or the higher isoelectric point of the proteins (10.07 for NP and 8.91 for RBD), which makes the proteins positively charged at the near-neutral pH of the assay buffers. Some of the commercial tests for detecting anti-NP antibodies use modified recombinant antigens, for example, the Euroimmun NCP ELISA employs a modified NP that contains only the relevant epitopes in order to prevent background binding. The use of such a truncated NP or other modified viral antigens might also reduce non-specific binding in our NP and/or RBD assay. An alternative to the use of native or recombinant SARS-CoV-2 protein antigen is to employ synthetic peptides that are derived from distinct linear epitope sites of the different SARS-CoV-2 antigens. An increasing number of linear epitopes have been described resulting from immunoinformatic analysis [42], studies with peptide-based ELISA [43] and proteome microarrays [44].

The Surfix photonic biosensor platform enables multiplex detection of antibodies that target viral antigens. The results obtained for three different SARS-CoV-2 antigens (SP, RBD, and NP) were found to correlate well with tests performed with the different CE-IVD marked reference methods (Figure 8). A multiplexing approach opens possibilities for advanced clinical analysis such as: (1) ruling out cross-reactivity with antibodies targeted against other coronaviruses, e.g., the different common cold viruses, to avoid false positive results; (2) simultaneously testing for antibodies against multiple viral antigens may lead to a better reliability of the test; (3) estimating disease severity in COVID-19 patients by using certain peptide epitopes that serve as a disease severity marker [43]; and (4) differentiation and detection of emerging SARS-CoV-2 variants-of-concern.

The presented work shows the potential of the Surfix photonic biosensor for further development into a POC IVD platform. To achieve this, several improvements are currently being implemented. Current developments are focusing on further miniaturization and cost reduction of the photonic chip itself, but also integration of the chip in a microfluidic cartridge to facilitate liquid handling and improve the user-friendliness of the system. Moreover, the read-out instrument and the user interface are being redesigned to meet the requirements of a practical and manufacturable POC IVD platform. In this paper, we have presented results on the sensitive detection of anti-SARS-CoV-2 antibodies in human plasma that target one or more viral antigens. Obviously, by immobilizing different bioreceptors on the sensor waveguides, the aMZI chips can easily be reconfigured for the detection of other targets such as nucleic acids, carbohydrates, viruses, bacteria, as well as small molecules. Hence, the Surfix photonic biosensor is truly a versatile platform technology that can be used in many different application areas. To facilitate the development of devices and applications based on this technology, an R&D system for assay development is being developed in parallel to an IVD system.

Author Contributions: Conceptualization, A.S.-T., A.v.A., G.B. and L.S.; data curation, A.S.-T. and G.B.; formal analysis, G.B., J.V. and M.V.; investigation, A.G., A.v.d.M., A.S.-T., E.L., G.B., H.D., J.V., K.E., M.V. and R.S.; methodology, A.S.-T., G.B., J.V., L.S. and W.K.; project administration, A.S.-T. and G.B.; resources, A.S.-T., G.B. and L.S.; supervision, A.S.-T., G.B. and L.S.; validation, A.G. and E.L.; G.B. and J.V.; visualization, G.B., J.V. and M.V.; writing—original draft preparation, G.B.; writing—review and editing, all authors. All authors have read and agreed to the published version of the manuscript.

Funding: This research received no external funding.

Institutional Review Board Statement: Not applicable.

Informed Consent Statement: Not applicable.

Data Availability Statement: The authors confirm that the data supporting the findings of this study are available within the article.

Acknowledgments: The authors thank Jan Wichers (Wageningen Food & Biobased Research, Wageningen, The Netherlands) for his valuable advice regarding the use and processing of proteins. Furthermore, the authors thank Erik Schreuder and Arnoud Everhardt (LioniX International, Enschede, The Netherlands) for providing the photo material for Figure 1, and for their technical advice regarding the chips and related issues.

Conflicts of Interest: A.v.d.M., A.S.-T., G.B., H.D., J.V., K.E., L.S., M.V., R.S. and W.K. are employees of Surfix Diagnostics. L.S. is founder and minority shareholder of Surfix Diagnostics. A.G. is founder and shareholder of Innatoss. A.v.A. and E.L. declare no conflict of interest.

References

1. Bahadir, E.B.; Sezgintürk, M.K. Applications of Commercial Biosensors in Clinical, Food, Environmental, and Biothreat/Biowarfare Analyses. *Anal. Biochem.* **2015**, *478*, 107–120. [CrossRef] [PubMed]
2. Jafari, S.; Guercetti, J.; Geballa-Koukoula, A.; Tsagkaris, A.S.; Nelis, J.L.D.; Marco, M.P.; Salvador, J.P.; Gerssen, A.; Hajslova, J.; Elliott, C.; et al. Assured Point-of-Need Food Safety Screening: A Critical Assessment of Portable Food Analyzers. *Foods* **2021**, *10*, 1399. [CrossRef] [PubMed]
3. Heidt, B.; Siqueira, W.F.; Eersels, K.; Diliën, H.; van Grinsven, B.; Fujiwara, R.T.; Cleij, T.J. Point of Care Diagnostics in Resource-Limited Settings: A Review of the Present and Future of PoC in Its Most Needed Environment. *Biosensors* **2020**, *10*, 133. [CrossRef] [PubMed]
4. Wang, C.; Liu, M.; Wang, Z.; Li, S.; Deng, Y.; He, N. Point-of-Care Diagnostics for Infectious Diseases: From Methods to Devices. *Nano Today* **2021**, *37*, 101092. [CrossRef]
5. Lim, W.Y.; Lan, B.L.; Ramakrishnan, N. Emerging Biosensors to Detect Severe Acute Respiratory Syndrome Coronavirus 2 (SARS-CoV-2): A Review. *Biosensors* **2021**, *11*, 434. [CrossRef]
6. Cui, F.; Zhou, H.S. Diagnostic Methods and Potential Portable Biosensors for Coronavirus Disease 2019. *Biosens. Bioelectron.* **2020**, *165*, 112349. [CrossRef]
7. Tantuoyir, M.M.; Rezaei, N. Serological Tests for COVID-19: Potential Opportunities. *Cell Biol. Int.* **2021**, *45*, 740–748. [CrossRef]
8. Hamady, A.; Lee, J.J.; Loboda, Z.A. Waning Antibody Responses in COVID-19: What Can We Learn from the Analysis of Other Coronaviruses? *Infection* **2022**, *50*, 11–25. [CrossRef]
9. Semmler, G.; Traugott, M.T.; Graninger, M.; Hoepler, W.; Seitz, T.; Kelani, H.; Karolyi, M.; Pawelka, E.; de La Cruz, S.A.; Puchhammer-Stöckl, E.; et al. Assessment of S1-, S2-, and NCP-Specific IgM, IgA, and IgG Antibody Kinetics in Acute SARS-CoV-2 Infection by a Microarray and Twelve Other Immunoassays. *J. Clin. Microbiol.* **2021**, *59*, e02890-20. [CrossRef]
10. Pinotti, F.; Obolski, U.; Wikramaratna, P.; Giovanetti, M.; Paton, R.; Klenerman, P.; Thompson, C.; Gupta, S.; Lourenço, J. Real-Time Seroprevalence and Exposure Levels of Emerging Pathogens in Infection-Naive Host Populations. *Sci. Rep.* **2021**, *11*, 5825. [CrossRef]
11. FIND Test Directory. Available online: https://www.finddx.org/covid-19/test-directory/ (accessed on 23 June 2022).
12. Gong, F.; Wei, H.X.; Li, Q.; Liu, L.; Li, B. Evaluation and Comparison of Serological Methods for COVID-19 Diagnosis. *Front. Mol. Biosci.* **2021**, *8*, 682405. [CrossRef] [PubMed]
13. Rasmi, Y.; Li, X.; Khan, J.; Ozer, T.; Choi, J.R. Emerging Point-of-Care Biosensors for Rapid Diagnosis of COVID-19: Current Progress, Challenges, and Future Prospects. *Anal. Bioanal. Chem.* **2021**, *413*, 4137–4159. [CrossRef] [PubMed]
14. Flores-Contreras, E.A.; González-González, R.B.; Rodríguez-Sánchez, I.P.; Yee-De León, J.F.; Iqbal, H.M.N.; González-González, E. Microfluidics-Based Biosensing Platforms: Emerging Frontiers in Point-of-Care Testing SARS-CoV-2 and Seroprevalence. *Biosensors* **2022**, *12*, 179. [CrossRef] [PubMed]
15. Manmana, Y.; Kubo, T.; Otsuka, K. Recent Developments of Point-of-Care (POC) Testing Platform for Biomolecules. *TrAC—Trends Anal. Chem.* **2021**, *135*, 116160. [CrossRef]
16. Taleghani, N.; Taghipour, F. Diagnosis of COVID-19 for Controlling the Pandemic: A Review of the State-of-the-Art. *Biosens. Bioelectron.* **2021**, *174*, 112830. [CrossRef]

17. Gauglitz, G. Critical Assessment of Relevant Methods in the Field of Biosensors with Direct Optical Detection Based on Fibers and Waveguides Using Plasmonic, Resonance, and Interference Effects. *Anal. Bioanal. Chem.* **2020**, *412*, 3317–3349. [CrossRef]
18. Shen, Y.; Anwar, T.B.; Mulchandani, A. Current Status, Advances, Challenges and Perspectives on Biosensors for COVID-19 Diagnosis in Resource-Limited Settings. *Sens. Actuators Rep.* **2021**, *3*, 100025. [CrossRef]
19. Estevez, M.C.; Alvarez, M.; Lechuga, L.M. Integrated Optical Devices for Lab-on-a-Chip Biosensing Applications. *Laser Photonics Rev.* **2011**, *6*, 463–487. [CrossRef]
20. Djaileb, A.; Hojjat Jodaylami, M.; Coutu, J.; Ricard, P.; Lamarre, M.; Rochet, L.; Cellier-Goetghebeur, S.; MacAulay, D.; Charron, B.; Lavallée, É.; et al. Cross-Validation of ELISA and a Portable Surface Plasmon Resonance Instrument for IgG Antibody Serology with SARS-CoV-2 Positive Individuals. *Analyst* **2021**, *146*, 4905–4917. [CrossRef]
21. Schasfoort, R.B.M.; van Weperen, J.; van Amsterdam, M.; Parisot, J.; Hendriks, J.; Koerselman, M.; Karperien, M.; Mentink, A.; Bennink, M.; Krabbe, H.; et al. Presence and Strength of Binding of IgM, IgG and IgA Antibodies against SARS-CoV-2 during CoViD-19 Infection. *Biosens. Bioelectron.* **2021**, *183*, 113165. [CrossRef]
22. Calvo-Lozano, O.; Sierra, M.; Soler, M.; Estévez, M.C.; Chiscano-Camón, L.; Ruiz-Sanmartin, A.; Ruiz-Rodriguez, J.C.; Ferrer, R.; González-López, J.J.; Esperalba, J.; et al. Label-Free Plasmonic Biosensor for Rapid, Quantitative, and Highly Sensitive COVID-19 Serology: Implementation and Clinical Validation. *Anal. Chem.* **2022**, *94*, 975–984. [CrossRef] [PubMed]
23. Syed Nor, S.N.; Rasanang, N.S.; Karman, S.; Zaman, W.S.W.K.; Harun, S.W.; Arof, H. A Review: Surface Plasmon Resonance-Based Biosensor for Early Screening of SARS-CoV2 Infection. *IEEE Access* **2022**, *10*, 1228–1244. [CrossRef]
24. Qu, J.H.; Leirs, K.; Maes, W.; Imbrechts, M.; Callewaert, N.; Lagrou, K.; Geukens, N.; Lammertyn, J.; Spasic, D. Innovative FO-SPR Label-Free Strategy for Detecting Anti-RBD Antibodies in COVID-19 Patient Serum and Whole Blood. *ACS Sens.* **2022**, *7*, 477–487. [CrossRef] [PubMed]
25. Dzimianski, J.V.; Lorig-Roach, N.; O'Rourke, S.M.; Alexander, D.L.; Kimmey, J.M.; DuBois, R.M. Rapid and Sensitive Detection of SARS-CoV-2 Antibodies by Biolayer Interferometry. *Sci. Rep.* **2020**, *10*, 21738. [CrossRef]
26. Donato, L.J.; Theel, E.S.; Baumann, N.A.; Bridgeman, A.R.; Blommel, J.H.; Wu, Y.; Karon, B.S. Evaluation of the Genalyte Maverick SARS-CoV-2 Multi-Antigen Serology Panel. *J. Clin. Virol. Plus* **2021**, *1*, 100030. [CrossRef]
27. Ikegami, S.; Benirschke, R.C.; Fakhrai-Rad, H.; Motamedi, M.H.; Hockett, R.; David, S.; Lee, H.K.; Kang, J.; Gniadek, T.J. Target Specific Serologic Analysis of COVID-19 Convalescent Plasma. *PLoS ONE* **2021**, *16*, e0249938. [CrossRef]
28. Asghari, A.; Wang, C.; Yoo, K.M.; Rostamian, A.; Xu, X.; Shin, J.D.; Dalir, H.; Chen, R.T. Fast, Accurate, Point-of-Care COVID-19 Pandemic Diagnosis Enabled through Advanced Lab-on-Chip Optical Biosensors: Opportunities and Challenges. *Appl. Phys. Rev.* **2021**, *8*, 031313. [CrossRef]
29. Roy, L.; Buragohain, P.; Borse, V. Strategies for Sensitivity Enhancement of Point-of-Care Devices. *Biosens. Bioelectron. X* **2022**, *10*, 100098. [CrossRef]
30. Chatzipetrou, M.; Gounaridis, L.; Tsekenis, G.; Dimadi, M.; Vestering-Stenger, R.; Schreuder, E.F.; Trilling, A.; Besselink, G.; Scheres, L.; van der Meer, A.; et al. A Miniature Bio-Photonics Companion Diagnostics Platform for Reliable Cancer Treatment Monitoring in Blood Fluids. *Sensors* **2021**, *21*, 2230. [CrossRef]
31. Geuzebroek, D.H.; Besselink, G.A.J.; Schreuder, F.; Falke, F.; Leinse, A.; Heideman, R.G. Silicon-Nitride Biophotonic Sensing Platform. In *Integrated Optics: Devices, Materials, and Technologies XXIII, Proceedings of the SPIE, San Francisco, CA, USA, 2–7 February 2009*; García-Blanco, M., Cheben, P., Eds.; The International Society for Optical Engineering: Bellingham, WA, USA, 2019; p. 10921. [CrossRef]
32. Knoben, W.; Besselink, G.; Roeven, E.; Zuilhof, H.; Schütz-Trilling, A.; van der Meer, A.; Scheres, L.; Leeuwis, H.; Falke, F.; Schreuder, F.; et al. Highly Sensitive Integrated Optical Biosensing Platform Based on an Asymmetric Mach-Zehnder Interferometer and Material-Selective (Bio)Functionalization. In Proceedings of the 22nd International Conference on Miniaturized Systems for Chemistry and Life Sciences (MicroTAS 2018), Kaohsiung, Taiwan, 11–15 November 2018; Volume 2.
33. Chalyan, T.; Potrich, C.; Schreuder, E.; Falke, F.; Pasquardini, L.; Pederzolli, C.; Heideman, R.; Pavesi, L. AFM1 Detection in Milk by Fab' Functionalized Si3N4 Asymmetric Mach-Zehnder Interferometric Biosensors. *Toxins* **2019**, *11*, 409. [CrossRef]
34. Chalyan, T.; Guider, R.; Pasquardini, L.; Zanetti, M.; Falke, F.; Schreuder, E.; Heideman, R.G.; Pederzolli, C.; Pavesi, L. Asymmetric Mach-Zehnder Interferometer Based Biosensors for Aflatoxin M1 Detection. *Biosensors* **2016**, *6*, 1. [CrossRef] [PubMed]
35. Fernández-Gavela, A.; Herranz, S.; Chocarro, B.; Falke, F.; Schreuder, E.; Leeuwis, H.; Heideman, R.G.; Lechuga, L.M. Full Integration of Photonic Nanoimmunosensors in Portable Platforms for On-Line Monitoring of Ocean Pollutants. *Sens. Actuators B Chem.* **2019**, *297*, 126758. [CrossRef]
36. Goodwin, M.J.; Besselink, G.A.J.; Falke, F.; Everhardt, A.S.; Cornelissen, J.J.L.M.; Huskens, J. Highly Sensitive Protein Detection by Asymmetric Mach-Zehnder Interferometry for Biosensing Applications. *ACS Appl. Bio Mater.* **2020**, *3*, 4566–4572. [CrossRef] [PubMed]
37. Wörhoff, K.; Heideman, R.G.; Leinse, A.; Hoekman, M. TriPleX: A Versatile Dielectric Photonic Platform. *Adv. Opt. Technol.* **2015**, *4*, 189–207. [CrossRef]
38. Besselink, G.A.J.; Heideman, R.G.; Schreuder, E.; Wevers, L.S.; Falke, F.; Van den Vlekkert, H.H. Performance of Arrayed Microring Resonator Sensors with the TriPleX Platform. *J. Biosens. Bioelectron.* **2016**, *7*, 1000209. [CrossRef]
39. Gajos, K.; Szafraniec, K.; Petrou, P.; Budkowski, A. Surface Density Dependent Orientation and Immunological Recognition of Antibody on Silicon: TOF-SIMS and Surface Analysis of Two Covalent Immobilization Methods. *Appl. Surf. Sci.* **2020**, *518*, 146269. [CrossRef]

40. Kozma, P.; Kehl, F.; Ehrentreich-Förster, E.; Stamm, C.; Bier, F.F. Integrated Planar Optical Waveguide Interferometer Biosensors: A Comparative Review. *Biosens. Bioelectron.* **2014**, *58*, 287–307. [CrossRef]
41. Lichtenberg, J.Y.; Ling, Y.; Kim, S. Non-Specific Adsorption Reduction Methods in Biosensing. *Sensors* **2019**, *19*, 2488. [CrossRef]
42. Oliveira, S.C.; de Magalhães, M.T.Q.; Homan, E.J. Immunoinformatic Analysis of SARS-CoV-2 Nucleocapsid Protein and Identification of COVID-19 Vaccine Targets. *Front. Immunol.* **2020**, *11*, 587615. [CrossRef]
43. Amrun, S.N.; Lee, C.Y.P.; Lee, B.; Fong, S.W.; Young, B.E.; Chee, R.S.L.; Yeo, N.K.W.; Torres-Ruesta, A.; Carissimo, G.; Poh, C.M.; et al. Linear B-Cell Epitopes in the Spike and Nucleocapsid Proteins as Markers of SARS-CoV-2 Exposure and Disease Severity. *eBioMedicine* **2020**, *58*, 102911. [CrossRef]
44. Wang, H.; Wu, X.; Zhang, X.; Hou, X.; Liang, T.; Wang, D.; Teng, F.; Dai, J.; Duan, H.; Guo, S.; et al. SARS-CoV-2 Proteome Microarray for Mapping COVID-19 Antibody Interactions at Amino Acid Resolution. *ACS Cent. Sci.* **2020**, *6*, 2238–2249. [CrossRef] [PubMed]

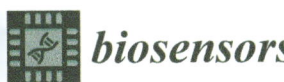

Article

Measurements of Anti-SARS-CoV-2 Antibody Levels after Vaccination Using a SH-SAW Biosensor

Chia-Hsuan Cheng [1], Yu-Chi Peng [1,2], Shu-Min Lin [3], Hiromi Yatsuda [1], Szu-Heng Liu [1], Shih-Jen Liu [4], Chen-Yen Kuo [5] and Robert Y. L. Wang [2,5,6,7,*]

1 Tst Biomedical Electronics Co., Ltd., Taoyuan 324403, Taiwan
2 Biotechnology Industry Master and Ph.D. Program, Chang Gung University, Taoyuan 33302, Taiwan
3 Department of Thoracic Medicine, Chang Gung Memorial Hospital, Linkou 33305, Taiwan
4 National Institute of Infectious Diseases and Vaccinology, Taoyuan 33302, Taiwan
5 Division of Pediatric Infectious Diseases, Department of Pediatrics, Chang Gung Memorial and Children's Hospital, Linkou 33305, Taiwan
6 Department of Biomedical Sciences, College of Medicine, Chang Gung University, Taoyuan 33302, Taiwan
7 Kidney Research Center and Department of Nephrology, Chang Gung Memorial Hospital, Linkou 33305, Taiwan
* Correspondence: yuwang@mail.cgu.edu.tw; Tel.: +886-3-211-8800 (ext. 3691)

Abstract: To prevent the COVID-19 pandemic that threatens human health, vaccination has become a useful and necessary tool in the response to the pandemic. The vaccine not only induces antibodies in the body, but may also cause adverse effects such as fatigue, muscle pain, blood clots, and myocarditis, especially in patients with chronic disease. To reduce unnecessary vaccinations, it is becoming increasingly important to monitor the amount of anti-SARS-CoV-2 S protein antibodies prior to vaccination. A novel SH-SAW biosensor, coated with SARS-CoV-2 spike protein, can help quantify the amount of anti-SARS-CoV-2 S protein antibodies with 5 µL of finger blood within 40 s. The LoD of the spike-protein-coated SAW biosensor was determined to be 41.91 BAU/mL, and the cut-off point was determined to be 50 BAU/mL (Youden's J statistic = 0.94733). By using the SH-SAW biosensor, we found that the total anti-SARS-CoV-2 S protein antibody concentrations spiked 10–14 days after the first vaccination (p = 0.0002) and 7–9 days after the second vaccination (p = 0.0116). Furthermore, mRNA vaccines, such as Moderna or BNT, could achieve higher concentrations of total anti-SARS-CoV-2 S protein antibodies compared with adenovirus vaccine, AZ (p < 0.0001). SH-SAW sensors in vitro diagnostic systems are a simple and powerful technology to investigate the local prevalence of COVID-19.

Keywords: SARS-CoV-2; SH-SAW biosensor; vaccine; antibody

Citation: Cheng, C.-H.; Peng, Y.-C.; Lin, S.-M.; Yatsuda, H.; Liu, S.-H.; Liu, S.-J.; Kuo, C.-Y.; Wang, R.Y.L. Measurements of Anti-SARS-CoV-2 Antibody Levels after Vaccination Using a SH-SAW Biosensor. *Biosensors* 2022, 12, 599. https://doi.org/10.3390/bios12080599

Received: 15 July 2022
Accepted: 2 August 2022
Published: 4 August 2022

Publisher's Note: MDPI stays neutral with regard to jurisdictional claims in published maps and institutional affiliations.

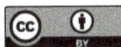

Copyright: © 2022 by the authors. Licensee MDPI, Basel, Switzerland. This article is an open access article distributed under the terms and conditions of the Creative Commons Attribution (CC BY) license (https://creativecommons.org/licenses/by/4.0/).

1. Introduction

Severe acute respiratory syndrome coronavirus 2 (SARS-CoV-2) is the cause of the 2019 coronavirus (COVID-19) pandemic [1]. It is an enveloped, positive-sense, and single-stranded RNA virus, which is transmitted through surface contamination, aerosol, and the fecal-oral route. The SARS-CoV-2 genome encodes four structural proteins including nucleocapsid (N) protein, spike (S) protein, membrane (M) protein, and envelop (E) protein [2,3]. The S and N proteins are the most immunogenic proteins of SARS-CoV-2 [4]. Recently, there are several COVID-19 vaccines in development for pandemic control and prevention of COVID-19. The vaccines include adenoviral-vectored vaccines, nucleic acid vaccines, subunit protein vaccines, and whole-cell inactivated virus vaccines [5,6]. The available COVID-19 vaccines in Taiwan are ChAdOx1 nCoV-19 by AstraZeneca/Oxford, BNT-162b2 by BioNTech/Pfizer, mRNA-1273 by Moderna, and MVC-COV1901 by Medigen. ChAdOx1 nCoV-19 is the adenoviral-vectored vaccine. Both BNT-162b2 and mRNA-1273 are mRNA vaccines. MVC-COV1901 is a recombinant protein subunit vaccine [6,7].

Follow-up measurements of anti-SARS-CoV-2 antibodies after vaccination are a potential surrogate marker of protection [5,8]. The general anti-SARS-CoV-2 antibody detection methods include enzyme-linked immunosorbent assay (ELISA) and lateral flow immunoassay (LFIA). ELISA is characterized by high throughput and high sensitivity. It needs to be performed in a conditioned laboratory due to the complexity of the operation steps. The measurement time of LFIA is short and some interfering factors may lead to false positive results [9,10]. Surface acoustic wave (SAW) biosensors have been used to detect various biomarkers with high selectivity, high sensitivity, and low cost [11,12]. Our previous study showed that shear-horizontal surface acoustic wave (SH-SAW) biosensors can measure anti-SARS-CoV-2 N protein antibodies with good sensitivity [13]. The SH-SAW biosensor contains an input and output interdigital transducer (IDT), a sensing area coated with antibodies or antigens of the target molecules, and a reflector. When the measurement starts, the incoming electrical signal is converted into surface acoustic waves by the input IDT. The wave then propagates along the sensing zone and is reflected through the reflector to the output IDT. Finally, the wave is converted into an electrical signal. The output signal is associated with the binding of the sensing zone. As the target molecules bind to the sensing region, the velocity and amplitude of the wave attenuate. The more the target molecules bind to the sensing region, the larger the signal it produces [12,14,15].

In this study, we demonstrated the performance of an S-protein coated SH-SAW biosensor and established a 4PL curve. Afterwards, we compared the antibody responses to each vaccine (AstraZeneca/Oxford, BioNTech/Pfizer, Moderna, and Medigen). In addition, we investigated the kinetic properties of total anti-SARS-CoV-2 S protein antibody levels in whole blood after vaccination. Our study showed that the concentrations of total anti-SARS-CoV-2 S protein antibodies spiked 10–14 days after the first vaccination. The concentration of total anti-SARS-CoV-2 S protein antibodies could reach 322.9 ± 614.4 BAU/mL at 29–56 days after the first vaccination. The concentration of total anti-SARS-CoV-2 S protein antibodies spiked and peaked 7–9 days after the second vaccination. This SH-SAW sensor system can easily confirm the amount of anti-S antibodies before additional injections of COVID-19 vaccine. This must be very effective for additional vaccination decisions.

2. Materials and Methods
2.1. Materials

iProtin immunoassay reader and SH-SAW biosensor chips were supplied by tst biomedical electronics Co., Ltd. (Taoyuan, Taiwan). Hellmanex III (259304) was purchased from Hellma Analytics (Munich, Germany). Dithiobis [succinimidyl propionate] (DSP) (VI309258) and dimethyl sulfoxide (DMSO) (TH270381) were obtained from Thermo Fisher Scientific (Waltham, MA, USA). The SARS-CoV-2 trimeric S protein coated on the capture channel of the SH-SAW biosensor chip was from the National Health Research Institutes. Casein (97062-926) was purchased from VWR (Radnor, PA, USA). Phosphate buffered saline (CWFF0613) and bovine albumin serum (FUBSA001.100) were bought from Bio-Future company (BioFuture biotech, Taoyuan, Taiwan). The first WHO International Standard for anti-SARS-CoV-2 immunoglobulin (human) (NIBSC code: 20/136) was purchased from the National Institute for Biological Standards and Control. The stabilizer was prepared by adding 15 µL of Tween 20 to 10% sucrose (BCBV9208, Sigma, St. Louis, MO, USA).

In this study, we used a 3 mm × 5 mm dual-channel SH-SAW biosensor chip; one channel for reference and the other for capture. Each channel on the chip has an IDT, a reflector, and a sensing zone between them. The dual-channel SH-SW biosensor chip mounted on a printed circuit board (PCB) is shown in Figure 1.

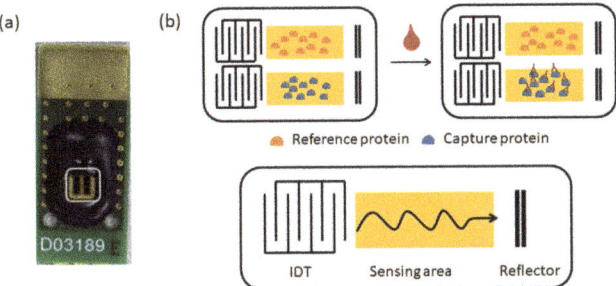

Figure 1. The dual-channel SH-SAW sensor chip. (**a**) Photograph of SH-SAW sensor chip; (**b**) schematic coated proteins in the dual-channel SH-SAW sensor chip.

2.2. Fabrication of SH-SAW Biosensor Chips Coated with S Protein

First, the sensing area of the SH-SAW biosensor chip was cleaned with O_2 plasma for 10 min. 2% of Hellmanex III was added and incubated for 20 min. Then, the chip was rinsed twice with double distilled water. We then added 0.4 mg/mL of DSP solution (in DMSO) and incubated for 20 min. After that, the chip was rinsed with DMSO. The chip was then washed with double distilled water and air dried. The reference and capture channels were coated with 10% bovine albumin serum (in double distilled water) and 0.45 mg/mL of SARS-CoV-2 trimeric S protein, respectively. After that, the chips were blocked with 2% casein pH 7.4 (in PBS). Finally, stabilizer was added and the chips were blown dry. The chips were labeled and stored in the dry carbinet.

2.3. Establishment of the 4PL Standard Curve

The WHO International Standard for anti-SARS-CoV-2 immunoglobulin (human) was used as the standard. The standard was serially diluted and mixed with whole blood. The standards were measured and a 4PL standard curve was established; the equation for the 4PL standard curve is as follows:

$$y = d + \frac{a-d}{1+\left(\frac{x}{c}\right)^b}$$

where a, b, c, and d are coefficients. X is the titre of anti-SARS-CoV-2 S protein total antibody. Anti-SARS-CoV-2 S protein total antibody levels were quantified in BAU/mL.

2.4. Measurement of Total Anti-S Protein Antibody Using SH-SAW Biosensor

Total anti-SARS-CoV-2 trimeric S protein antibodies were measured by iProtin immunoassay and SARS-CoV-2 S protein-coated SH-SAW sensor chips (Figure 2). After the iProtin immunoassay was pre-warmed, the QR code containing the 4PL standard curve was scanned. The SARS-CoV-2 S protein assay cassette was inserted into the slot of the iProtin immunoassay reader. Then, 5 µL of whole blood was dropped onto the chip. After 3 min of incubation, the antibody level was displayed on the screen of the iProtin immunoassay reader.

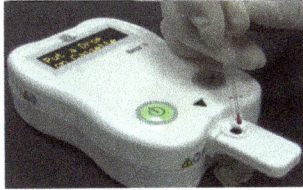

Figure 2. Physical photograph of the iProtin immunoassay and SH-SAW sensor chip coated with SARS-CoV-2 S protein.

2.5. Clinical Trial

Participants in this study included subjects who had received a SARS-CoV-2 vaccine. The study protocol was reviewed and approved by the Institutional Review Board (IRB2108130013). Inclusion criteria were adults between the ages of 20 and 65 years. Subjects diagnosed with metabolic disorders or immunodeficiency diseases were excluded. Whole blood was collected from participants who consented to participate in this study.

2.6. Statistical Analysis

Quantitative data were expressed as means ± standard deviation (SD) and compared using the Student's t-test. A p-value < 0.05 was considered statistically significant. Statistical analyses were performed using SPSS statistics 17 (SPSS, Chicago, IL, USA).

3. Results

3.1. Characterization of S Protein Coated SAW Biosensor

To establish the standard curve, the SAW signals for different concentrations of total anti-S protein antibodies are plotted in Figure 3 and fitted with the following four-parameter logistics (4PL) equation (Figure 4):

$$\text{SAW signal} = A + (B - A)/\{1 + ([\text{Anti-S tAb}]/C)^D\}$$

where A = 0.9199, B = 0.0255, C = 1066.4, and D = 1.5054 are the coefficients for the SAW biosensor chip with a coefficient of correlation (R) of 0.9947; [Anti-S tAb] is the concentration of the first WHO international standard for anti-SARS-CoV-2 immunoglobulin (human).

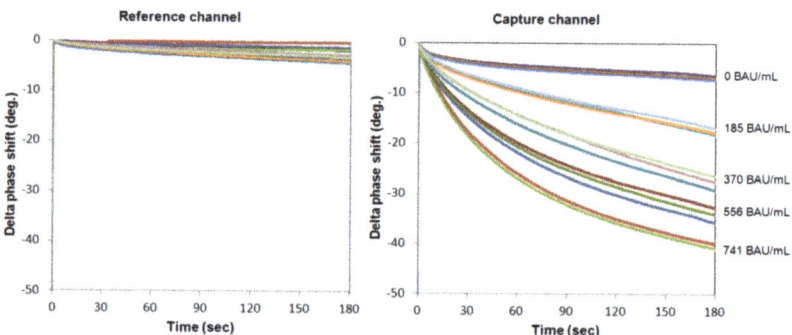

Figure 3. Real-time measurement of various concentrations of total anti-S protein antibodies in the reference and capture channels.

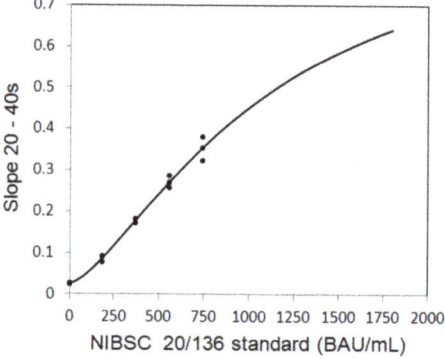

Figure 4. Establishment of four parameter logistics (4PL) standard curve.

3.2. Performance of S Protein Coated SAW Biosensor

To determine the limit of detection (LoD) of the S protein-coated SAW biosensor, the LoD was determined by the mean (Mean$_{BLK}$) of 60 blank samples plus 1.645 times (σ) the standard deviation of the 60 lowest concentrations, with the following equation:

$$\text{LoD} = \text{Mean}_{BLK} + 1.645\, \sigma_{lowest\ conce.}$$

The LoD of the S protein-coated SAW biosensor was determined to be 41.91 BAU/mL. From a linearity study, the S protein-coated SAW biosensor was tested between 48.3 to 1597.2 BAU/mL, with a linear regression of 0.9935. According to the receiver operating characteristic (ROC) analysis shown in Figure 5, when the cut-off point was determined to be 50 BAU/mL, the Youden's J statistic was 0.94733.

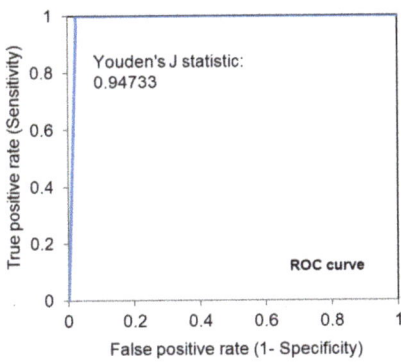

Figure 5. Receiver operating characteristic (ROC) analysis of S protein coated SAW biosensors.

3.3. Epidemiologic Surveillance of the Total Anti-SARS-CoV-2 S Protein Antibodies after Vaccination

A total of 25 subjects participated in the follow-up measurements of total anti-SARS-CoV-2 S protein antibodies after vaccination from July 2021 to February 2022, as shown in Figure 6. Among them, 16 subjects received the AZ vaccine, 4 subjects received BNT, 1 subject received Medigen, and 4 subjects received Moderna in the first vaccination; 10 subjects received AZ, 4 subjects received BNT, 1 subject received Medigen, and 5 subjects received Moderna in the second vaccination. Subsequently, 2 subjects received a third dose of Medigen vaccine, and 5 subjects received a third dose of Moderna vaccine in the third vaccination.

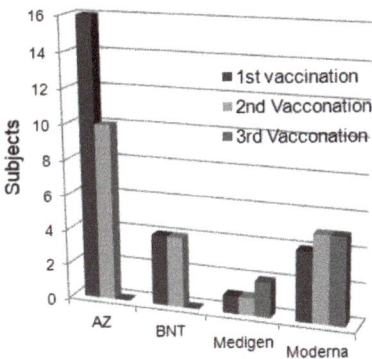

Figure 6. Distribution of vaccine brands received by subjects.

3.4. Quantitative Analysis of the Total Anti-SARS-CoV-2 S Protein Antibodies

The concentrations of total anti-SARS-CoV-2 S protein antibodies after vaccination with different brands of vaccines were analyzed (Figure 7). First, we collected and measured the antibodies after the vaccination, regardless of the brand, and found that the concentrations of total anti-SARS-CoV-2 S protein antibodies in the second vaccination samples were much higher than the first vaccination (Figure 7a,b). Interestingly, we found that mRNA vaccines, such as Moderna or BNT, could achieve higher concentrations of total anti-SARS-CoV-2 S protein antibodies than the adenovirus vaccine, AZ ($p < 0.0001$) (Figure 7c). Moreover, the concentrations of total anti-SARS-CoV-2 S protein antibodies could reach more than 3000.5 ± 0.71 BAU/mL after two BNT vaccinations, which was higher than that of two Moderna vaccinations (1708.5 ± 632.39 BAU/mL, $p = 0.03$) (Figure 7d).

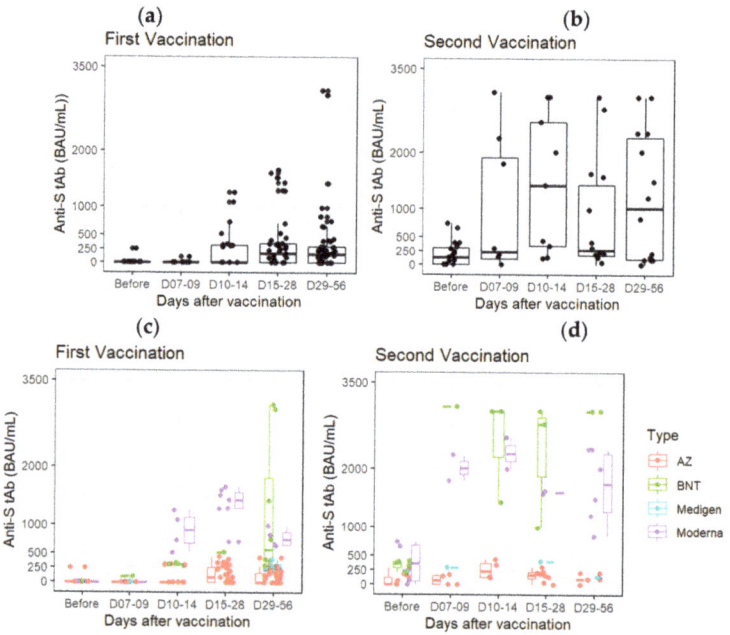

Figure 7. Follow-up and comparison of total anti-SARS-CoV-2 S protein antibody concentrations after the first (**a**,**c**) and second (**b**,**d**) vaccination. (**a**,**b**) All brands of vaccines; (**c**,**d**) different brands of vaccines.

3.5. Follow-Up Measurements of Total Anti-SARS-CoV-2 S Protein Antibodies after Vaccination

In all vaccinated subjects, the concentrations of total anti-SARS-CoV-2 S protein antibodies spiked 10–14 days after the first vaccination ($p = 0.0002$, compared with pre-inoculation antibody concentrations) (Figure 8a). The concentration of total anti-SARS-CoV-2 S protein antibodies could reach 322.9 ± 614.4 BAU/mL at 29–56 days after the first vaccination (Figure 8a). The concentration of total anti-SARS-CoV-2 S protein antibodies spiked and peaked 7–9 days after the second vaccination ($p = 0.0116$, compared with the pr-inoculation antibody concentration) (Figure 8b).

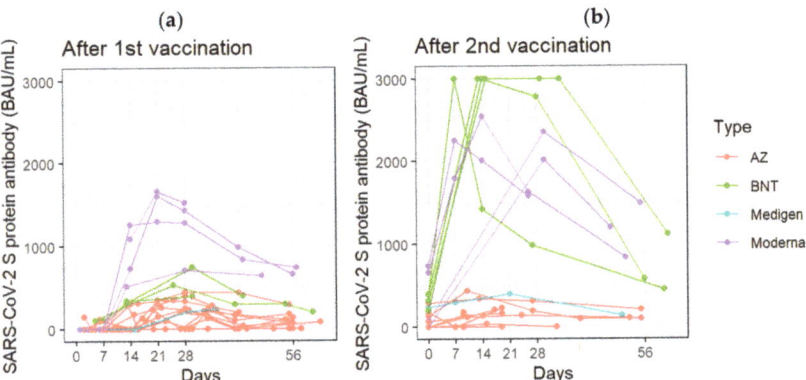

Figure 8. Follow-up measurements of anti-SARS-CoV-2 S protein total antibodies (**a**) at the indicated days after the first vaccination (**b**) at the indicated days after the second vaccination. Each line represents the concentration of antibodies in the blood continuously measured after receiving one brand of vaccine on the specified date.

4. Discussion

The SH-SAW biosensor measures the phase shifts of the output signal based on binding event on the sensing region. After dropping the sample, the target antibody in the sample is bound to the S proteins on the surface of the chip. Since all anti-S antibodies, such as IgA, IgM, and IgG, bind to S proteins on the surface, the SH-SAW biosensor detects total anti-S antibodies. To establish the calibration curve, the WHO international SARS-CoV-2 antibody standard (20/136) was used. The electrical phase shifts of the output signal were measured 3 min after dropping the sample. The data were analyzed. As shown in Figure 3, for the range of concentrations to be measured, the concentration can be estimated by the time rate of the phase shifts for tens of seconds after the sample drop. We confirmed that a 40 s measurement time is good enough and have performed a number of experiments using a 40 s measurement time.

This study showed the kinetic properties of total anti-SARS-CoV-2 S protein antibodies after vaccination. The results showed that total anti-SARS-CoV-2 S protein antibodies spiked on days 10 to 14 after the first dose, and on days 7 to 9 after the second dose. For the mRNA vaccines, some studies showed that the vaccine-induced antibody production occurred within 2 weeks after the first dose. Additionally, antibody levels increase to a peak within a week after the second dose [1,5]. Anti-SARS-CoV-2 S protein antibodies were detectable 14 days after the first dose of AZ vaccine and peaked at 28 days. Additionally, antibody levels increase to a peak at 14 days after the second dose of AZ vaccine [6,16].

The results of this study also suggested that there are individual differences in the antibody response to vaccination. Potential factors are age, gender, and genetics [17]. Several studies have shown that women and men have an overall similar antibody response after vaccination, however some women have a faster decrease in antibody levels. In contrast, women have an overall stronger immune response after vaccination than men [18,19]. The antibody responses after vaccination were lower and antibody levels decreased more rapidly in older adults. A study showed that there were significant differences in vaccine-initiated antibody responses between older and younger people after BNT vaccination [19,20].

The SH-SAW biosensor-based anti-SARS-CoV-2 S protein antibody assay has many advantages. First, the operation procedure is simple. No labeling and washing process is required. Furthermore, the SAW platform assay does not require secondary antibodies or antibody-conjugated gold nanoparticles to enhance the signal. Secondly, it takes only forty seconds to achieve quantitative results, which is much faster than other immunoassays such as ELISA or high sensitivity chemiluminescence enzyme immunoassay (HISCL) [21].

Forty seconds of measurement time constitutes a great benefit for practical applications in clinics. Third, the exact volume of the sample is not required, and the sample can be whole blood, plasma, serum, or saliva [22]. Even for whole blood samples with blood cells and many different proteins, the binding event between the capture protein causes a change in the SAW velocity and the concentration estimated. On our SH-SAW biosensor platform, a physician can apply around 5 micro-liters of finger-pricked blood on the sensor chip and then obtain a quantitative result after 40 s. Compared to electrochemistry methods, it greatly simplifies the procedure and avoids the pain of venipuncture [23]. Finally, the SH-SAW biosensor can measure antibodies against SARS-CoV-2 total S protein. Much has been reported about the increase of IgA, IgM, IgG, and other antibody levels after SARS-CoV-2 infection. During the infection phase, the dynamics of the different antibody isotypes are different. Over time, IgG becomes dominant compared with IgA and IgM [24]. When total antibody levels are measured, it can be assumed that they are almost exclusively IgG antibody levels. Total anti-S antibodies measurement is valid for true commercial use.

Neutralization levels were highly predictive of immune protection, with 50% protection at a neutralization level equivalent to 20.2% of the mean convalescent level [25]. Moreover, the presence of RBD- or S protein-directed antibodies correlated with the level of neutralization of SARS-CoV-2, which strongly suggests that monitoring of anti-RBD and anti-S protein antibody responses could be a reliable and high-throughput compatible alternative to neutralization assays [26]. Therefore, a reliable quantitative method of SARS-CoV-2 antibody detection is needed to identify possible vaccine failure and estimate the duration of protection. The SAW platform can be used as a rapid and convenient method to determine vaccine immune protection and to help control future epidemiological trajectories.

Although we now have access to a variety of quantitative assays with CE marked antibodies against viral spike proteins, their results are not interchangeable, even when converted to BAU per milliliter using the NIBSC WHO international standard for SARS-CoV-2 immunoglobulin [27]. It is better to track one's antibody levels with the same quantitative assay, and the palm-sized iProtin immunoassay reader is a good device for long-term monitoring of the number of antibodies after vaccination. To date, all good quantitative assays of relevance are for informational purposes only, the assay still needs to provide a cut-off point for determining the presence of antibodies to the SARS-CoV-2 S protein.

We are now developing a two-in-one kit for COVID anti-S and anti-N antibodies. The test kit has three channels; the first channel is coated with S proteins, the second channel is coated with N proteins, and the third channel is coated with blocking proteins. The third channel is used as a reference. The test kit informs us whether we are infected or not, as well as the amount of the anti-S antibodies at the same time. It is very useful in commercial applications.

5. Conclusions

It is important for us to know the amount of anti-SARS-CoV-2 S protein antibodies produced after vaccination, and it is also important to know if we have been infected. If we measure anti-SARS-CoV-2 N protein antibodies, we know whether we have previously been infected. The SH-SAW sensor system is useful to investigate the local prevalence of COVID-19. The simple test procedure of placing a drop of whole blood from the fingertip on the test kit, and then getting the results after 40 s provides more opportunities to obtain big data. In addition, we can easily confirm the amount of anti-S and anti-N antibodies before additional booster injections of COVID-19 vaccines. This information is very effective for additional vaccination decisions.

Author Contributions: Conceptualization, H.Y., S.-J.L.; methodology, H.Y., S.-H.L. and C.-Y.K.; formal analysis, Y.-C.P. and C.-H.C.; investigation, R.Y.L.W. and S.-J.L.; resources, H.Y., S.-J.L., C.-Y.K. and S.-M.L.; data curation, Y.-C.P. and C.-H.C.; writing—original draft preparation, Y.-C.P. and C.-H.C.; writing—review and editing, R.Y.L.W., H.Y., C.-Y.K. and S.-H.L.; supervision, R.Y.L.W.; funding acquisition, R.Y.L.W. and S.-H.L. All authors have read and agreed to the published version of the manuscript.

Funding: This research was funded in part by grants from the Ministry of Science and Technology, Taiwan (MOST-110-2320-B-182-029) and the Chang Gung Memorial Hospital Research Fund (CMRPD1M0421, CMRPD1K0252 and CMRPD1L0061) to RW, and the APC was funded by Chang Gung University (BMRBP16).

Institutional Review Board Statement: The study protocol was reviewed and approved by the Institutional Review Board (IRB2108130013) of Chang Gung Memorial Hospital, Linkou, Taiwan.

Informed Consent Statement: Informed consent was obtained from all subjects involved in the study.

Conflicts of Interest: The authors declare no conflict of interest.

References

1. Wheeler, S.E.; Shurin, G.V.; Yost, M.; Anderson, A.; Pinto, L.; Wells, A.; Shurin, M.R. Differential Antibody Response to mRNA COVID-19 Vaccines in Healthy Subjects. *Microbiol. Spectr.* **2021**, *9*, e0034121. [CrossRef] [PubMed]
2. Zeng, W.; Liu, G.; Ma, H.; Zhao, D.; Yang, Y.; Liu, M.; Mohammed, A.; Zhao, C.; Yang, Y.; Xie, J.; et al. Biochemical characterization of SARS-CoV-2 nucleocapsid protein. *Biochem. Biophys. Res. Commun.* **2020**, *527*, 618–623. [CrossRef] [PubMed]
3. Harrison, A.G.; Lin, T.; Wang, P. Mechanisms of SARS-CoV-2 Transmission and Pathogenesis. *Trends Immunol.* **2020**, *41*, 1100–1115. [CrossRef] [PubMed]
4. Van Elslande, J.; Decru, B.; Jonckheere, S.; Van Wijngaerden, E.; Houben, E.; Vandecandelaere, P.; Indevuyst, C.; Depypere, M.; Desmet, S.; Andre, E.; et al. Antibody response against SARS-CoV-2 spike protein and nucleoprotein evaluated by four automated immunoassays and three ELISAs. *Clin. Microbiol. Infect.* **2020**, *26*, 1557.e1–1557.e7. [CrossRef] [PubMed]
5. Kaneko, S.; Kurosaki, M.; Sugiyama, T.; Takahashi, Y.; Yamaguchi, Y.; Nagasawa, M.; Izumi, N. The dynamics of quantitative SARS-CoV-2 antispike IgG response to BNT162b2 vaccination. *J. Med. Virol.* **2021**, *93*, 6813–6817. [CrossRef] [PubMed]
6. Sadarangani, M.; Marchant, A.; Kollmann, T.R. Immunological mechanisms of vaccine-induced protection against COVID-19 in humans. *Nat. Rev. Immunol.* **2021**, *21*, 475–484. [CrossRef]
7. Hsieh, S.M.; Liu, M.C.; Chen, Y.H.; Lee, W.S.; Hwang, S.J.; Cheng, S.H.; Ko, W.C.; Hwang, K.P.; Wang, N.C.; Lee, Y.L.; et al. Safety and immunogenicity of CpG 1018 and aluminium hydroxide-adjuvanted SARS-CoV-2 S-2P protein vaccine MVC-COV1901: Interim results of a large-scale, double-blind, randomised, placebo-controlled phase 2 trial in Taiwan. *Lancet Respir. Med.* **2021**, *9*, 1396–1406. [CrossRef]
8. Xu, Q.Y.; Xue, J.H.; Xiao, Y.; Jia, Z.J.; Wu, M.J.; Liu, Y.Y.; Li, W.L.; Liang, X.M.; Yang, T.C. Response and Duration of Serum Anti-SARS-CoV-2 Antibodies After Inactivated Vaccination Within 160 Days. *Front. Immunol.* **2021**, *12*, 786554. [CrossRef]
9. Song, Q.; Sun, X.; Dai, Z.; Gao, Y.; Gong, X.; Zhou, B.; Wu, J.; Wen, W. Point-of-care testing detection methods for COVID-19. *Lab Chip* **2021**, *21*, 1634–1660. [CrossRef]
10. D'Cruz, R.J.; Currier, A.W.; Sampson, V.B. Laboratory Testing Methods for Novel Severe Acute Respiratory Syndrome-Coronavirus-2 (SARS-CoV-2). *Front. Cell Dev. Biol.* **2020**, *8*, 468. [CrossRef]
11. Lee, J.; Choi, Y.S.; Lee, Y.; Lee, H.J.; Lee, J.N.; Kim, S.K.; Han, K.Y.; Cho, E.C.; Park, J.C.; Lee, S.S. Sensitive and simultaneous detection of cardiac markers in human serum using surface acoustic wave immunosensor. *Anal. Chem.* **2011**, *83*, 8629–8635. [CrossRef] [PubMed]
12. Toma, K.; Miki, D.; Kishikawa, C.; Yoshimura, N.; Miyajima, K.; Arakawa, T.; Yatsuda, H.; Mitsubayashi, K. Repetitive Immunoassay with a Surface Acoustic Wave Device and a Highly Stable Protein Monolayer for On-Site Monitoring of Airborne Dust Mite Allergens. *Anal. Chem.* **2015**, *87*, 10470–10474. [CrossRef]
13. Peng, Y.C.; Cheng, C.H.; Yatsuda, H.; Liu, S.H.; Liu, S.J.; Kogai, T.; Kuo, C.Y.; Wang, R.Y.L. A Novel Rapid Test to Detect Anti-SARS-CoV-2 N Protein IgG Based on Shear Horizontal Surface Acoustic Wave (SH-SAW). *Diagnostics* **2021**, *11*, 1838. [CrossRef] [PubMed]
14. Jeng, M.J.; Sharma, M.; Li, Y.C.; Lu, Y.C.; Yu, C.Y.; Tsai, C.L.; Huang, S.F.; Chang, L.B.; Lai, C.S. Surface Acoustic Wave Sensor for C-Reactive Protein Detection. *Sensors* **2020**, *20*, 6640. [CrossRef]
15. Lo, X.C.; Li, J.Y.; Lee, M.T.; Yao, D.J. Frequency Shift of a SH-SAW Biosensor with Glutaraldehyde and 3-Aminopropyltriethoxysilane Functionalized Films for Detection of Epidermal Growth Factor. *Biosensors* **2020**, *10*, 92. [CrossRef] [PubMed]
16. Ewer, K.J.; Barrett, J.R.; Belij-Rammerstorfer, S.; Sharpe, H.; Makinson, R.; Morter, R.; Flaxman, A.; Wright, D.; Bellamy, D.; Bittaye, M.; et al. T cell and antibody responses induced by a single dose of ChAdOx1 nCoV-19 (AZD1222) vaccine in a phase 1/2 clinical trial. *Nat. Med.* **2021**, *27*, 270–278. [CrossRef]

17. Anastassopoulou, C.; Antoni, D.; Manoussopoulos, Y.; Stefanou, P.; Argyropoulou, S.; Vrioni, G.; Tsakris, A. Age and sex associations of SARS-CoV-2 antibody responses post BNT162b2 vaccination in healthcare workers: A mixed effects model across two vaccination periods. *PLoS ONE* **2022**, *17*, e0266958. [CrossRef]
18. Zhang, J.; Xing, S.; Liang, D.; Hu, W.; Ke, C.; He, J.; Yuan, R.; Huang, Y.; Li, Y.; Liu, D.; et al. Differential Antibody Response to Inactivated COVID-19 Vaccines in Healthy Subjects. *Front. Cell Infect. Microbiol.* **2021**, *11*, 791660. [CrossRef]
19. Kang, Y.M.; Minn, D.; Lim, J.; Lee, K.D.; Jo, D.H.; Choe, K.W.; Kim, M.J.; Kim, J.M.; Kim, K.N. Comparison of Antibody Response Elicited by ChAdOx1 and BNT162b2 COVID-19 Vaccine. *J. Korean Med. Sci.* **2021**, *36*, e311. [CrossRef]
20. Zimmermann, P.; Curtis, N. Factors That Influence the Immune Response to Vaccination. *Clin. Microbiol. Rev.* **2019**, *32*, e00084-18. [CrossRef]
21. Noda, K.; Matsuda, K.; Yagishita, S.; Maeda, K.; Akiyama, Y.; Terada-Hirashima, J.; Matsushita, H.; Iwata, S.; Yamashita, K.; Atarashi, Y.; et al. A novel highly quantitative and reproducible assay for the detection of anti-SARS-CoV-2 IgG and IgM antibodies. *Sci. Rep.* **2021**, *11*, 5198. [CrossRef] [PubMed]
22. Taylor, J.J.; Jaedicke, K.M.; van de Merwe, R.C.; Bissett, S.M.; Landsdowne, N.; Whall, K.M.; Pickering, K.; Thornton, V.; Lawson, V.; Yatsuda, H.; et al. A Prototype Antibody-based Biosensor for Measurement of Salivary MMP-8 in Periodontitis using Surface Acoustic Wave Technology. *Sci. Rep.* **2019**, *9*, 11034. [CrossRef] [PubMed]
23. Mojsoska, B.; Larsen, S.; Olsen, D.A.; Madsen, J.S.; Brandslund, I.; AlZahra'a Alatraktchi, F. Rapid SARS-CoV-2 Detection Using Electrochemical Immunosensor. *Sensors* **2021**, *21*, 390. [CrossRef] [PubMed]
24. Galipeau, Y.; Greig, M.; Liu, G.; Driedger, M.; Langlois, M.A. Humoral Responses and Serological Assays in SARS-CoV-2 Infections. *Front. Immunol.* **2020**, *11*, 610688. [CrossRef] [PubMed]
25. Khoury, D.S.; Cromer, D.; Reynaldi, A.; Schlub, T.E.; Wheatley, A.K.; Juno, J.A.; Subbarao, K.; Kent, S.J.; Triccas, J.A.; Davenport, M.P. Neutralizing antibody levels are highly predictive of immune protection from symptomatic SARS-CoV-2 infection. *Nat. Med.* **2021**, *27*, 1205–1211. [CrossRef]
26. Peterhoff, D.; Gluck, V.; Vogel, M.; Schuster, P.; Schutz, A.; Neubert, P.; Albert, V.; Frisch, S.; Kiessling, M.; Pervan, P.; et al. A highly specific and sensitive serological assay detects SARS-CoV-2 antibody levels in COVID-19 patients that correlate with neutralization. *Infection* **2021**, *49*, 75–82. [CrossRef]
27. Perkmann, T.; Perkmann-Nagele, N.; Koller, T.; Mucher, P.; Radakovics, A.; Marculescu, R.; Wolzt, M.; Wagner, O.F.; Binder, C.J.; Haslacher, H. Anti-Spike Protein Assays to Determine SARS-CoV-2 Antibody Levels: A Head-to-Head Comparison of Five Quantitative Assays. *Microbiol. Spectr.* **2021**, *9*, e0024721. [CrossRef]

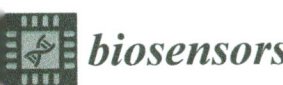

Article

A Rapid and Sensitive Microfluidics-Based Tool for Seroprevalence Immunity Assessment of COVID-19 and Vaccination-Induced Humoral Antibody Response at the Point of Care

Kritika Srinivasan Rajsri [1,2], Michael P. McRae [1], Glennon W. Simmons [1], Nicolaos J. Christodoulides [1], Hanover Matz [3], Helen Dooley [3], Akiko Koide [4], Shohei Koide [5] and John T. McDevitt [1,6,*]

1. Department of Molecular Pathobiology, Division of Biomaterials, Bioengineering Institute, New York University College of Dentistry, New York, NY 10010, USA
2. Vilcek Institute of Graduate Biomedical Sciences, New York University School of Medicine, New York, NY 10016, USA
3. Department of Microbiology and Immunology, Institute of Marine and Environmental Technology, University of Maryland School of Medicine, Baltimore, MD 21202, USA
4. Department of Medicine, NYU Grossman School of Medicine, New York, NY 10016, USA
5. Department of Biochemistry and Molecular Pharmacology, NYU Grossman School of Medicine, New York, NY 10016, USA
6. Department of Chemical and Biomolecular Engineering, NYU Tandon School of Engineering, Brooklyn, NY 11201, USA
* Correspondence: mcdevitt@nyu.edu

Citation: Rajsri, K.S.; McRae, M.P.; Simmons, G.W.; Christodoulides, N.J.; Matz, H.; Dooley, H.; Koide, A.; Koide, S.; McDevitt, J.T. A Rapid and Sensitive Microfluidics-Based Tool for Seroprevalence Immunity Assessment of COVID-19 and Vaccination-Induced Humoral Antibody Response at the Point of Care. *Biosensors* **2022**, *12*, 621. https://doi.org/10.3390/bios12080621

Received: 9 July 2022
Accepted: 6 August 2022
Published: 10 August 2022

Publisher's Note: MDPI stays neutral with regard to jurisdictional claims in published maps and institutional affiliations.

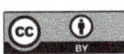

Copyright: © 2022 by the authors. Licensee MDPI, Basel, Switzerland. This article is an open access article distributed under the terms and conditions of the Creative Commons Attribution (CC BY) license (https://creativecommons.org/licenses/by/4.0/).

Abstract: As of 8 August 2022, SARS-CoV-2, the causative agent of COVID-19, has infected over 585 million people and resulted in more than 6.42 million deaths worldwide. While approved SARS-CoV-2 spike (S) protein-based vaccines induce robust seroconversion in most individuals, dramatically reducing disease severity and the risk of hospitalization, poorer responses are observed in aged, immunocompromised individuals and patients with certain pre-existing health conditions. Further, it is difficult to predict the protection conferred through vaccination or previous infection against new viral variants of concern (VoC) as they emerge. In this context, a rapid quantitative point-of-care (POC) serological assay able to quantify circulating anti-SARS-CoV-2 antibodies would allow clinicians to make informed decisions on the timing of booster shots, permit researchers to measure the level of cross-reactive antibody against new VoC in a previously immunized and/or infected individual, and help assess appropriate convalescent plasma donors, among other applications. Utilizing a lab-on-a-chip ecosystem, we present proof of concept, optimization, and validation of a POC strategy to quantitate COVID-19 humoral protection. This platform covers the entire diagnostic timeline of the disease, seroconversion, and vaccination response spanning multiple doses of immunization in a single POC test. Our results demonstrate that this platform is rapid (~15 min) and quantitative for SARS-CoV-2-specific IgG detection.

Keywords: COVID-19; SARS-CoV-2; seroprevalence; humoral immunity; diagnostics; point of care; microfluidics; clinical decision support tool

1. Introduction

Vaccines and testing play parallel roles in the COVID-19 pandemic response and containment. Multiple studies have indicated that serum binding antibodies to SARS-CoV-2 spike receptor binding domain (RBD) and S proteins and neutralizing antibodies from COVID-19 convalescent plasma are maintained from 6 months to 1 year [1–4]. Additionally, studies have shown the presence of these antibodies correlates with protection against COVID-19 [5,6]. Conversely, other studies have shown that vaccination of otherwise healthy individuals elicited B cell antibody seroconversion, neutralizing antibodies, and

T cell response-based immunity against reinfection and, importantly, protection against exhibiting severe COVID-19 for at least 6 months [7]. Although there is insufficient data on antibody titer thresholds that might indicate protection from infection, substantial evidence suggests that the immune response after infection plus vaccination typically leads to higher antibody titers [5,8–10]. These effects are not as robust in aging and immunocompromised individuals. Studies suggest that a smaller percentage of individuals seroconvert and sustain the neutralizing antibodies, making this population vulnerable to infection and potentially severe disease [11].

With at least 585 million people known to have been infected with SARS-CoV-2 worldwide to date and likely many more undetected/unreported cases, antibody responses could be measured across this population [12–14] to determine seroconversion against existing and rapidly mutating viral antigens. With the emergence of constantly mutating strains of COVID-19—some termed VoC—understanding infection history, the vaccination response, and the antibody response elicited becomes important and adds value to vaccine reception and dosage [15–17]. Thus, understanding and quantitatively screening the immune response is highly valuable, not just in immunocompromised individuals. Serosurveillance has insightful applications in diagnostics relating to COVID vaccination and/or infection elicited immune response [5,18].

There is currently significant interest in screening and understanding both humoral and cellular immunity [5,19], as our study also represents. The humoral or B cell antibody response demonstrates a significant aspect of the immunity conferred against SARS-CoV-2, being evaluated with significant importance [19–23]. Multiple labs are also assessing the cellular or T cell response to evaluate immunity induced by vaccination and/or infection [24,25]. These studies signify immense value to the understanding of immunity but have a high turnaround time, high cost, and need for skilled personnel to run an assay in a centralized lab involving stimulation of T cells and RNA purification steps prior to running an elaborate qPCR assessment of the T cell gene expression [24]. Importantly, all these immunity assessment studies represent time-consuming procedures not suitable for POC settings. Across studies, the S protein is shown to be highly immunogenic in eliciting a robust humoral response and is quite conserved among human coronaviruses [26,27]. Further, their interaction with the host cells has made them, and the less conserved RBD subunit, indispensable targets for diagnostics, vaccines, and therapeutic neutralizing antibodies [26]. Due to varying antibody levels based on individual immunity dynamics and the timeline of sample collection, the sensitivity of antibody tests may be variable, being more sensitive as the infection progresses and in individuals with established postinfection and postvaccine seroconversion [11,15,16]. Although IgM may have an early serological appearance, it usually has a low affinity to the target antigen. In contrast, IgG antibodies, which appear later, have higher titers and better affinities, making them better candidates for a detection test [28]. The enzyme-linked immunosorbent assay (ELISA) techniques commonly used in centralized clinical lab settings provide accurate and sensitive quantitative results but require long processing to result time, which delays onsite testing [29].

Over the last year, multiple microfluidics POC technologies have been reported, each quantifying viral proteins and antibodies with good precision and ease of use compared with traditional benchtop technologies [30]. Some integrated microfluidic detection systems have explored enhanced detection of SARS-CoV-2 nucleic acid compared with lateral flow assays, most based on the RT-LAMP technology [31–33]. Other POC devices with alternative microfluidics approaches—through fluorescence-based detection [34], impedance-based sensors [35], electrochemical-based sensors [36], and colorimetric detection [37]—have been reported in the past with application in infectious diseases and potential utility in the COVID-19 detection trail. Recently, some multiplexed SARS-CoV-2 antibody detection systems of interest have also been reported [38,39], although none of these have simultaneous rapid POC and quantitative capabilities.

In accordance with multiple studies demonstrating the significant value in assessing the SARS-CoV-2 antibody response in mitigating COVID-19 [19,22,40] and the ability to develop a rapidly (<20 min) quantitative and inexpensive antibody screen utilizing the anti-S RBD IgG at a POC setting, we have strived to develop an integrated lab-on-a-chip platform-based methodology that is rapid, quantitative and accurate while being easily accessible. This information, when available in quantitative, rapidly measurable POC settings, can help clinicians and scientists strategize evaluating the immune response after each vaccine dose and can also add insight toward the timing of subsequent boosts, ensure robust seroconversion in highly vulnerable patient populations and the selection of convalescent plasma donors and therapeutics to mitigate disease risk, and add essential value to vaccine perception and reception [41]. Critically, POC antibody tests are viable options for scaling up in community screening—being fast, easily accessible, and convenient.

We have recently published a general framework for implementing a POC clinical decision support system [42] that was adapted to the task of predicting mortality in cardiac patients with COVID-19 [43]. Additionally, a two-tiered system for evaluating COVID-19 prognosis in inpatient and outpatient settings was developed using data from a diverse population of patients across the New York City metropolitan area and externally validated using data from hospitals in Wuhan, China. Building upon this work, we present here the development and initial validation of a POC strategy for quantitative COVID-19 seroprevalence screening involving a SARS-CoV-2 antibody (IgG) test that covers the entire seroconversion timeline of the infection and vaccination response spanning across single and multidose vaccines—all over a single POC test. The work presented here is an important step forward toward completing the development of an integrated, accessible, and quantitative immunity screener, aiding the monitoring of seroconversion for epidemiological, preventive, and therapeutic applications at POC.

2. Materials and Methods

2.1. Immunoreagents and Buffers

All reagents used in the immunoassay were prepared with phosphate-buffered saline (PBS) buffer (Thermo Fisher Scientific Inc., Waltham, MA, USA). Additionally, a 3% bovine serum albumin (BSA) (Sigma-Aldrich, Burlington, MA, USA) solution was used for reagent stability and blocking nonspecific binding, and a sample carrier spiked in a dose-dependent manner with the analyte was also used. The RBD protein was produced in Expi293F cells transfected with the vector pCAGGS SARS-CoV-2 RBD (BEI Resources #NR-52309) following the methods of Stadlbauer et al., 2020, but using PEI as the transfection reagent, then supplementing the media with valproic acid as per Fang et al., 2017; protein purification was performed by gravity flow using Ni Sepharose excel resin (Cytiva, Marlborough, MA, USA). Antibody anti-Spike protein (RBD) (Sb#15), human IgG1-Fc fusion—Absolute antibody #ab02013-10.159, US and Canada, and nucleocapsid (NP) antigen (2019-nCoV—NP-His recombinant protein #40588-V08B, Beijing, China), and a goat antihuman IgG (H + L) cross-adsorbed secondary antibody Alexa fluor 488 (#A-11013, Invitrogen, Waltham, MA, USA) were procured. Human serum (Sigma-Aldrich; human male AB plasma, sterile-filtered) was utilized as a sample and tested spiked with or without the anti-RBD IgG antibody in different predetermined concentrations. Once acquired, the serum was tested to have not contained any pre-existing human COVID antibodies using clinical laboratory-based ELISA. For concerns of safety and toxicity of the human serum, each donor was tested and found nonreactive for HIV and hepatitis B and C antibodies by ELISA. Furthermore, the sterile-filtered human serum was heat inactivated at 56 °C for 30 min. Nevertheless, each reagent of human origin or otherwise used for this work was considered potentially infectious and handled safely with complete BSL-2 compliance.

2.2. Fabrication of the Microfluidic Cartridge

Assays were performed using prototype microfluidic cartridges and custom instrumentation and software, as described previously [44,45]. The base form of the cartridges, injection-molded polymethyl methacrylate (PMMA) prototype cartridges, were designed in-house and manufactured by Protolabs (USA). The top layers of the cartridges are constructed with 3M 9500PC double-sided adhesive and 3M AF4300 polyethylene terephthalate (3M Company, Maplewood, MN, USA) laminates, while the bottom layer utilizes Adhesives Research ARflow® 93049 material, bound to the PMMA using a table-top hydraulic lab press (Carver, Inc). This specialty adhesive is hydrophilic and wicks the sample fluid into the cartridge via capillary action. Glass fiber pads (EMD Millipore, Burlington, MA, USA) were cut into 2 × 15 mm rectangles with SummaCut D75 and used to store detecting antibodies in the card. Agarose beads sensors were contained in a modular chip that features a 4 × 5 array of hexagon-shaped wells, cast using a UV-curable photopolymer (Norland Products Inc., East Windsor, NJ, USA) on a custom machined aluminum mold and cured for 30 min. Air vents were built into the card using hydrophobic SurePVDF membranes (EMD Millipore, USA) to mitigate bubble formation. To address the concerns of toxicity through the process of fabrication of these synthetic supplies, the entire process was performed in the presence of an industry-standard filter and fume extractor (BOFA™). Additionally, all assembly was performed with the use of appropriate personal protective equipment (PPE).

2.3. Immunoassay, Imaging, and Analysis

Initial reagent validation and proof-of-concept assays were performed with Transwell membrane plates and inserts (Corning HTS Transwell—24-well permeable units w/0.4 and 3 μm polycarbonate membrane, USA) (Supplementary Figure S1). A volume of 10 μL of in-house activated conjugated agarose beads (250–300 μm size) was placed onto a polycarbonate membrane support. The phosphate-buffered saline (PBS) solution and 3% normal goat serum buffer sample (with or without anti-RBD antibody) were dispensed to the beads and incubated for 1 h while being mixed at low speed on a plate mixer. A wash was performed with 200 μL of PBS, and the beads were resuspended in the detection antibody and incubated before a final wash in PBS. After the beads settled on the membrane, they were imaged by fluorescence microscopy. The total assay time was about 4 h performed on a plate mixer. Imaging was performed using an Olympus BXFM fluorescent microscope. Images were analyzed using ImageJ (NIH) software using a region of interest (ROI) that encompassed the outer 10% of the bead sensor, calculating the corrected total cell/bead fluorescence method described in a protocol [46].

More integrated testing was completed on assay cartridges. Here, images were captured after each assay step using 5× magnification on a modified Olympus BXFM epifluorescent microscope (exposure at 1500 ms). Images were analyzed using software previously described [45], which averages the fluorescence intensity within an annular region of interest between the bead outer diameter and 90% of the bead radius. Calibration curves for the assays were completed and fit to a four-parameter logistic regression with MyCurveFit and SigmaPlot software. Unknown concentrations for samples were interpreted from the standard curve using spiked sampling methodology: 0 (Blank), 2.5, 12.8, 64, 320, and 1600, 8000, 40,000, and 200,000 ng of anti-RBD IgG/mL. Limit-of-detection (LOD) values were calculated using blank control replicates (average signal intensity plus three standard deviations). In the final stages of these studies, the complete set of chip-based measurements was completed using the fully integrated instrumentation

3. Results and Discussion

3.1. Assay Development

In order to produce lab-quality results in near-patient settings, it is necessary to have access to a testing platform that can complete all the sample processing, analyte capture, signal generation, and data processing within an integrated diagnostic platform. Using our previously described programmable bio-nano-chip (p-BNC) platform [47,48], we adapted this flexible tool to service the needs of a quantitative immunity screening device. Likewise, a quantitative microfluidics-based lab-on-a-chip POC antibody combination test was developed for the detection of anti-SARS-CoV-2 RBD IgG. Here, in-house fabricated agarose beads sensors (250–300 μm, 2% porosity), with the potential to host a variety of proteins and molecules, were utilized as the backbone for assay chemistry. Before moving these bead sensors into the final diagnostic cartridge, a surrogate method was used to optimize the bead sensor ensemble.

Likewise, the recombinant SARS-CoV-2 WA-1 RBD protein was conjugated in-house to the agarose bead sensors. Agarose beads hosting the antihuman IgG and nucleocapsid antigen were used as positive and negative controls, respectively. Initial reagent validation and proof of concept were performed with membrane plates and inserts (Supplementary Figure S1a) to serve as a surrogate test platform prior to the development of the microfluidic assays. The inserts allowed for the placement of the agarose beads onto the polycarbonate membrane while consistently being immersed in the sample buffer to allow the completion of different assay steps. Postwash beads were imaged under the fluorescence microscope by separating the inserts onto the imaging tray. The assay was performed in a sample (with and without antibody) titrated manner with appropriate controls (Supplementary Figure S1b). Images were captured on a fluorescent microscope on FITC, Cy5, and DAPI channels and stacked to generate image outputs used for analysis, followed by whole bead fluorescence measurements (Supplementary Figure S1c). A subsequent concentration vs. intensity curve was generated (Supplementary Figure S1d) to determine an initial detection range.

3.2. Assay Optimization and Instrumentation

Reagent and assay validation on the Transwell plates with inserts permitted the transition to validation and optimization of assays on the cartridge. The assay system is a fully integrated microfluidic network that functions as a portable diagnostic cartridge/reader system applicable for POC testing of a wide variety of clinical interest areas. The disposable injection-molded cartridge system consists of interconnected individual segments for parsing the various immunoassay steps, including sample and reagent introduction and delivery, fluid mixing, bubbles and debris removal, and dedicated analyte image capture through optical fluorescence signal readout. The cartridge functions through fluid/buffer delivery via three blisters and robust dual waste collection. The multilayer microfluidics immunoassay cartridge is a lab-on-a-chip platform featuring a network of microfluidic channels for sample delivery and metering, with detecting reagents embedded within the fluidic network and delivered through a series of flow steps. Additionally, mixers are patterned into the cartridge layer's channels to ensure homogenous reagent delivery of fluids across the bead array (Figure 1A). Any bubbles entrained in flow are captured by the hydrophobic filter membrane material designed specifically as bubble trap structures. The analyte capture segment houses the 4×5 format bead array, with each vertically tapering well able to house a 250–300 µm agarose bead (Figure 1B), which accommodates the immunocomplex (Figure 1C). This design allows for connected fluid/buffer transport over the beads, allowing robust analyte capture across the 3D matrix of the porous agarose sensors and subsequent ease of quantitation. In addition, the reader features advanced optics, a complementary metal oxide semiconductor (CMOS) camera, a focus actuator, blister actuators, an external and internal code scanner, an integrated computer, display, and software to support automated analysis (Figure 1D). This evolution of this instrumentation system is summarized in Supplementary Figure S2.

This unified mini-sensor system allows for multiplexing biomarker detection and quantification of analyte and parallel immunoassay platforms while simultaneously helping translate tedious benchtop chemistry steps to POC. Each of these microporous ensemble beads hosts a network of 'nano net' structures that significantly increase the signal capture footprint and directly influence the assay timeline while being sensitive microsponge-like mediums. Recently, some groups have also shown significant applications of other nanotechnology and similar hydrogel-like materials; in diagnostics, vaccine delivery, and therapeutics, including polyanhydride, chitosan, poly(lactic-co-glycolic acid), and gold nanoparticles, among others [49]. Our novel biomimetic 'nano net' adapters resemble hydrogels and demonstrate a uniquely advanced application of nanotechnology in diagnostic applications, the other exception being gold nanoparticles capped with antisense oligonucleotide for detecting viral RNA in a sample [49].

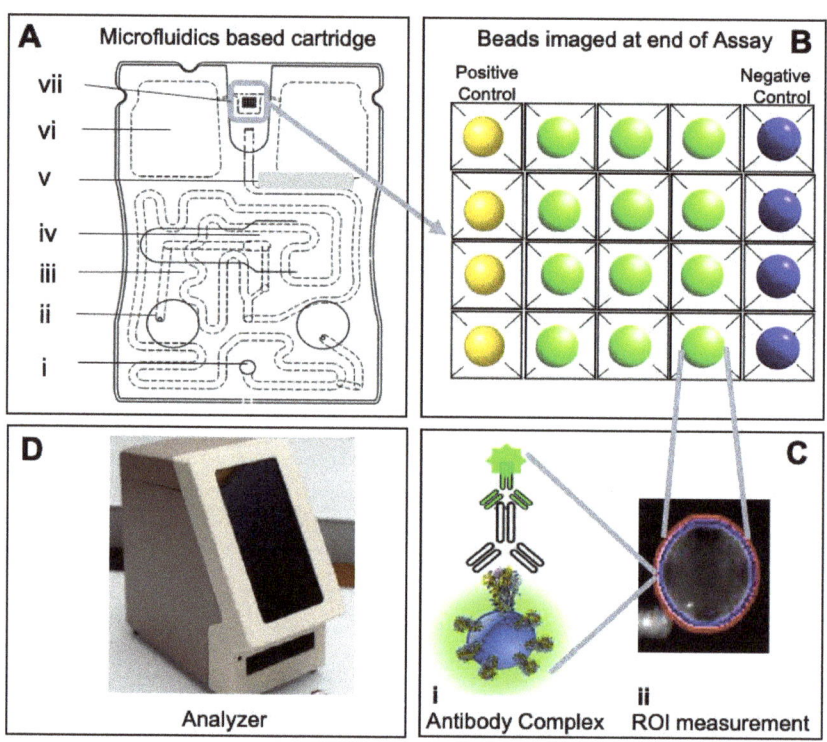

Figure 1. The point-of-care microfluidics-based combination antigen/antibody assay cartridge and analyzer. Illustration of assay cartridge (**A**) with sample input port (i), syringe pump adapter port (ii), sample loop (iii), glass fiber pad slot for detection reagent (iv), bubble trap (v), waste reservoir chamber (vi), and 4 × 5 bead array chamber (vii) shows an array of 20 programmable agarose bead sensors (**B**), with control and antibody capture beads imaged at steps 6 of the assay. The bead sensor serves as a high surface area substrate for developing programmable immunoassays for COVID-19 antibody detection and houses the immunocomplex (**C.i**). Image analysis for each individual bead sensor is performed by measuring 95% region of interest (ROI) on the bead (**C.ii**), capturing the many optimally stained and washed immune complexes formed over the bead. The integrated assay is completed in an automated fashion housed in the analyzer with optics, camera, actuator, blister actuators, integrated computer and display, and software to support automated analysis (**D**). While initial development work was completed with the aid of a commercial microscope, the final implementation was completed using the integrated instrumentation shown here.

3.3. Assay Execution and Integration

The cartridge design allows for key immunoassay complexes to form on programmable 3D agarose bead sensors contained in the bead chip, integrated into the microfluidic environment, which aids optimal analyte capture and immunoassay completion and achieves low limits of detection. The spatial arrangement and redundancy of predefined beads and controls permit multiplexing and robust quantitative measurements. After the initial sample delivery to the bead array is completed via activation of flow pumps attached to the cartridge, subsequent incubation allows the capture of the analyte to the 3D bead sensor containing the capture reagent. The sample is delivered by pushing flow in through the right fluid input, which displaces the sample fluid to the bead sensors. Here the target-specific antibody present in the sample binds to the SARS-CoV-2 spike RBD bound to the bead sensor. After the sample is depleted, the composition of the flow grades to PBS buffer, automatically initiating a wash step to remove unbound analytes. In the next step, PBS buffer is delivered through the middle fluid input, which reconstitutes and releases the detecting reagent from the glass reagent pad. The detection reagent binds to the anti-SARS-CoV-2 antibody, which yields a fluorescent signal. Any unbound material is removed in a final wash step that removes all debris and analytes not specifically captured by the beads. All assay steps are summarized in Figure 2.

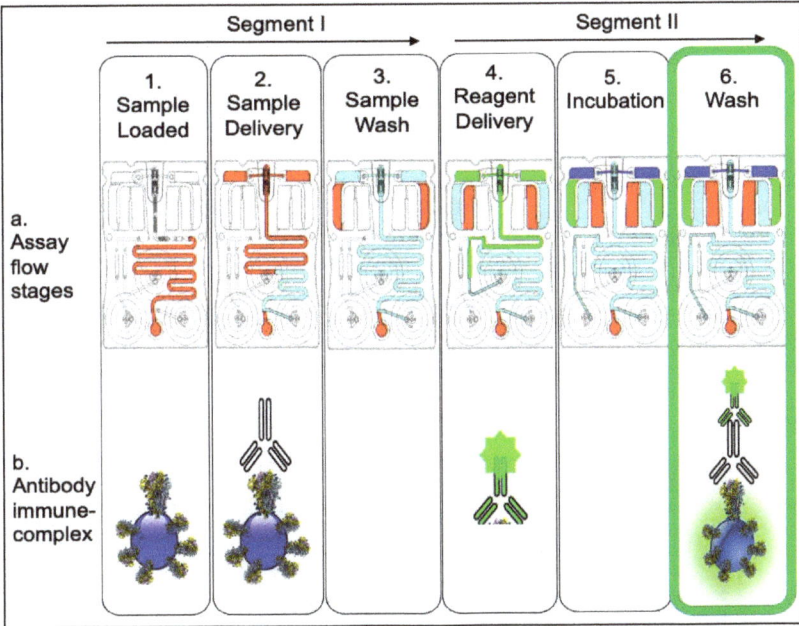

Figure 2. The COVID-19 antibody assay sequence. Step 1 shows the sample (+/− antibody) loaded to the cartridge input port, followed by sample delivery over the bead array through buffer flow via right blister (Step 2) and finished with a wash step (Step 3). Step 4 shows introduction of the antibody detection reagent conjugated to Alexa Fluor 488 that is eluted from the reagent pad over the bead array, followed by final incubation (Step 5) and final wash (Step 6) steps. In the presence of SARS-CoV-2 IgG1 antibody in the sample, the postassay completion image shows the antibody capture beads fluorescing as a result of the antibody immune complex formation (Step 6b).

Here a 100 µL total sample volume (human serum spiked with or without the antibody) was introduced to the input port of the cartridge. The detection antibodies were deposited on the glass reagent pad. Agarose beads functionalized with capture reagents (recombinant SARS-CoV-2 WA-1 RBD protein) were placed in the 4 × 5 wells, with four-fold redundancy per analyte, permitting robust variance measurement and spatial identification while multiplexing. Positive (conjugated with antihuman IgG) and negative control beads (conjugated with NP antigen beads) were placed in the first and fifth columns, respectively. The positive and negative controls represent internal quality assurance and quality control beads in which the response parameters can be used as the basis for run rejection in the event of an error. A standard protocol was developed using automated fluid routing to control buffer flow across priming, sample/reagent delivery and incubation, and wash for sample (segment I: stages 1–3) and reagent (segment II: stages 4–6) introduction (Figure 2).

By actuating two different fluidic streams, approximately 350 µL of PBS was passed over the beads during each segment of the assay. Total time for each assay segment was approx. 5 min, and the total assay time was 15 min. For these initial experiments, the bead sensor priming, sample delivery, reagent incubation, and wash steps were performed using syringe pumps attached to the cartridge platform and imaged under the fluorescent microscope. Importantly, these lab-based research tools have been shown to produce nearly identical results as the fully integrated single push of the button point-of-care instrumentation described previously [44]. Integrated measurements that replicate the function and performance of the microscope and external syringe pump measurements were also completed for the studies presented here (see below). The formation of completed immune complexes (Figure 2—6b) over the 3D beads allows them to fluoresce in the FITC channel, captured under consistent imaging settings across samples.

After the initial validation and optimization studies were complete, standard curves for the antibody (anti-spike RBD) were completed with the five-fold serially diluted anti-RBD IgG-spiked sample buffer (Figure 3A), covering a range from very high Ig titers (200 µg IgG per ml) to very low titers (2 ng IgG per ml), as indicated in the recent literature [13,14,50]. Image analysis extracts the fluorescent intensity of the beads (Figure 3B), generating data sets to measure variances and signal-to-noise ratios. The resulting standard curves show increases in fluorescence intensity proportional to target analyte (IgG) concentration, with intra-assay precision ranging from 10–20%, encompassing a wide range required to cover the potential physiological range of anti-RBD antibody detection (Figure 3C). The limit-of-detection (LOD) calculations suggest 47 ng/mL for anti-SARS-CoV-2 IgG antibody detection, consistent with the lower biological threshold that would indicate positive SARS-CoV-2 antibody detection. Assay functionality was further demonstrated by the signal-to-noise ratio (SNR), showing a robust monotonic increase from low to high loads (SNR ~1 to 15, respectively) (Figure 3D).

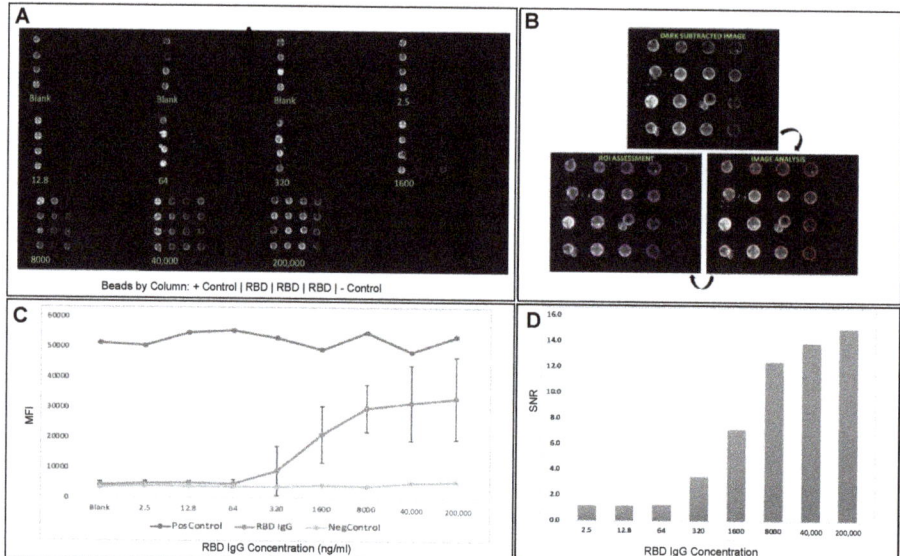

Figure 3. Fluorescent images show bead sensor arrangement and captured analyte, with variation in signal intensity at various concentrations (**A**). Image analysis was performed by measuring 95% ROI on sensor beads on a dark subtracted image captured during last stage of assay (**B**). The SARS-CoV-2 antibody concentration was assessed on the McDevitt lab point-of-care quantitative immunity scoring assay tool, and the dose curve here depicts a dynamic range between 10^0 and 10^5 (with potential to capture titers up to ~10^6); all values depicted in the curve are represented by mean and error bars—standard deviation (**C**). Subsequently, signal-to-noise ratio (SNR) was calculated to indicate assay robustness and functionality (**D**).

Following the completion of the assay development and initial validation, it will be necessary to develop and clinically model the sample collection methodology that will be used within an integrated POC setting. A critical part of this process is to translate the assay parameters to completely integrated metrics, and we have most recently demonstrated a successful integration and validation of the immunity screening assay onto the existing p-BNC technology, as seen in Figure 4. The initial developments described here pave the pathway for the movement of immunity screening methods into real-world clinical practice. These integrated tests have the potential to reduce the time and costs associated with currently available approaches that target antibody detection via clinical lab-based tests, helping to address unmet needs in community settings and, in doing so, address concerns about the current gaps in testing associated with remote laboratory testing. This also reduces plastic waste and infectious material waste, which is better for the environment and reduces cost. In comparing this technology with other microfluidics-based POC tests [51], we demonstrate the advances and advantages of our technology and instrumentation in the ease of handling, including minimal training to run the assay, high sensitivity while being quantitative, and a potential capability to be coupled with smart devices and cloud services for ease of data transmission and tether patient history and other datasets for comprehensive diagnostic reporting, demonstrated in our previous work [43,52,53].

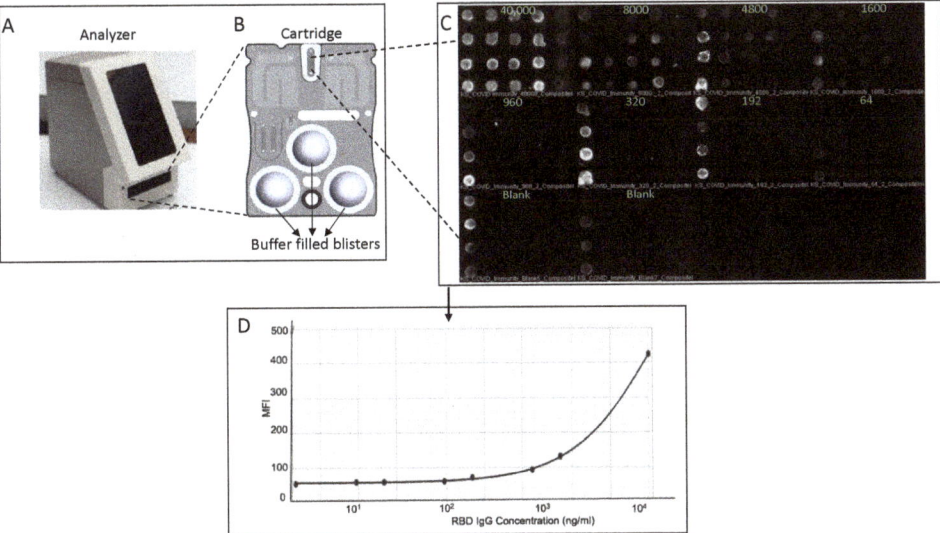

Figure 4. Initial proof of concept and reagent validation demonstration in an integrated POC format. The analyzer (**A**) with inserted blister mounted cartridge (**B**) allows for assay automation through integration of blister actuation, imaging, and data analysis, with visual engagement of each step through the touchscreen interface. Blank (no antibody) and positive (antibody present) sample assays were run on the integrated platform, and images were captured postassay run (**C**), followed by bead-to-bead fluorescent intensity measurement, data analysis followed by generation of dose–response curve (**D**).

3.4. Development of Immunity Assessment

Having developed a robust assay and having shown its functionality in both lab-based and integrated instrumentation, our next step involved the exploration of how these assays might be used in the context of a clinical decision support tool. To explore this area, we also combined data sets from the recent literature that observe seroconversion responses, allowing us to model and compare antibody responses, including naïve and vaccinated data points (Figure 5A). This data helped generate a foundation for the immunity screening range, indicating individuals demonstrating no immunity at the lower end, partially immune moderate antibody response, and fully immune antibody titers at the highest range, corroborating with vaccination status and/or history of previous infection with vaccination adding a booster response. We have then overlaid these reference ranges to our standard curve, indicating the coverage of this range on our platform, as well as the ability to quantitatively report the antibody response (Figure 5B).

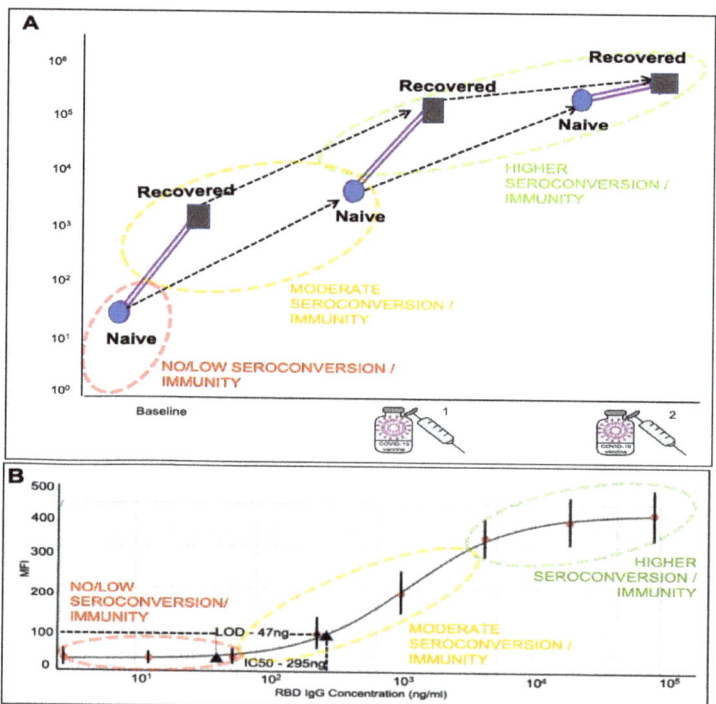

Figure 5. Median SARS-CoV-2 spike antibody titers compared in COVID-19 naïve (round blue end dots) vs. recovered square gray end dots) individuals—prevaccination and postvaccination, across six study data sets (Samanovic et al., Saadat et al., Stamatatos et al., Krammer et al., Rishi R. Goel et al., Joseph E. Ebinger et al.) (**A**). Panel (**B**) shows a standard curve from Figure 3C now depicting the SARS-CoV-2 antibody concentrations assessed on the McDevitt lab point-of-care quantitative immunity scoring assay tool, fitting the physiological range for anti-spike IgG antibody response, as seen above.

Backing the concept of a POC immunity screen, recent studies have made suggestions that individuals with prior infection exposure, leading to seroconversion, may achieve high antibody titers post one vaccine dosage compared with previously noninfected individuals [15]. In one study, the median baseline IgG antibody titers were 3–4 logs higher in the SARS-CoV-2 recovered compared with SARS-CoV-2 naïve individuals [54]. In the postvaccination, infection-recovered individuals were able to maintain a 1-to-2-log higher IgG titer than infection-naïve individuals only after the dose [13,55]. However, the booster (2nd) dose was able to raise the IgG tiers in infection-naïve individuals to the same levels as infection-recovered individuals. Surprisingly, the increase in IgG tiers was significantly improved in infection-naïve individuals after both doses but seemed to plateau after the first dose in infection-recovered subjects [12–14,54–57]. Other studies have shown similar results, with infection-recovered individuals showing higher antibody titers post the first dose but infection-naïve individuals requiring a second dose to improve their antibody titers to match that of the former (data points from these studies have been summarized and modeled in Figure 5A) [12,13,50,54–56].

Recent studies indicate that vaccination elicits distinct B cell and T cell responses between infection-recovered and -naïve subjects, pointing toward a robust antibody recall post the first dose of vaccine in the former group [54,55,58]. Thus, this indicates the importance for previously seropositive individuals to require vaccination to achieve significantly increased seroconversion with each vaccine dose. Serological testing alongside vaccination may add significant value in assessing prior and currently infected individuals who remain undiagnosed or undocumented [59], aiding in disease prevention, the assessment of potential convalescent plasma donors [60], and seroprevalence and serosurveillance studies [5]. Further, with a constant evolutionary race between the virus and host response, screening antibody titers in post vaccinated individuals may also provide insight into the efficacy and robust seroconversion against the newer VoC. Our tool can be tailored and multiplexed rapidly to sensitively screen antibody responses from the newer viral mutations. Antibody/seroconversion screening will potentially be utilized in upcoming months by epidemiological, healthcare, and various governing bodies, tailoring guidelines toward bringing societal normalcy and, importantly, managing immunocompromised and aging individuals [12–14,50,61].

The POC tools with enhanced diagnostic accuracy could be used in easily accessible settings with the potential to have a dramatic influence on community screening and immunity profiling alongside safe management of COVID-19 spread. With the advent of COVID-19 vaccinations playing a role in disease prevention, robust immune responses in individuals postvaccination will not only play a protective role individually but also achieve herd immunity [5]. Continuous improvements in diagnostic tests are essential for rapid detection of patients, surveillance, and healthcare preparedness, both in high- and low-resource settings. While these kits are not currently available for widespread use, public and private organizations worldwide are working on prototypes, with over 50 currently in development [62]. To date, these new diagnostic tests have been developed outside an integrated screening procedure. The development and customization of diagnostic tests is a key priority alongside its use with gated patient screening and risk-based triage procedures. None of the existing diagnostic tests cover the initial screening process, comprehensive POC diagnostic testing, as well as immunity screening for community risk assessment.

A significant challenge faced in the development of various tests in the diagnostic menu, including antibody-specific assays, relates to the highly evolving viral strain and cross-reactivity between other coronaviruses (SARS-CoV, MERS), as well as lowered sensitivity due to epitope changes/mismatches [63]. These issues can be mitigated through optimization of reagent sources, subtypes, blocking strategies, assay flow rates, and volumes. Further, limitations of this testing strategy include obtaining negative results in patients during the early incubation period of an ongoing infection later becoming infectious. Cost, complexity, and supply chain shortages are bottlenecks for scaling SARS-CoV-2 immunity screening. This work serves to demonstrate a new technology for assessing antibodies to screen immunity associated with COVID-19 and vaccination. This promising tool can be implemented in high-risk settings requiring rapid, cost-effective, convenient, and accurate screening results. The next steps of this study will explore the analytical performance of this system and will involve the assessment of qualitative performance (sensitivity and specificity) and blinded validation of the combinatorial format with the "spiked sera" and "patient samples" compared with control samples, confirmed by RT-PCR and lab-based serological testing methods. Data from these studies will be collected to the end of precision studies and clinical validation, including logistic regression modeling, to generate ROC curves and correlation assessment. Additionally, longitudinal, multi-time point assessments will be made to assess changes in immunity across horizontal timelines. Establishing sensitivity and specificity for POC tests is a critical step in establishing their efficiency as a diagnostic screening tool. Either in the current assay state, progressing toward initial clinical validation, or introducing evidence-based changes into the assay format (that is, swapping reagents or adding additional data points for improving testing efficiency) would entail rigorous reagent assessment through validation, optimization, and quantitation—requiring a robust supply chain of working reagents. The use of a programmable diagnostics platform, as described in this study already, allows for an agile approach well suited for this dynamically changing infectious disease target.

4. Conclusions

In closing, we have developed a novel application of a programmable microfluidic platform for rapid, accurate, and quantitative detection of SARS-CoV-2-specific humoral response to assess seroprevalence and humoral immunity. These new integrated medical microdevice systems have the potential to help profile the immune status of individuals, informing public health strategies: risk stratification of individuals, particularly in the aging and immune-compromised population, to isolate the variables contributing to increased morbidity and mortality, rational designing and deployment of vaccine doses, rapid identification of a convalescent plasma donor, a better understanding of the mechanisms of immunity, facilitate individual or institutional decision-making, and epidemiological monitoring of seroconversion. We believe that understanding the specific role of the humoral response to SARS-CoV-2, gathered in a rapid quantitative POC setting, can complement the lab-based cellular and humoral immune response assessments to further mitigate our vulnerability to the virus.

Supplementary Materials: The following supporting information can be downloaded at: https://www.mdpi.com/article/10.3390/bios12080621/s1, Figure S1: Immunoassay on Transwell plates with inserts (a) were performed for initial proof of concept and reagent validation studies. Antibody titration was also performed alongside controls and imaged under a fluorescent microscope (b). The images were examined with the ImageJ (NIH) software and individual beads analyzed with whole bead fluorescence intensity measurement method (c), and intensity vs. concentration dataset generated (d). Figure S2: This illustration shows the evolution of instrumentation and the fluidics system that were used to capture the measurements completed in this manuscript.

Author Contributions: Conceptualization, K.S.R. and J.T.M.; methodology, K.S.R., M.P.M., G.W.S., N.J.C., H.D., S.K. and J.T.M.; software, K.S.R., M.P.M. and J.T.M.; validation, K.S.R. and J.T.M.; formal analysis, K.S.R. and J.T.M.; investigation, K.S.R., M.P.M., G.W.S., N.J.C. and J.T.M.; resources, K.S.R., H.M., H.D., A.K., S.K. and J.T.M.; data curation, K.S.R., M.P.M., G.W.S., N.J.C. and J.T.M.; writing—original draft preparation, K.S.R.; writing—review and editing, K.S.R., M.P.M., G.W.S., N.J.C., H.D., S.K. and J.T.M.; visualization, K.S.R., M.P.M., G.W.S. and J.T.M.; supervision, H.D., S.K. and J.T.M.; project administration, K.S.R., G.W.S. and J.T.M.; funding acquisition, J.T.M. All authors have read and agreed to the published version of the manuscript.

Funding: This research was funded by the Renaissance Health Service Corporation and Delta Dental of Michigan. Funding was also provided by the NIH through the National Institute on Drug Abuse (NIH grant no. R42DA041959). The content is solely the responsibility of the authors and does not necessarily represent or reflect the views of the funding agencies.

Institutional Review Board Statement: Not applicable.

Informed Consent Statement: Not applicable.

Data Availability Statement: Data is contained within the article and Supplementary Material. The data presented in this study are available across the Figures and Supplementary Figure S1 in this manuscript. Further information and data presented in this study are available on request from the corresponding author.

Acknowledgments: Malvin Janal is thanked for his comments on the manuscript. Mike Murray, Steve Dietl, Bob Mehalso, Todd Haran, Roger Markham, Dwight Petruchik, and Bob Altavela of SensoDx are thanked for their contributions to the development of the integrated immunoassay infrastructure shown in Supplementary Figure S2C.

Conflicts of Interest: J.T.M., M.P.M., N.J.C. and K.S.R. have a patent pending based in part on the work presented in this manuscript. M.P.M. has served as a paid consultant for SensoDx and has a provisional patent pending. N.J.C. has a provisional patent pending. J.T.M. has a provisional patent pending. In addition, he has an ownership position and an equity interest in SensoDx II LLC and OraLiva, Inc. All other authors declare no competing interest.

References

1. L'Huillier, A.G.; Meyer, B.; Andrey, D.O.; Arm-Vernez, I.; Baggio, S.; Didierlaurent, A.; Eberhardt, C.S.; Eckerle, I.; Grasset-Salomon, C.; Huttner, A.; et al. Antibody Persistence in the First 6 Months Following SARS-CoV-2 Infection among Hospital Workers: A Prospective Longitudinal Study. *Clin. Microbiol. Infect.* **2021**, *27*, 784.e1–784.e8. [CrossRef] [PubMed]
2. Wang, H.; Yuan, Y.; Xiao, M.; Chen, L.; Zhao, Y.; Zhang, H.; Long, P.; Zhou, Y.; Xu, X.; Lei, Y.; et al. Dynamics of the SARS-CoV-2 Antibody Response up to 10 Months after Infection. *Cell. Mol. Immunol.* **2021**, *18*, 1832–1834. [CrossRef]
3. Wu, J.; Liang, B.; Chen, C.; Wang, H.; Fang, Y.; Shen, S.; Yang, X.; Wang, B.; Chen, L.; Chen, Q.; et al. SARS-CoV-2 Infection Induces Sustained Humoral Immune Responses in Convalescent Patients Following Symptomatic COVID-19. *Nat. Commun.* **2021**, *12*, 1813. [CrossRef] [PubMed]
4. Pirofski, L. Disease Severity and Durability of the Severe Acute Respiratory Syndrome Coronavirus 2 (SARS-CoV-2) Antibody Response: A View Through the Lens of the Second Year of the Pandemic. *Clin. Infect. Dis.* **2021**, *73*, e1345–e1347. [CrossRef] [PubMed]
5. National Center for Immunization and Respiratory Diseases (NCIRD); Division of Viral Diseases Science Brief. SARS-CoV-2 Infection-Induced and Vaccine-Induced Immunity. Available online: https://www.cdc.gov/coronavirus/2019-ncov/science/science-briefs/vaccine-induced-immunity.html (accessed on 18 May 2022).
6. Dan, J.M.; Mateus, J.; Kato, Y.; Hastie, K.M.; Yu, E.D.; Faliti, C.E.; Grifoni, A.; Ramirez, S.I.; Haupt, S.; Frazier, A.; et al. Immunological Memory to SARS-CoV-2 Assessed for up to 8 Months after Infection. *Science* **2021**, *371*, eabf4063. [CrossRef] [PubMed]
7. Radbruch, A.; Chang, H.-D. A Long-Term Perspective on Immunity to COVID. *Nature* **2021**, *595*, 359–360. [CrossRef]
8. Hall, V.; Foulkes, S.; Insalata, F.; Kirwan, P.; Saei, A.; Atti, A.; Wellington, E.; Khawam, J.; Munro, K.; Cole, M.; et al. Protection against SARS-CoV-2 after COVID-19 Vaccination and Previous Infection. *N. Engl. J. Med.* **2022**, *386*, 1207–1220. [CrossRef]
9. Bates, T.A.; McBride, S.K.; Leier, H.C.; Guzman, G.; Lyski, Z.L.; Schoen, D.; Winders, B.; Lee, J.-Y.; Lee, D.X.; Messer, W.B.; et al. Vaccination before or after SARS-CoV-2 Infection Leads to Robust Humoral Response and Antibodies That Effectively Neutralize Variants. *Sci. Immunol.* **2022**, *7*, eabn8014. [CrossRef]
10. Walls, A.C.; Sprouse, K.R.; Bowen, J.E.; Joshi, A.; Franko, N.; Navarro, M.J.; Stewart, C.; Cameroni, E.; McCallum, M.; Goecker, E.A.; et al. SARS-CoV-2 Breakthrough Infections Elicit Potent, Broad, and Durable Neutralizing Antibody Responses. *Cell* **2022**, *185*, 872–880.e3. [CrossRef]
11. Bergman, P.; Blennow, O.; Hansson, L.; Mielke, S.; Nowak, P.; Chen, P.; Söderdahl, G.; Österborg, A.; Smith, C.I.E.; Wullimann, D.; et al. Safety and Efficacy of the MRNA BNT162b2 Vaccine against SARS-CoV-2 in Five Groups of Immunocompromised Patients and Healthy Controls in a Prospective Open-Label Clinical Trial. *eBioMedicine* **2021**, *74*, 103705. [CrossRef]
12. Saadat, S.; Tehrani, Z.R.; Logue, J.; Newman, M.; Frieman, M.B.; Harris, A.D.; Sajadi, M.M. Single Dose Vaccination in Healthcare Workers Previously Infected with SARS-CoV-2. In *Infectious Diseases (except HIV/AIDS)*; Elsevier: Amsterdam, The Netherlands, 2021.
13. Krammer, F.; Srivastava, K.; the PARIS Team; Simon, V. Robust Spike Antibody Responses and Increased Reactogenicity in Seropositive Individuals after a Single Dose of SARS-CoV-2 MRNA Vaccine. In *Allergy and Immunology*; Elsevier: Amsterdam, The Netherlands, 2021.
14. Samanovic, M.I.; Cornelius, A.R.; Gray-Gaillard, S.L.; Allen, J.R.; Karmacharya, T.; Wilson, J.P.; Hyman, S.W.; Tuen, M.; Koralov, S.B.; Mulligan, M.J.; et al. Robust Immune Responses after One Dose of BNT162b2 MRNA Vaccine Dose in SARS-CoV-2 Experienced Individuals. In *Infectious Diseases (except HIV/AIDS)*; Elsevier: Amsterdam, The Netherlands, 2021.
15. Bates, T.A.; McBride, S.K.; Winders, B.; Schoen, D.; Trautmann, L.; Curlin, M.E.; Tafesse, F.G. Antibody Response and Variant Cross-Neutralization After SARS-CoV-2 Breakthrough Infection. *JAMA* **2022**, *327*, 179. [CrossRef] [PubMed]
16. Feikin, D.R.; Higdon, M.M.; Abu-Raddad, L.J.; Andrews, N.; Araos, R.; Goldberg, Y.; Groome, M.J.; Huppert, A.; O'Brien, K.L.; Smith, P.G.; et al. Duration of Effectiveness of Vaccines against SARS-CoV-2 Infection and COVID-19 Disease: Results of a Systematic Review and Meta-Regression. *Lancet* **2022**, *399*, 924–944. [CrossRef]
17. Andrews, N.; Stowe, J.; Kirsebom, F.; Toffa, S.; Rickeard, T.; Gallagher, E.; Gower, C.; Kall, M.; Groves, N.; O'Connell, A.-M.; et al. COVID-19 Vaccine Effectiveness against the Omicron (B.1.1.529) Variant. *N. Engl. J. Med.* **2022**, *386*, 1532–1546. [CrossRef] [PubMed]
18. CDC Cases, Data, and Surveillance. Available online: https://www.cdc.gov/coronavirus/2019-ncov/covid-data/seroprevalance-surveys-tell-us.html (accessed on 29 June 2022).
19. Wyllie, D.; Jones, H.E.; Mulchandani, R.; Trickey, A.; Taylor-Phillips, S.; Brooks, T.; Charlett, A.; Ades, A.; EDSAB-HOME investigators; Moore, P.; et al. SARS-CoV-2 Responsive T Cell Numbers and Anti-Spike IgG Levels Are Both Associated with Protection from COVID-19: A Prospective Cohort Study in Keyworkers. In *Infectious Diseases (except HIV/AIDS)*; Elsevier: Amsterdam, The Netherlands, 2020.

20. Hu, C.; Li, D.; Liu, Z.; Ren, L.; Su, J.; Zhu, M.; Feng, Y.; Wang, Z.; Liu, Q.; Zhu, B.; et al. Exploring Rapid and Effective Screening Methods for Anti-SARS-CoV-2 Neutralizing Antibodies in COVID-19 Convalescent Patients and Longitudinal Vaccinated Populations. *Pathogens* **2022**, *11*, 171. [CrossRef]
21. Khoury, D.S.; Cromer, D.; Reynaldi, A.; Schlub, T.E.; Wheatley, A.K.; Juno, J.A.; Subbarao, K.; Kent, S.J.; Triccas, J.A.; Davenport, M.P. Neutralizing Antibody Levels Are Highly Predictive of Immune Protection from Symptomatic SARS-CoV-2 Infection. *Nat. Med.* **2021**, *27*, 1205–1211. [CrossRef]
22. Wang, Z.; Schmidt, F.; Weisblum, Y.; Muecksch, F.; Barnes, C.O.; Finkin, S.; Schaefer-Babajew, D.; Cipolla, M.; Gaebler, C.; Lieberman, J.A.; et al. MRNA Vaccine-Elicited Antibodies to SARS-CoV-2 and Circulating Variants. *Nature* **2021**, *592*, 616–622. [CrossRef]
23. Cromer, D.; Juno, J.A.; Khoury, D.; Reynaldi, A.; Wheatley, A.K.; Kent, S.J.; Davenport, M.P. Prospects for Durable Immune Control of SARS-CoV-2 and Prevention of Reinfection. *Nat. Rev. Immunol.* **2021**, *21*, 395–404. [CrossRef]
24. Schwarz, M.; Torre, D.; Lozano-Ojalvo, D.; Tan, A.T.; Tabaglio, T.; Mzoughi, S.; Sanchez-Tarjuelo, R.; Le Bert, N.; Lim, J.M.E.; Hatem, S.; et al. Rapid, Scalable Assessment of SARS-CoV-2 Cellular Immunity by Whole-Blood PCR. *Nat. Biotechnol.* **2022**, 1–10. [CrossRef]
25. Moss, P. The T Cell Immune Response against SARS-CoV-2. *Nat. Immunol.* **2022**, *23*, 186–193. [CrossRef]
26. Amanat, F.; Krammer, F. SARS-CoV-2 Vaccines: Status Report. *Immunity* **2020**, *52*, 583–589. [CrossRef]
27. Yang, Y.; Du, L. SARS-CoV-2 Spike Protein: A Key Target for Eliciting Persistent Neutralizing Antibodies. *Signal Transduct. Target. Ther.* **2021**, *6*, 95. [CrossRef] [PubMed]
28. Peeling, R.W.; Heymann, D.L.; Teo, Y.-Y.; Garcia, P.J. Diagnostics for COVID-19: Moving from Pandemic Response to Control. *Lancet* **2022**, *399*, 757–768. [CrossRef]
29. Amanat, F.; Stadlbauer, D.; Strohmeier, S.; Nguyen, T.H.O.; Chromikova, V.; McMahon, M.; Jiang, K.; Arunkumar, G.A.; Jurczyszak, D.; Polanco, J.; et al. A Serological Assay to Detect SARS-CoV-2 Seroconversion in Humans. *Nat. Med.* **2020**, *26*, 1033–1036. [CrossRef] [PubMed]
30. Song, Q.; Sun, X.; Dai, Z.; Gao, Y.; Gong, X.; Zhou, B.; Wu, J.; Wen, W. Point-of-Care Testing Detection Methods for COVID-19. *Lab. Chip* **2021**, *21*, 1634–1660. [CrossRef] [PubMed]
31. Huang, W.E.; Lim, B.; Hsu, C.; Xiong, D.; Wu, W.; Yu, Y.; Jia, H.; Wang, Y.; Zeng, Y.; Ji, M.; et al. RT-LAMP for Rapid Diagnosis of Coronavirus SARS-CoV-2. *Microb. Biotechnol.* **2020**, *13*, 950–961. [CrossRef]
32. Ganguli, A.; Mostafa, A.; Berger, J.; Aydin, M.Y.; Sun, F.; de Ramirez, S.A.S.; Valera, E.; Cunningham, B.T.; King, W.P.; Bashir, R. Rapid Isothermal Amplification and Portable Detection System for SARS-CoV-2. *Proc. Natl. Acad. Sci. USA* **2020**, *117*, 22727–22735. [CrossRef]
33. Dao Thi, V.L.; Herbst, K.; Boerner, K.; Meurer, M.; Kremer, L.P.; Kirrmaier, D.; Freistaedter, A.; Papagiannidis, D.; Galmozzi, C.; Stanifer, M.L.; et al. A Colorimetric RT-LAMP Assay and LAMP-Sequencing for Detecting SARS-CoV-2 RNA in Clinical Samples. *Sci. Transl. Med.* **2020**, *12*, eabc7075. [CrossRef]
34. Seia, M.A.; Pereira, S.V.; Fontán, C.A.; De Vito, I.E.; Messina, G.A.; Raba, J. Laser-Induced Fluorescence Integrated in a Microfluidic Immunosensor for Quantification of Human Serum IgG Antibodies to Helicobacter Pylori. *Sens. Actuators B Chem.* **2012**, *168*, 297–302. [CrossRef]
35. Valera, E.; Berger, J.; Hassan, U.; Ghonge, T.; Liu, J.; Rappleye, M.; Winter, J.; Abboud, D.; Haidry, Z.; Healey, R.; et al. A Microfluidic Biochip Platform for Electrical Quantification of Proteins. *Lab. Chip* **2018**, *18*, 1461–1470. [CrossRef]
36. Pereira, S.V.; Raba, J.; Messina, G.A. IgG Anti-Gliadin Determination with an Immunological Microfluidic System Applied to the Automated Diagnostic of the Celiac Disease. *Anal. Bioanal. Chem.* **2010**, *396*, 2921–2927. [CrossRef]
37. Sanjay, S.T.; Dou, M.; Sun, J.; Li, X. A Paper/Polymer Hybrid Microfluidic Microplate for Rapid Quantitative Detection of Multiple Disease Biomarkers. *Sci. Rep.* **2016**, *6*, 30474. [CrossRef] [PubMed]
38. Rodriguez-Moncayo, R.; Cedillo-Alcantar, D.F.; Guevara-Pantoja, P.E.; Chavez-Pineda, O.G.; Hernandez-Ortiz, J.A.; Amador-Hernandez, J.U.; Rojas-Velasco, G.; Sanchez-Muñoz, F.; Manzur-Sandoval, D.; Patino-Lopez, L.D.; et al. A High-Throughput Multiplexed Microfluidic Device for COVID-19 Serology Assays. *Lab. Chip* **2021**, *21*, 93–104. [CrossRef] [PubMed]
39. Lin, Q.; Wen, D.; Wu, J.; Liu, L.; Wu, W.; Fang, X.; Kong, J. Microfluidic Immunoassays for Sensitive and Simultaneous Detection of IgG/IgM/Antigen of SARS-CoV-2 within 15 Min. *Anal. Chem.* **2020**, *92*, 9454–9458. [CrossRef] [PubMed]
40. Hansen, C.B.; Jarlhelt, I.; Pérez-Alós, L.; Hummelshøj Landsy, L.; Loftager, M.; Rosbjerg, A.; Helgstrand, C.; Bjelke, J.R.; Egebjerg, T.; Jardine, J.G.; et al. SARS-CoV-2 Antibody Responses Are Correlated to Disease Severity in COVID-19 Convalescent Individuals. *J. Immunol.* **2021**, *206*, 109–117. [CrossRef]
41. Cheng, M.P.; Yansouni, C.P.; Basta, N.E.; Desjardins, M.; Kanjilal, S.; Paquette, K.; Caya, C.; Semret, M.; Quach, C.; Libman, M.; et al. Serodiagnostics for Severe Acute Respiratory Syndrome–Related Coronavirus 2: A Narrative Review. *Ann. Intern. Med.* **2020**, *173*, 450–460. [CrossRef]
42. McRae, M.P.; Simmons, G.; Wong, J.; McDevitt, J.T. Programmable Bio-Nanochip Platform: A Point-of-Care Biosensor System with the Capacity to Learn. *Acc. Chem. Res.* **2016**, *49*, 1359–1368. [CrossRef]
43. McRae, M.P.; Simmons, G.W.; Christodoulides, N.J.; Lu, Z.; Kang, S.K.; Fenyo, D.; Alcorn, T.; Dapkins, I.P.; Sharif, I.; Vurmaz, D.; et al. Clinical Decision Support Tool and Rapid Point-of-Care Platform for Determining Disease Severity in Patients with COVID-19. *Lab. Chip* **2020**, *20*, 2075–2085. [CrossRef]

44. Shadfan, B.H.; Simmons, A.R.; Simmons, G.W.; Ho, A.; Wong, J.; Lu, K.H.; Bast, R.C.; McDevitt, J.T. A Multiplexable, Microfluidic Platform for the Rapid Quantitation of a Biomarker Panel for Early Ovarian Cancer Detection at the Point-of-Care. *Cancer Prev. Res.* **2015**, *8*, 37–48. [CrossRef]
45. McRae, M.P.; Simmons, G.W.; Wong, J.; Shadfan, B.; Gopalkrishnan, S.; Christodoulides, N.; McDevitt, J.T. Programmable Bio-Nano-Chip System: A Flexible Point-of-Care Platform for Bioscience and Clinical Measurements. *Lab. Chip* **2015**, *15*, 4020–4031. [CrossRef]
46. Measuring Cell Fluorescence Using ImageJ—The Open Lab Book v1.0. Available online: https://theolb.readthedocs.io/en/latest/imaging/measuring-cell-fluorescence-using-imagej.html (accessed on 29 June 2022).
47. McRae, M.P.; Bozkurt, B.; Ballantyne, C.M.; Sanchez, X.; Christodoulides, N.; Simmons, G.; Nambi, V.; Misra, A.; Miller, C.S.; Ebersole, J.L.; et al. Cardiac ScoreCard: A Diagnostic Multivariate Index Assay System for Predicting a Spectrum of Cardiovascular Disease. *Expert Syst. Appl.* **2016**, *54*, 136–147. [CrossRef]
48. Christodoulides, N.; De La Garza, R.; Simmons, G.W.; McRae, M.P.; Wong, J.; Newton, T.F.; Smith, R.; Mahoney, J.J., III; Hohenstein, J.; Gomez, S.; et al. Application of Programmable Bio-Nano-Chip System for the Quantitative Detection of Drugs of Abuse in Oral Fluids. *Drug Alcohol Depend.* **2015**, *153*, 306–313. [CrossRef] [PubMed]
49. Rashidzadeh, H.; Danafar, H.; Rahimi, H.; Mozafari, F.; Salehiabar, M.; Rahmati, M.A.; Rahamooz-Haghighi, S.; Mousazadeh, N.; Mohammadi, A.; Ertas, Y.N.; et al. Nanotechnology against the Novel Coronavirus (Severe Acute Respiratory Syndrome Coronavirus 2): Diagnosis, Treatment, Therapy and Future Perspectives. *Nanomedicine* **2021**, *16*, 497–516. [CrossRef] [PubMed]
50. Stamatatos, L.; Czartoski, J.; Wan, Y.-H.; Homad, L.J.; Rubin, V.; Glantz, H.; Neradilek, M.; Seydoux, E.; Jennewein, M.F.; MacCamy, A.J.; et al. A Single MRNA Immunization Boosts Cross-Variant Neutralizing Antibodies Elicited by SARS-CoV-2 Infection. In *Infectious Diseases (Except HIV/AIDS)*; Elsevier: Amsterdam, The Netherlands, 2021.
51. Kumar, A.; Parihar, A.; Panda, U.; Parihar, D.S. Microfluidics-Based Point-of-Care Testing (POCT) Devices in Dealing with Waves of COVID-19 Pandemic: The Emerging Solution. *ACS Appl. Bio Mater.* **2022**, *5*, 2046–2068. [CrossRef] [PubMed]
52. McRae, M.P.; Dapkins, I.P.; Sharif, I.; Anderman, J.; Fenyo, D.; Sinokrot, O.; Kang, S.K.; Christodoulides, N.J.; Vurmaz, D.; Simmons, G.W.; et al. Managing COVID-19 With a Clinical Decision Support Tool in a Community Health Network: Algorithm Development and Validation. *J. Med. Internet Res.* **2020**, *22*, e22033. [CrossRef]
53. McRae, M.P.; Modak, S.S.; Simmons, G.W.; Trochesset, D.A.; Kerr, A.R.; Thornhill, M.H.; Redding, S.W.; Vigneswaran, N.; Kang, S.K.; Christodoulides, N.J.; et al. Point-of-care Oral Cytology Tool for the Screening and Assessment of Potentially Malignant Oral Lesions. *Cancer Cytopathol.* **2020**, *128*, 207–220. [CrossRef]
54. Goel, R.R.; Apostolidis, S.A.; Painter, M.M.; Mathew, D.; Pattekar, A.; Kuthuru, O.; Gouma, S.; Hicks, P.; Meng, W.; Rosenfeld, A.M.; et al. Distinct Antibody and Memory B Cell Responses in SARS-CoV-2 Naïve and Recovered Individuals after MRNA Vaccination. *Sci. Immunol.* **2021**, *6*, eabi6950. [CrossRef]
55. Angyal, A.; Longet, S.; Moore, S.C.; Payne, R.P.; Harding, A.; Tipton, T.; Rongkard, P.; Ali, M.; Hering, L.M.; Meardon, N.; et al. T-Cell and Antibody Responses to First BNT162b2 Vaccine Dose in Previously Infected and SARS-CoV-2-Naive UK Health-Care Workers: A Multicentre Prospective Cohort Study. *Lancet Microbe* **2022**, *3*, e21–e31. [CrossRef]
56. Ebinger, J.E.; Fert-Bober, J.; Printsev, I.; Wu, M.; Sun, N.; Prostko, J.C.; Frias, E.C.; Stewart, J.L.; Van Eyk, J.E.; Braun, J.G.; et al. Antibody Responses to the BNT162b2 MRNA Vaccine in Individuals Previously Infected with SARS-CoV-2. *Nat. Med.* **2021**, *27*, 981–984. [CrossRef]
57. Krammer, F.; Srivastava, K.; Alshammary, H.; Amoako, A.A.; Awawda, M.H.; Beach, K.F.; Bermúdez-González, M.C.; Bielak, D.A.; Carreño, J.M.; Chernet, R.L.; et al. Antibody Responses in Seropositive Persons after a Single Dose of SARS-CoV-2 MRNA Vaccine. *N. Engl. J. Med.* **2021**, *384*, 1372–1374. [CrossRef]
58. Painter, M.M.; Mathew, D.; Goel, R.R.; Apostolidis, S.A.; Pattekar, A.; Kuthuru, O.; Baxter, A.E.; Herati, R.S.; Oldridge, D.A.; Gouma, S.; et al. Rapid Induction of Antigen-Specific CD4 + T Cells Guides Coordinated Humoral and Cellular Immune Responses to SARS-CoV-2 MRNA Vaccination. *Immunology* **2021**, *54*, 2133–2142.e3.
59. Reese, H.; Iuliano, A.D.; Patel, N.N.; Garg, S.; Kim, L.; Silk, B.J.; Hall, A.J.; Fry, A.; Reed, C. Estimated Incidence of Coronavirus Disease 2019 (COVID-19) Illness and Hospitalization—United States, February–September 2020. *Clin. Infect. Dis.* **2021**, *72*, e1010–e1017. [CrossRef] [PubMed]
60. Wang, H.E.; Ostrosky-Zeichner, L.; Katz, J.; Wanger, A.; Bai, Y.; Sridhar, S.; Patel, B. Screening Donors for COVID-19 Convalescent Plasma. *Transfusion* **2021**, *61*, 1047–1052. [CrossRef]
61. Fujimoto, A.B.; Yildirim, I.; Keskinocak, P. Significance of SARS-CoV-2 Specific Antibody Testing during COVID-19 Vaccine Allocation. In *Infectious Diseases (Except HIV/AIDS)*; Elsevier: Amsterdam, The Netherlands, 2021.
62. Kubina, R.; Dziedzic, A. Molecular and Serological Tests for COVID-19. A Comparative Review of SARS-CoV-2 Coronavirus Laboratory and Point-of-Care Diagnostics. *Diagnostics* **2020**, *10*, 434. [CrossRef] [PubMed]
63. Zhou, D.; Dejnirattisai, W.; Supasa, P.; Liu, C.; Mentzer, A.J.; Ginn, H.M.; Zhao, Y.; Duyvesteyn, H.M.E.; Tuekprakhon, A.; Nutalai, R.; et al. Evidence of Escape of SARS-CoV-2 Variant B.1.351 from Natural and Vaccine-Induced Sera. *Cell* **2021**, *184*, 2348–2361.e6. [CrossRef] [PubMed]

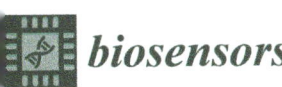

Review

Challenges in the Detection of SARS-CoV-2: Evolution of the Lateral Flow Immunoassay as a Valuable Tool for Viral Diagnosis

Nayeli Shantal Castrejón-Jiménez [1], Blanca Estela García-Pérez [2], Nydia Edith Reyes-Rodríguez [1], Vicente Vega-Sánchez [1], Víctor Manuel Martínez-Juárez [1] and Juan Carlos Hernández-González [1,*]

1. Área Académica de Medicina Veterinaria y Zootecnia, Instituto de Ciencias Agropecuarias, Universidad Autónoma del Estado de Hidalgo, Av. Universidad km 1 Exhacienda de Aquetzalpa A.P. 32, Tulancingo 43600, Mexico
2. Department of Microbiology, Instituto Politécnico Nacional, Escuela Nacional de Ciencias Biológicas Prolongación de Carpio y Plan de Ayala S/N, Col. Santo Tomás, México City 11340, Mexico
* Correspondence: juan_hernandez8281@uaeh.edu.mx; Tel.: +52-775-756-0308

Abstract: SARS-CoV-2 is an emerging infectious disease of zoonotic origin that caused the coronavirus disease in late 2019 and triggered a pandemic that has severely affected human health and caused millions of deaths. Early and massive diagnosis of SARS-CoV-2 infected patients is the key to preventing the spread of the virus and controlling the outbreak. Lateral flow immunoassays (LFIA) are the simplest biosensors. These devices are clinical diagnostic tools that can detect various analytes, including viruses and antibodies, with high sensitivity and specificity. This review summarizes the advantages, limitations, and evolution of LFIA during the SARS-CoV-2 pandemic and the challenges of improving these diagnostic devices.

Keywords: lateral flow immunoassay; biosensors; COVID-19; SARS-CoV-2; diagnosis; antibodies

1. Introduction

In December 2019, in Wuhan, China, a severe outbreak of acute respiratory illness caused by a novel beta-coronavirus identified as SARS-CoV-2 (severe acute respiratory syndrome associated coronavirus-2) was reported. The virus spread rapidly, and on 11 March 2020, the World Health Organization (WHO) declared COVID-19 (coronavirus disease-19) as a pandemic causing high severe morbidity and mortality worldwide. The reported cases globally exceed 596 million, and deaths are nearly 6.4 million as of 24 August 2022 [1].

Accurate diagnostic tests to identify the causative agent of COVID-19 are essential to prevent the spread of the virus in the population, provide prompt and timely treatment, and avoid future viral variants. The WHO recommends viral gene detection by reverse transcription-polymerase chain reaction (RT-PCR) as the gold standard for diagnosing a SARS-CoV-2 infection [2,3]. However, RT-PCR demands trained personnel, laboratory equipment, and expensive reagents, limiting its implementation in point-of-care testing (POC) in the field [4,5]. Moreover, inadequate collection of clinical specimens or poor handling of a sample during testing can result in false-negative RT-PCR [6].

The pandemic SARS-CoV-2 represents an unprecedented emergency globally, and its dissemination in the future leaves an uncertain path forward. The immunization expressed the hope for COVID-19 control and possible eradication [7]. The WHO reported that the new variant B.1.1.529, also known as omicron, has a deletion in the S gene, which can cause failure in some RT-PCR assays. Other PCR methods are proposed in these cases, such as Single Nucleotide Polymorphism (SNP) [8]. SNP assays enable the detection of single nucleotide changes within the SARS-CoV-2 genome to detect variants of concern as a complement to whole genome sequencing [8]. However, this diagnostic resource implies a high cost of specialized equipment and trained personnel.

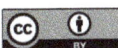

Recent advances in nanotechnology and biotechnology have enabled the development of biosensors for disease diagnosis. A conventional biosensor device consists of a bioreceptor where an immobilized biological component is supported in nanomaterials, a site that recognizes the analyte in the sample. The transducer confers classification to a biosensor by the type of signal (electric current, thermal changes, magnetic fields, etc.), which sends analog data to the processing system that converts them into digital data [9]. The biosensors developed in the diagnosis of COVID-19, according to the target molecule identified in the sample, can detect high specificity antibodies in serum or high-affinity molecules of the SARS-CoV-2 virus [10–12]. Biosensor development for SARS-CoV-2 diagnostic is a challenge to researchers. Biosensors with transducers have demonstrated superior specificity and sensitivity to other diagnostic techniques, but only under controlled laboratory conditions (known virus concentration in buffered solution or hyperimmune sera produced in laboratory animals) [13,14]. Most of these devices show poor performance when tested in clinical practice due to contaminants abundant in enzymes in pharyngeal swabs, mucus, and cellular detritus, among others. The difficulties in clinical aspects are threshold (cut-off value), qualitative or quantitative reader, and others [15]. Sometimes, the material that makes up the biosensor is not easy to obtain and manipulate, as is the case of graphene, which requires nanotechnology facilities. These devices for SARS-CoV-2 diagnostic are in the experimental phase, and most are not commercially available.

Recent decades' development of rapid test biosensors represents a remarkably effective tool for diagnosis, including SARS-CoV-2, as they are fast, sensitive, and inexpensive. The simplest biosensors (without transducer) are paper-based and do not require multiple steps or the addition of any solution other than the patient sample [16]. The lateral flow immunoassay (LFIA) is the most representative and commercially available among the different types of biosensors. LFIAs have been widely recognized as fast biosensors with point of care (POC) status [17–19]. LFIA test detects the target molecule on an absorbent membrane with antibodies aligned to form the test and control lines; the signal is analyzed qualitatively in a visual or semi-quantitative reading [18,20] (Figure 1). LFIA is a valuable tool that has been used for detecting, diagnosing, and monitoring various viruses such as human immunodeficiency virus (HIV), human adenovirus, influenza A H1N1 virus, and SARS-CoV-2 [21–23].

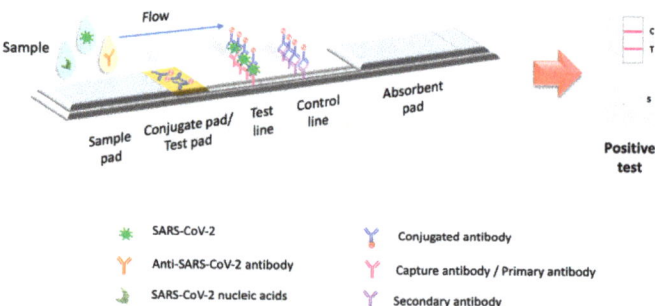

Figure 1. Principle of LFIA test. LFIA test detects the target molecule on an absorbent membrane with antibodies aligned to form the test and control lines. The sample is placed on a sample pad, then migrates to the conjugate pad, which contains the immobilized conjugate, usually made of nanoparticles (colloidal gold, colored or fluorescent latex, colored cellulose) conjugated to antibodies or antigens. The sample interacts with the conjugate, and both migrate to the next section of the strip, where the biological components of the assay (proteins/antibodies/antigens) are immobilized. In this section, the analyte and conjugate are captured. Excess reagent passes through the capture lines and accumulates on the absorbent pad. The results are interpreted on the nitrocellulose membrane as the presence or absence of the test and control lines.

During the pandemic, LFIA has been used as a mass test of POC for early detection of SARS-CoV-2 globally, in contrast to RT-PCR testing [24]. LFIA diagnostic tests have a dual function: on the one hand, they can detect the patient's antibodies to determine protection against SARS-CoV-2, and on the other hand, they can detect viral antigens for early diagnosis of infection, including asymptomatic people. This review analyzes the evolution of the LFIA biosensor for the early diagnosis of SARS-CoV-2, highlighting its improvements since the pandemic began.

2. SARS-CoV-2 Overview

Coronaviruses are a large family of well-established pathogens of various hosts, including domestic animals, wild animals, and humans [25]. Viruses that caused previous outbreaks in humans, causing severe respiratory illness, lung injury, and death, are SARS-CoV (severe acute respiratory syndrome coronavirus) in 2003 and MERS-CoV (Middle East respiratory syndrome coronavirus) in 2012 [26]. Recent genome analysis with various bioinformatics tools demonstrated that SARS-CoV-2 has a highly similar genome as the Bat coronavirus and receptor-binding domain (RBD) of spike glycoprotein as Malayan pangolin coronavirus [27]. This evidence indicates that the horseshoe bat is the natural reservoir, and primary evidence suggests that the Malayan pangolin is an intermediate host [27].

SARS-CoV-2 is an enveloped virus with a positive-sense single-stranded RNA. The genome size of this pathogen varies from 29.8 kb to 29.9 kb [28]. The virus encodes at least 29 proteins. The structural proteins are spike (S), membrane (M), envelope (E), and nucleocapsid (NP) proteins [29]. The non-structural proteins (nsps) have functions required for replication and transcription in the virus life cycle [30]. The viral particle size ranges from 80 to 120 nm [31].

The mechanism of viral infection in humans is through droplets and aerosols, which can travel through the air [32]. Infection occurs in cells that express ACE2 (angiotensin-converting enzyme 2) and TMPRSS2 (transmembrane serine protease 2) [33]. The coronavirus S protein binds to the ACE2, the primary receptor for SARS-CoV-2 that mediates virus entry into cells, and TMPRSS2 cleaves the S protein (into S1 and S2 subunits) of SARS-CoV-2 facilitating the fusion of SARS-CoV-2 and cellular membrane [33–35]. Moreover, it has been demonstrated that the endosomal cysteine proteases cathepsin B and cathepsin L can also contribute to this process [34,36,37]. In the respiratory tract, ACE2 and TMPRSS2 are expressed in the secretory and ciliated cells in the nose, secretory and ciliated cells in the conductive airways, in the type II alveolar cells in the lung as well as in corneal conjunctiva in the eye [38–41].

The etiological virus of the pandemic has continuously evolved, with many variants emerging worldwide. Variants are categorized as the variant of interest, variant of concern, and variant under monitoring [42]. There are five SARS-CoV-2 lineages designated as the variant of concern alpha, beta, gamma, delta, and omicron variants [43]. These variants increase transmissibility compared to the original virus and potentially increase disease severity [44].

3. Immune Response against SARS-CoV-2 in Brief

The SARS-CoV-2 infection involves diverse stages in the individual: start of infection, disease development, recovery, or systemic compromise. Each infection stage triggers and modulates innate and adaptative immune system mechanisms. Although SARS-CoV-2 is a virus that humanity is learning about, the immune response is equipped with mechanisms capable of dealing with this new threat. In the initial phase of SARS-CoV-2 infection, the individual presents a presymptomatic phase lasting up to 5 days, in which a high viral load is present [45]. In these early days of infection, antibodies may not have been produced. Therefore, innate immunity is the first activated. The innate immune response comprises soluble and cellular components that respond nonspecifically against the virus. The cellular compounds include dendritic cells (DC), monocytes, macrophages, neutrophils, natural killer (NK) cells, and other innate lymphoid cells (ILCs) [46]. Whereas soluble components include complement systems, soluble proteins, interferons, chemokines, and naturally occurring antibodies [47]. Immune response cells recognize pathogen-associated molecular patterns (PAMPs) of SARS-CoV-2 through pattern recognition receptors (PRRs) such as Toll-like receptors (TLR), RIG-I-like receptors (RLR), and melanoma differentiation-associated protein 5 (MDA5). The viral sensing triggers the activation of signaling pathways which induce the production of immune mediators to generate an antiviral state mainly mediated by type I (IFN-α/β) and type III (IFN-λ) interferons (IFNs) [48]. Reports have described that robust IFNs production during the early stage of infection is required to have a protective innate immune response against the virus [49]. On the contrary, an inadequate and slow response to type I and type III IFNs due to virus evasion mechanisms, host comorbidities, or genetic defects cause an exacerbated immune response. This inadequate response induces elevated levels of chemokines (CCL2, CCL8, CXCL2, CXCL8, CXCL9, and CXCL16), high expression of proinflammatory cytokines such as IL-6, IL-10, IL-1, and TNF, in addition to activation, and recruitment of immune cells [50,51]. The called "cytokine storm" leads to unbalanced levels of proinflammatory and antiviral mediators that remain the leading cause of ARDS and multi-organ failure [49,50,52].

On the other hand, the adaptive immune response is orchestrated by CD8+ T lymphocytes, TCD4+, and B lymphocytes, responsible for immunological memory. In response to SARS-CoV-2 infection, it has been shown that non-severe patients or patients with mild symptoms have a low viral load and may not have produced antibodies [53,54]. In contrast, antibodies have been detected by immunoassay tests and biosensors in patients with severe symptoms or cases [53,55]. Patients with a high viral load activate the humoral immune response in the first two weeks of infection [56]. The first seroconversion of antibodies is against protein N, followed by protein S of SARS-CoV-2 in patients with disease symptoms [57]. Immunoglobulins IgA and IgM begin to be detected within the first ten days of infection; however, both antibodies can cross-react with protein N, which is highly conserved among coronaviruses [58,59]. Moreover, high levels of IgG1 and IgG3 are expressed ten to fourteen days after infection in patients with disease symptoms [60,61]. Older adults and seriously ill individuals reach high specificity antibodies concentrations against SARS-CoV-2 S protein.

Due to the urgency of reducing thousands of people's cases and deaths, scientists have developed several vaccines against COVID-19. Efforts are being made to apply vaccines with emergency use authorization to the world population. Vaccination elicits immune responses capable of potently neutralizing SARS-CoV-2. However, the available data show that most approved COVID-19 vaccines protect against severe disease but do not prevent the clinical manifestation of COVID-19 [62]. Instead, it has been demonstrated that new variants with mutations in the spike, the main target of neutralizing antibodies, can escape the neutralization of humoral immunity [63,64].

4. SARS-CoV-2 Detection

Molecular tests or biosensors are the tools for detecting SARS-CoV-2 nucleic acids/antigens/antibodies against the virus (Figure 1). In the early part of the illness, viral particles and their subunits can be detected; beyond the first two weeks of illness onset, antibodies against the virus could be detected [65]. The SARS-CoV-2 infection stage is highly correlated to the diagnostic technique recommended for the pandemic. Early diagnosis of the disease and isolation of infected people is key to controlling the transmission of SARS-CoV-2 [66,67]. In the initial phase of SARS-CoV-2 infection, the individual presents a presymptomatic phase lasting up to 5 days, in which a high viral load is present [45]. During these early days of infection, antibodies may not be detected. Therefore, since the pandemic began, the diagnostic method has been based on detecting viral genes using the molecular PCR technique, the gold standard worldwide [2,3,68]. The pandemic has exceeded the ability to identify the virus in laboratories using molecular techniques; this has motivated the development of new technologies for the rapid detection of SARS-CoV-2 that are easy to perform compared to molecular tests in clinical laboratories. LFIA has been the unique device approved and available to use in mass worldwide. Biosensors with transducers are developing in SARS-CoV-2 diagnostic. However, most nanomaterials used in these biosensors present interferences with contaminants in human samples compared to performance under experimental conditions. It is important to emphasize that LFIAs have the unique properties of availability, accessibility, economy, and POC (including home use), these characteristics that are not shared by all biosensors with a transducer. In addition, biosensors with transducers require exclusive handling in laboratories certified under the Clinical Laboratory Improvement Amendments of 1998 [69,70]. The FDA have to date approved only one piezoelectric biosensor [69] (Figure 1).

5. Lateral Flow Immunoassay Evolution in the Pandemic

LFIAs are devices with features designed into POC testing technologies that fulfill AS-SURED criteria (affordable, sensitive, specific, user-friendly, rapid and robust, equipment-free, deliverable to end-user) [71]. LFIAs have been widely used to diagnose bacterial and viral infections, including SARS-CoV-2. At the beginning of the pandemic, in North America and Europe, patients with symptoms consistent with COVID-19 but negative for SARS-CoV-2 by RT-PCR could be diagnosed by serological testing using LFIA [72]. Furthermore, these rapid detection tests were approved for emergency to detect serum antibodies in symptomatic patients [69]. However, the start of vaccination stimulated the production of protective antibodies in the world population, so the LFIA that detected antibodies became obsolete for early diagnosis of the disease.

Only LFIAs that detect viral antigens have been approved worldwide for the diagnosis of COVID-19 [69,73]. The manufacture of LFIAs continues to be developed to increase their sensitivity and specificity, implementing nanomaterials for their manufacture and advanced technology in chromatography. The future of these devices makes them as efficient as biosensors in diagnosing SARS-CoV-2, maintaining their application as a complementary test to PCR.

5.1. Lateral Flow Immunoassay Antibody Testing in COVID-19 Pandemic

At the beginning of 2020, LFIAs biosensors were commercially available to be used in mass to detect IgM/IgG antibodies against the new SARS-CoV-2 virus [3]. These devices were recommended in patients with clinical symptoms of SARS-CoV-2. Their main advantages were used at the POC, with qualitative outcomes in just 15 min or less, reaching a larger population without saturating the capacity of laboratories [74]. The pressing need to diagnose COVID-19 rushed manufacturing of large-scale, accurate, and affordable diagnostic immunoassays, including LFIA [69] (Figure 2). As of 2020, after evaluating five immunoassays and one lateral flow immunochromatography for anti-SARS-CoV-2 antibodies detection, FDA-EUA (Food and Drug Administration—Emergency Use Authorization) approved only two manufacturers of LFIAs to detect IgG/IgM anti-SARS-CoV-2 [3]. At the moment, forty-eight LFIAs manufacturing laboratories were granted EUA authorization to apply for SARS-CoV-2 diagnostic [69]. The marketing was exceptionally authorized without prior evaluation in the interest of world public health. Whereas the pandemic started, LFIAs tests showed variable performance when assessing test sensitivity and specificity towards the main immunogenic structures of the virus. In pediatric age (2 months to 18 years), COVID-19 symptoms are generally less severe than in adults, and a low level of antibodies is produced [75]. This immune response is associated with a low yield of sensitivity of LFIA antibody detection (about 70%); this value was lower in the second week after disease onset. [76]. In England, LFIA was applied twice per week to the general population, including asymptomatic individuals. False-positive results caused unnecessary isolation involving the cost of shutting down entire economic sectors [77].

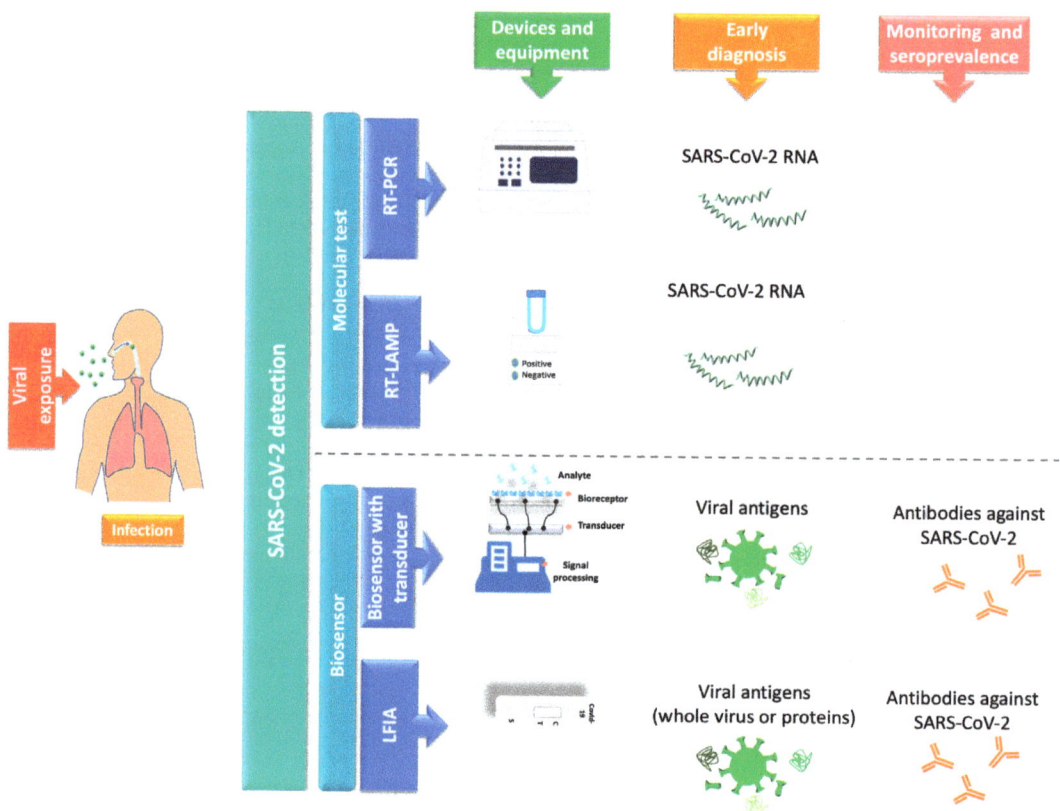

Figure 2. Main methods for detecting SARS-CoV-2. Currently, the detection of SARS-CoV-2 is carried out using molecular tests and biosensors. RT-PCR is the gold standard for detecting SARS-CoV-2 viral RNA. There are other available molecular tests used based on RT-LAMP. Biosensors with transducers have been developed to detect viral antigens or antibodies. LFIA is the representative test for mass diagnosis of SARS-CoV-2 in POC and antibody prevalence studies worldwide. These biosensors have been widely marketed because they can be applied at the POC and are inexpensive, fast, and easy to read.

LFIA Is a Quantitative Tool for Detecting Antibodies against SARS-CoV-2

Serological tests detect the presence of antibodies in the blood from the adaptive immune response to an infection. LFIAs as diagnostic serological tests for COVID-19, are designed to absorb a blood drop sample obtained by puncture onto a nitrocellulose membrane that captures and detects IgG antibodies or IgM/IgG antibodies [78–81]. The result is visualized by precipitation of usually gold nanoparticles or other colored nanoparticles to generate colored lines on the membrane [82]. Early in the pandemic, the FDA granted emergency clearance to LFIAs that detect IgG/IgM antibodies to diagnose COVID-19. Some of these tests did not meet the clinical serologic performance estimates required to meet EUA efficacy and risk/benefit standards, so they were revoked [3]. This evidence contributed to the withdrawal of most LFIA antibody screening tests for the diagnosis of COVID-19.

In 2021, the need for LFIAs antibody tests to detect with high sensitivity and/or quantitative mode neutralizing antibodies in individuals immunized or recovered from natural COVID-19 illness resurfaced [83–85]. The novel vaccines manufactured against SARS-CoV-2 make it necessary to assess the efficiency of immunization to produce neutralizing antibodies against SARS-CoV-2 and how long they last in the vaccinated individual [84,86]. The speed and affordability of the LFIA test allow timely detection of individuals who show a short or absent humoral immune response. On the other hand, in 2020, the USA approved an emergency authorization to use plasma therapy as part of treatment in patients with COVID-19 [87]. This process consists of obtaining convalescent plasma from patients recovered from COVID-19, abundant in neutralizing antibodies, to treat patients. [88]. LFIA is an effective tool in both cases because of its speed and lack of laboratory equipment requirements. LFIAs have shifted from COVID-19 diagnosis to monitoring post-infection or post-vaccination antibody production in the global population. However, LFIA tests had to improve sensitivity and a positive cut-off threshold limit for post-vaccination antibody detection and/or convalescent patients. COVID-19 being a newly emerging disease, it was necessary to determine the exact disease stage in which the LFIA antibody tests should be applied to the global population. It was necessary to analyze the humoral immune response in the world population at different stages of the disease (uninfected, asymptomatic, symptomatic, convalescent, and reinfected) [89–92]. Other factors such as age, sex, comorbidities, or high risk in healthcare personnel are involved in the variations of the humoral response [93]. On the other hand, the manufacture of LFIAs focused its development on the incorporation of new nanomaterials and biomaterials, which in conjunction with the highly antigenic regions and/or subunits of the SARS-CoV-2 virus (S, N, or both), improved the affinity of the antibodies and/or increased the visible signal of antigen–antibody binding [94]. The main LFIA models for the detection of antibodies against SARS-CoV-2 have been designed in a competitive and sandwich type with antibodies coupled to colloidal gold nanoparticles (AuNPs), QDs, and fluorescent nanomaterials (FND) as visual reporters.

The LFIAs that use N (N-LFIA) viral antigen to detect IgG antibodies against SARS-CoV-2 contribute to identifying natural COVID-19 illness individuals that, once infected, produced high levels of neutralizing antibodies against N viral antigen up to two months after the onset of symptoms [95,96]. This time could be considered a diagnostic limit for the use of N-LFIA. Even it is possible that N-LFIA could detect SARS-CoV-2 in asymptomatic personnel at high risk. Nickel and colleagues (2022) carried out the N-LFIA serological test on at-risk healthcare workers and detected antibodies to the N viral protein with a sensitivity of >99%, indicating prior infection [86]. The early identification of individuals with antibodies against viral protein N could be considered a biomarker of the previous infection. The condition of the previous infection gives them an advantage from the first dose of vaccine (tested with Pfizer/BioNTech); they form antibodies against viral protein S, 2.7 times more than those not exposed to the virus [96]. Identifying anti-N antibody-negative individuals means there is no prior SARS-CoV-2 infection, so they will require a second dose of vaccine (Pfizer/BioNTech) to produce neutralizing antibodies against the antigenic S protein [96]. It has been proposed that in countries where vaccination against SARS-CoV-2 is of low availability, the N-LFIAs that detect previous SARS-CoV-2 infected individuals allow identifying naturally immunized individuals who could receive the vaccine some weeks later [97].

In regions where other beta-coronaviruses are present, their N-terminal domain of the N antigen is highly conserved, which may cause N-LFIAs to give false-positive results and/or fail to detect true early sensitization [98]. LFIA targeting the S antigens does not distinguish between vaccine- and infection-induced antibodies [99] (Figure 3A). The incorporation of the ACE2 receptor as an immobilized protein in the test pad assay line enhanced the LFIA sensitivity. This improvement favored an increased detection of the serum antibody complex with the receptor binding domain (RBD) of the S1 subunit of the SARS-CoV-2 virus. If a neutralizing antibody were present, it would bind to AuNP-RBD and prevent the AuNP-RBD from being captured by the immobilized ACE2 protein, indicating the absence of a tag in the test line [100].

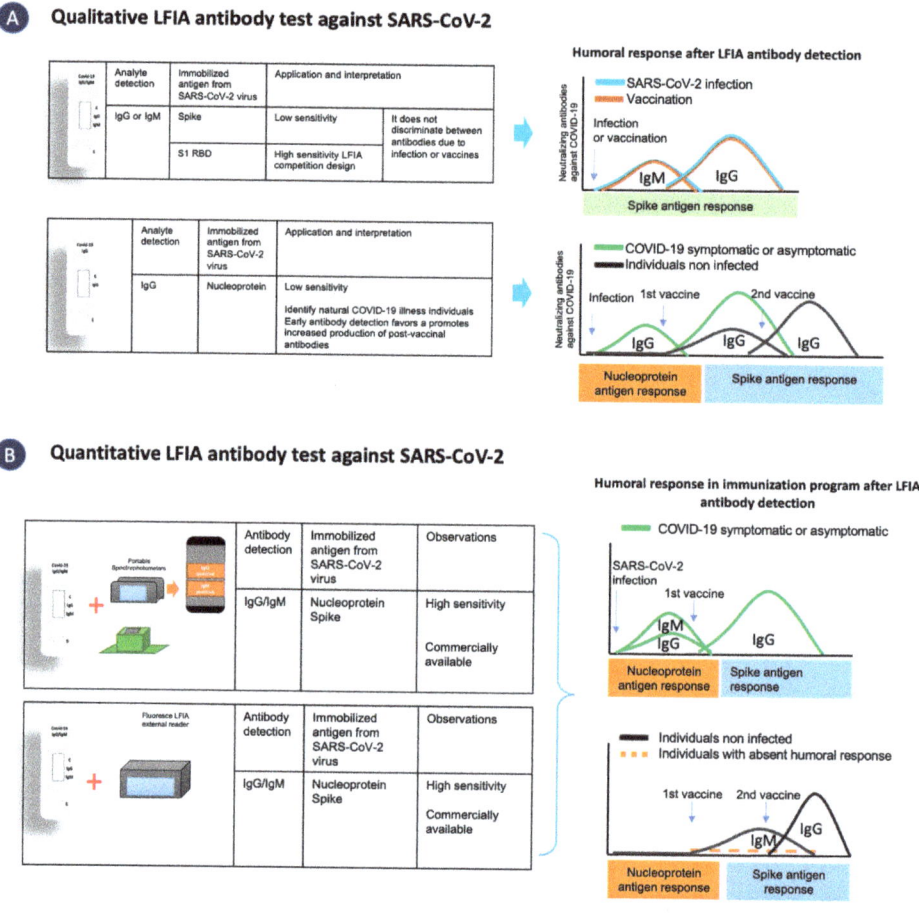

Figure 3. LFIAs detect IgG and/or IgM antibodies in asymptomatic, symptomatic, and immunized individuals. (**A**) LFIAs with qualitative readouts are available with the SARS-CoV-2 NP antigenic protein and the S protein. (**B**) LFIAs coupled to portable spectrophotometer have a greater sensitivity for evaluating the humoral response of convalescent, symptomatic, asymptomatic, and immunized individuals. The graphs on the right indicate the interpretation of LFIA results showing the humoral response in SARS-CoV-2 infected and uninfected individuals and those who have received at least the first dose of vaccine.

A qualitative positive LFIA result is when the test line region is observed with low to marked color intensity. If the test line is not marked, the result is declared negative. The test is only valid if the control line shows a visible color in all cases. In some cases, it is difficult to interpret the color band by the naked eye when the intensity is low [101]. The strategy to increase the sensitivity of LFIA to detect IgG/IgM against SARS-CoV-2 and a positive cut-off threshold limit has been to transform the qualitative reading with the naked eye for a quantitative measure with the help of a portable spectrophotometer [94,101,102]. It was also observed that depending on the format in which the LFIA was manufactured (sandwich or competition type) and the viral antigen immobilized in the conjugation pad region, the test's sensitivity could be improved. Chen and colleagues (2021) designed a combined LFIA with N and S antigens on the solid phase (conjugate pad) to recognize IgM/IgG from the serum sample. After antigen–antibody binding occurs, the complex migrates to the test line. A second binding is conjugated with colloidal gold-labeled anti-human IgM/IgG antibodies, evidencing the positive mark that a spectrophotometer quantifies. This LFIA coupled to a portable spectrophotometer detects a positive cut-off threshold of 0.5 ng/mL compared to 5–10 ng/mL detected by a qualitative LFIA. The LFIA spectrum analyzer uses a primary reflectance wavelength of 540–470 nm for samples with a low IgG concentration and a wavelength of 650 nm to reference IgG concentrations. The ratio between both wavelengths obtains the α value. A higher α value indicates a stronger reflection color intensity of the colloidal gold antibody-conjugated IgG and IgM complexes [94]. Hung and colleagues (2021) used an LFIA, with N protein as antigen in the conjugated pad, and anti-human IgG/IgM antibodies in the test line conjugate region [102]. The measure was performed using the same spectrophotometer as Chen and colleagues (2021) [94]. The authors reported an increase in the antibody detection limit to 186 pg/mL on these assays [102].

Chen and colleagues (2021) replaced colloidal gold with gap-enhanced Raman nanotags (GERTs) in an LFIA to detection of human IgM and IgG against SARS-CoV-2 recombinant antigens. The sensitivity was 1 ng/mL and 0.1 ng/mL for detection of IgM and IgG respectively [103]. Furthermore, in another study, Huang and colleagues (2022) included an LFIA with a competitive format, using the S antigen to detect IgG/IgM antibodies, a final capture in the test line region with the ACE-2 receptor, and the quantitative analysis was performed with a spectrophotometer [101]. The authors changed the antigen to detect neutralizing IgG/IgM antibodies in individuals vaccinated with the AstraZeneca COVID-19 vaccine. Moreover, they demonstrated that LFIA had efficient sensitivity and sensitivity as the ELISA assay (80 and 100%, respectively), with a Rho coefficient of 0.933. The LFIAs for detecting antibodies described here still require evaluating their efficacy with the new variants of the SARS-CoV-2 virus [101]. Pieri and colleagues (2022) used a kit that includes the LFIA sandwich-type (Affimedix Inc., Hayward, USA) that detects qualitative IgG neutralizing antibodies that recognize the S protein receptor-binding domain antigen. The cassette is placed in a RapidRead reader system (Affimedix Inc., Hayward, USA) for quantitative diagnosis of COVID-19 antibodies. The kit LFIA and reflective optical density reader have equal sensitivity to two chemiluminescence immunoassay methods [83].

The fluorescence LFIA (FLFIA) with a quantitative reading by a spectrofluorometer has high sensitivity to detect total antibodies. The evaluation of an FLFIA test with sandwich immunodetection method has included the N antigenic recombinant protein or S-RBD proteins as immobilized antigens. Both showed a high sensitivity (92–98.68%) to detect serum antibodies in SARS-CoV-2 symptomatic and asymptomatic patients. The authors recommend that these commercial tests assess binding and neutralizing antibody response after SARS-CoV-2 infection or vaccination (Figure 3B) [104,105].

Novel labeling nanomaterials can enhance fluorescence as a signal amplification label, improving the sensitivity of LFIA for detections of antibodies against SARS-CoV-2 antigens. Lanthanide-doped polystyrene nanoparticles (LNPs) can bind to mouse anti-human IgG antibodies, which are located on a conjugate pad as a fluorescent reporter. The readout was performed with a fluorescent reader, and the detection took 10 min. The test's sensitivity was comparable to RT-PCR in 51 human serum samples [106].

Quantum dots nanobeads (QBs) made with CdSe/ZnS can be coated with Octadecylamine, which gives them highly luminescent properties. These QBs linked to the recombinant SARS-CoV-2 spike protein are placed on the conjugated pad where antibodies in the serum can recognize them. In experimental conditions, the QB-LFIA has high sensitivity with positive samples up to 10 times higher than a traditional AuNP-LFIA. The QB-LFIA showed a sensitivity of 97.1% and a specificity of 100% in assays with serum samples, although analysis with whole blood is required [107].

All quantitative LFIAs require a portable device as a reader, which could compromise their POC status. On the other hand, the amount of reagents required is considerably less than with traditional LFIAs, which would justify the cost/benefit for mass implementation.

Moreover, the humoral immune response against SARS-CoV-2 can generate null or high antibody production, which must be considered for any antibody test. It is recommended that the results of LFIA be complemented with RT-PCR for greater sensitivity in the diagnosis of SARS-CoV-2, as the detection of IgM/IgG antibodies by ELISA has been shown to have higher sensitivity when combined with RT-PCR (98.6%) than RT-PCR alone (92.2%) [108].

5.2. Lateral Flow Immunoassay Viral Antigen Testing for COVID-19

In 2020, the manufacture of LFIAs that detect SARS-CoV-2 specific viral structures (SARS-CoV-2 protein antigens N and S) increased because COVID-19 infection remains present in the vaccinated population worldwide. At the pandemic's start, LFIA devices that detect the SARS-CoV-2 viral antigen were discarded and not recommended due to their limited reliability in patients with low viral load [108,109]. In regions of the world with a disease prevalence of less than 0.5%, antigen-based LFIAs were not recommended due asymptomatic individuals showed a positive predictive value of 11% to 28%, meaning that 7 out of 10 to 9 out of 10 positive results will be false positives, and 1 out of 2 to 1 out of 3 cases will be missed [109]. By increasing the spread of SARS-CoV-2 and turning it into a pandemic, the LFIAs were redesigned for the detection of SARS-CoV-2 antigens, highlighting that the S protein possessed the antigenicity that gave a remarkable improvement in the sensitivity and specificity of the test, although still below the standard test accepted worldwide, RT-PCR [104].

Improvements in LFIA testing led to clinical trials in Europe, Asia, and the USA, using various LFIA devices that showed high specificity (95–100%) while sensitivity was low (30–78%) [110]. The factors involved in the low sensitivity of the LFIAs tests that detect SARS-CoV-2 antigens were the time of infection, age, inadequate collection, sample conservation, and the quality of the product by the manufacturer. It has been determined that the time to detect the viral antigen with LFIA is in the first 7 days the patient develops symptoms because the highest viral load occurs in this period. Individuals with mild or asymptomatic symptoms or who exceed this time could have a low viral load [111]. In this disease period, LFIAs detect at least a Ct value < 25 (~100,000 RNA copies/mL), which is sufficiently accurate and helpful for mass population screening programs [112,113]. The WHO recommends using LFIAs, which meet the minimum performance requirements of $\geq$80% sensitivity and $\geq$97% specificity. To detect cases in symptomatic people suspected of being infected and asymptomatic people at high risk of COVID-19; for contact tracing; during outbreak investigations; and to monitor trends in disease incidence in communities [114]. The LFIAs are designed to take a nasopharyngeal swab sample. However, some researchers switched to saliva to reduce the risks of infection for the sampler. Saliva may affect the test due to the sample collection and storage technique, which could have implications for the low sensitivity of the assay [115,116]. These conditions have not yet been analyzed.

The main LFIA models for detecting SARS-CoV-2 antigen were competitive and sandwich types with antibodies coupled to AuNPs, quantum dots (QDs), and fluorescent nanodiamond (FND) as a visual reporter [117,118]. Afterward, LFIAs that detect viral antigens in the detection of SARS-CoV-2 focused the improvement of sensitivity on increasing the specificity of antibodies immobilized in the test, using nanomaterials as labels that increase the signal generated by antigen–antibody binding, and detection of nucleic acids (Figure 4).

The classical technology to produce monoclonal antibodies incorporated into LFIAs is insufficient to improve sensitivity against SARS-CoV-2 target proteins. Kim and colleagues (2021) resolved antibody affinity enhancement using phage display technology to develop an LFIA-based biosensor specific for SARS-CoV-2. Researchers generate phage-engineered monoclonal antibodies against SARS-CoV-2 NP. Newly developed antibodies specific for SARS-CoV-2 were conjugated to nanobead, with a sensitivity of 2 ng antigen protein and 2.5×10^4 pfu cultured virus. The new LFIA platform gives an outcome that can be confirmed with the naked eye in 20 min and has a sensitivity of 100%, detecting only SARS-CoV-2 NP, not NPs from MERS-CoV, SARS-CoV, or influenza H1N1 [17]. Another advantage of this new LFIA is that the outcome can be analyzed and quantified using a portable LFIA reader. The authors tested the diagnostic device in experimental laboratory conditions, and non-human samples were tested [17].

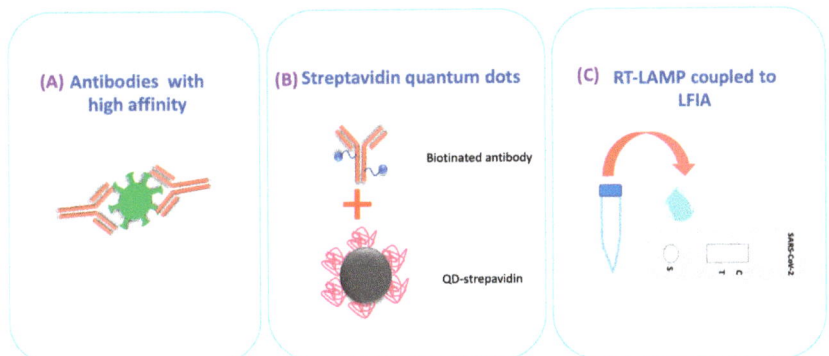

Figure 4. Strategies to improve the detection of SARS-CoV-2 antigens or nucleic acids by Lateral flow immunoassay. (**A**) The sensitivity of LFIAs focuses on developing high-affinity antibodies for the antigen. (**B**) Use of nanomaterials as markers that potentiate the antigen–antibody signal. (**C**) The detection of nucleic acids, incorporating different isothermal amplification techniques.

Concerning labels that amplify the antigen–antibody binding signal, copper coupled to antibodies has been used to amplify the chromatographic signal for a minimum detection limit in the sample of 10 pg/mL [119].

The fluorescence immunochromatographic (FIC) method uses antibodies conjugated to fluorochromes to detect SARS-CoV-2 viral antigens. This test requires an immunofluorescence analyzer for the quantitative results. Diao and colleagues (2021) developed an FIC with mouse polyclonal antibodies and labeled them with fluorescent europium microparticles to detect the antigenic protein N of SARS-CoV-2. The authors reported a sensitivity of 75.6% [120]. In India, using a commercially available FIC (Standard F, SD Biosensor) made with monoclonal antibodies did not improve the sensitivity and was reported to be 38% [121]. The FIC assay is slower and less convenient than LFIAs and requires a battery-powered immunofluorescence analyzer. Incubation time can be up to 30 min, which affects test performance at the POC. Europium, used in ICF, has a fluorescence stability limit. It has been established that the time limit for performing the hybridization process is 30 min. After this time, a positive sample by RT-PCR will give a false positive. The limit to the correct detection of positive and negative reference samples is 15 min [122].

The fluorescent signal can be amplified by magnetic QD tags (Fe_3O_4-QD) (MagTQD). When this nanomaterial is used to amplify fluorescence in an LFIA strip, the biosensor could simultaneously detect SARS-CoV-2 S/NP antigens with high sensitivity (0.5–1 pg/mL). The biosensor is not yet tested with clinical samples [123]. Interestingly, high-affinity peptides have been developed that detect the RBD protein of the SARS-CoV-2 virus at levels as low as 0.01 nM. These peptides are inexpensive and easy to synthesize and could be coupled to LFIA to improve their sensitivity and reduce costs [124].

5.3. LFIA Simultaneously Detects Antigens and Antibodies

The biotechnology applied at LFIA has succeeded in developing a biosensor that simultaneously detects the alpha and beta antigenic variants of SARS-CoV-2 and the neutralizing antibodies. This device uses an immobilized ACE2 receptor to detect antigenic variants of the SARS-CoV-2 S protein from the nasopharyngeal sample via color differences of substrates. Antibody detection is achieved by a competition LFIA, where a sample containing neutralizing antibodies binds to the RBD antigen blocking the binding to the ACE2 receptor; thus *t* (test) line is absent [125].

6. LFIA Detects Nucleic Acids of SARS-CoV-2

The sensitivity of LFIAs remained questionable because, unlike RT-PCR, they could not be designed to detect SARS-CoV-2 nucleic acid (NA). Interestingly, advances in biotechnology have made it possible for LFIAs to integrate new methods of NA detection. The main methods for this detection are new high-affinity monoclonal antibodies and coupling isothermal amplification methods (IAM), such as RT-PCR and LAMP.

The method called hybrid capture fluorescence immunoassay (HC-FIA) uses S9.6 monoclonal antibodies, which were used to capture the hybridization of nucleic acids (SARS-CoV-2 DNA and RNA probes) on a lateral flow strip and immunofluorescence analysis. The HC-FIA test showed 100% sensitivity and 99% specificity from throat swabs and sputum samples [122].

Avidin-carbon nanoparticles (CNPs) have been evaluated as a label in LFIA for NA detection. This method increases the contrast in the paper background after the nucleic acid-antibody complex union. The visual limit of detection is in the nanomolar range (2.2×10^{-2} pg μL^{-1}) without the assistance of any instrumentation. The advantages of CNPs are they are cheaper labels; the suspension is very stable and easy to modify. The critical point of this method is the double tagging of primers in the PCR procedure, which allows the posterior binding with Av-CNPs [126].

The IAM method tests Accula SARS-CoV-2 of Mesa Biotech combined RT-PCR and LFIA. The test cassette contains all reaction reagents and targets the N gene of SARS-CoV-2 from nasal and throat samples in 30 min, and the results are interpreted visually. The analytical sensitivity reported is 200 copies/mL (Mesa Biotech Inc., San Diego, USA, 2020). The clinical performance with 30 positive and 30 negative samples showed clinical sensitivity and specificity of 100% [3]. The disadvantage of this test is that it is limited to laboratories certified in EUA under the Clinical Laboratory Improvement Amendments of 1988 (CLIA). Still, where available, the test is considered POC (Mesa Biotech Inc., San Diego, USA, 2020). The methodology of combining LFIA and PCR implied a breakthrough in the fusion of reagents and biomaterials of both techniques. However, the complexity of manufacturing increased the risks of kit contamination. On 6 April 2022, Mesa Biotech, Inc. announced the recall of Accula SARS-CoV-2 tests due to possible contamination of the kit causing false positives in the individuals to which they are applied [127]. Agarwal and colleagues (2022) developed an LFIA that detects antigenic protein N in cDNA by combining RT-LAMP methodology [128]. In SARS-CoV-2 positive patients, the test demonstrated an accuracy of 81.66% and a minimum viral RNA detection limit of Ct < 33. The result of RT-LAMP in combination with LFA can be completed with a smartphone-based semi-quantitative data analysis [128]. The challenges of LFIA for nucleic acid detection are that isothermal amplification requires a complex primer design, and the signal can only be analyzed by portable readers [129,130].

7. Conclusions and Perspectives

LFIAs have been a very efficient tool during the pandemic due to their simplicity, speed, and cost-effectiveness. LFIAs can be used in low-resource field settings and in developing countries that cannot use other methods for SARS-CoV-2 detection. However, there are still some challenges to face. One of the main challenges is to develop their ultra-sensitivity, together with POC advantages, especially in samples that require more than one step to detect the virus. The improvement in LFIAs includes: (1) the synthesis of immobilized biomaterials, antigens, or antibodies in the conjugation region with high affinity to the analyte; (2) the use of new nanomaterials to label the antigen or antibody that is conjugated to the analyte; (3) quantitative analysis using an external device. It is important to highlight that current LFIAs' performances are comparable with ELISA and chemiluminescence immunoassay methods. The results can be quantitative and qualitative according to the epidemiological needs or the vaccination present in the region or country. In addition, the quantitative LFIAs could contribute to data digitization, allowing the monitoring, storage, and transmission of data, reducing interpretation and transcription errors, and thus ensuring the quality and control of the tests. LFIAs are highly adaptable devices. In the future, it has been proposed that LFIA will focus on detecting SARS-CoV-2 virus nucleic acids by incorporating isothermal amplification methods under non-laboratory conditions and novel labeling materials that amplify the signal. The implementation of low-cost handheld readers, including smartphones, will be able to match or even improve the efficiency of LFIA on par with the RT-PCR test.

Author Contributions: N.S.C.-J. and J.C.H.-G. are responsible for the conceptualization, research, analysis, writing, and editing of this review. B.E.G.-P. participated in the immunological concepts, editing, and analysis of this work. V.M.M.-J. participated in the literature search on the LFIA biosensor concepts of this work. N.E.R.-R. and V.V.-S. contributed to the review and analysis of this work. All authors have read and agreed to the published version of the manuscript.

Funding: The authors kindly acknowledge the financial support of the PRODEP (Programa para el Desarrollo Profesional Docente en Educación Superior). Universidad Autónoma del Estado de Hidalgo and Consejo Nacional de Ciencia y Tecnología (CONACyT).

Institutional Review Board Statement: Not applicable.

Informed Consent Statement: Not applicable.

Data Availability Statement: Not applicable.

Acknowledgments: N.S.C.J., J.C.H.G., B.E.G.P., N.E.R.R., and V.V.S. would also like to acknowledge the S.N.I. fellowship.

Conflicts of Interest: The authors declare no conflict of interest.

References

1. World Health Organization. Coronavirus (COVID-19) Dashboard. Available online: https://covid19.who.int (accessed on 29 August 2022).
2. World Health Organization. Laboratory Testing for 2019 Novel Coronavirus (2019-NCoV) in Suspected Human Cases. Available online: https://www.who.int/publications-detail-redirect/10665-331501 (accessed on 23 May 2022).
3. Ravi, N.; Cortade, D.L.; Ng, E.; Wang, S.X. Diagnostics for SARS-CoV-2 Detection: A Comprehensive Review of the FDA-EUA COVID-19 Testing Landscape. *Biosens. Bioelectron.* **2020**, *165*, 112454. [CrossRef] [PubMed]
4. Patel, R.; Babady, E.; Theel, E.S.; Storch, G.A.; Pinsky, B.A.; St George, K.; Smith, T.C.; Bertuzzi, S. Report from the American Society for Microbiology COVID-19 International Summit, 23 March 2020: Value of Diagnostic Testing for SARS–CoV-2/COVID-19. *mBio* **2020**, *11*, e00722-20. [CrossRef] [PubMed]
5. Lu, X.; Wang, L.; Sakthivel, S.K.; Whitaker, B.; Murray, J.; Kamili, S.; Lynch, B.; Malapati, L.; Burke, S.A.; Harcourt, J.; et al. US CDC Real-Time Reverse Transcription PCR Panel for Detection of Severe Acute Respiratory Syndrome Coronavirus 2. *Emerg. Infect. Dis.* **2020**, *26*, 1654–1665. [CrossRef] [PubMed]
6. Mouliou, D.S.; Gourgoulianis, K.I. False-Positive and False-Negative COVID-19 Cases: Respiratory Prevention and Management Strategies, Vaccination, and Further Perspectives. *Expert Rev. Respir. Med.* **2021**, *15*, 993–1002. [CrossRef]
7. Meo, S.A.; Meo, A.S.; Al-Jassir, F.F.; Klonoff, D.C. Omicron SARS-CoV-2 New Variant: Global Prevalence and Biological and Clinical Characteristics. *Eur. Rev. Med. Pharmacol. Sci.* **2021**, *25*, 8012–8018. [CrossRef]
8. World Health Organization. Weekly Operational Update on COVID-19—4 August 2021. Available online: https://www.who.int/publications/m/item/weekly-operational-update-on-covid-19---4-august-2021 (accessed on 1 June 2022).
9. Perumal, V.; Hashim, U. Advances in Biosensors: Principle, Architecture and Applications. *J. Appl. Biomed.* **2014**, *12*, 1–15. [CrossRef]
10. Abid, S.A.; Ahmed Muneer, A.; Al-Kadmy, I.M.S.; Sattar, A.A.; Beshbishy, A.M.; Batiha, G.E.-S.; Hetta, H.F. Biosensors as a Future Diagnostic Approach for COVID-19. *Life Sci.* **2021**, *273*, 119117. [CrossRef]
11. Drobysh, M.; Ramanaviciene, A.; Viter, R.; Chen, C.-F.; Samukaite-Bubniene, U.; Ratautaite, V.; Ramanavicius, A. Biosensors for the Determination of SARS-CoV-2 Virus and Diagnosis of COVID-19 Infection. *Int. J. Mol. Sci.* **2022**, *23*, 666. [CrossRef]
12. Adeel, M.; Asif, K.; Canzonieri, V.; Barai, H.R.; Rahman, M.d.M.; Daniele, S.; Rizzolio, F. Controlled, Partially Exfoliated, Self-Supported Functionalized Flexible Graphitic Carbon Foil for Ultrasensitive Detection of SARS-CoV-2 Spike Protein. *Sens. Actuators B Chem.* **2022**, *359*, 131591. [CrossRef]

13. Zhang, J.Z.; Yeh, H.-W.; Walls, A.C.; Wicky, B.I.M.; Sprouse, K.R.; VanBlargan, L.A.; Treger, R.; Quijano-Rubio, A.; Pham, M.N.; Kraft, J.C.; et al. Thermodynamically Coupled Biosensors for Detecting Neutralizing Antibodies against SARS-CoV-2 Variants. *Nat. Biotechnol.* **2022**, 1–5. [CrossRef]
14. Zamhuri, S.A.; Soon, C.F.; Nordin, A.N.; Ab Rahim, R.; Sultana, N.; Khan, M.A.; Lim, G.P.; Tee, K.S. A Review on the Contamination of SARS-CoV-2 in Water Bodies: Transmission Route, Virus Recovery and Recent Biosensor Detection Techniques. *Sens. Bio-Sens. Res.* **2022**, *36*, 100482. [CrossRef] [PubMed]
15. Prabowo, B.A.; Cabral, P.D.; Freitas, P.; Fernandes, E. The Challenges of Developing Biosensors for Clinical Assessment: A Review. *Chemosensors* **2021**, *9*, 299. [CrossRef]
16. Bissonnette, L.; Bergeron, M.G. Diagnosing Infections—Current and Anticipated Technologies for Point-of-Care Diagnostics and Home-Based Testing. *Clin. Microbiol. Infect.* **2010**, *16*, 1044–1053. [CrossRef] [PubMed]
17. Kim, H.-Y.; Lee, J.-H.; Kim, M.J.; Park, S.C.; Choi, M.; Lee, W.; Ku, K.B.; Kim, B.T.; Changkyun Park, E.; Kim, H.G.; et al. Development of a SARS-CoV-2-Specific Biosensor for Antigen Detection Using ScFv-Fc Fusion Proteins. *Biosens. Bioelectron.* **2021**, *175*, 112868. [CrossRef]
18. Antiochia, R. Paper-Based Biosensors: Frontiers in Point-of-Care Detection of COVID-19 Disease. *Biosensors* **2021**, *11*, 110. [CrossRef]
19. Chaimayo, C.; Kaewnaphan, B.; Tanlieng, N.; Athipanyasilp, N.; Sirijatuphat, R.; Chayakulkeeree, M.; Angkasekwinai, N.; Sutthent, R.; Puangpunngam, N.; Tharmviboonsri, T.; et al. Rapid SARS-CoV-2 Antigen Detection Assay in Comparison with Real-Time RT-PCR Assay for Laboratory Diagnosis of COVID-19 in Thailand. *Virol. J.* **2020**, *17*, 177. [CrossRef]
20. Anfossi, L.; Di Nardo, F.; Cavalera, S.; Giovannoli, C.; Baggiani, C. Multiplex Lateral Flow Immunoassay: An Overview of Strategies towards High-Throughput Point-of-Need Testing. *Biosensors* **2018**, *9*, 2. [CrossRef]
21. Martiskainen, I.; Juntunen, E.; Salminen, T.; Vuorenpää, K.; Bayoumy, S.; Vuorinen, T.; Khanna, N.; Pettersson, K.; Batra, G.; Talha, S.M. Double-Antigen Lateral Flow Immunoassay for the Detection of Anti-HIV-1 and -2 Antibodies Using Upconverting Nanoparticle Reporters. *Sensors* **2021**, *21*, 330. [CrossRef]
22. Wang, C.; Wang, C.; Wang, X.; Wang, K.; Zhu, Y.; Rong, Z.; Wang, W.; Xiao, R.; Wang, S. Magnetic SERS Strip for Sensitive and Simultaneous Detection of Respiratory Viruses. *ACS Appl. Mater. Interfaces* **2019**, *11*, 19495–19505. [CrossRef]
23. Nicol, T.; Lefeuvre, C.; Serri, O.; Pivert, A.; Joubaud, F.; Dubée, V.; Kouatchet, A.; Ducancelle, A.; Lunel-Fabiani, F.; Le Guillou-Guillemette, H. Assessment of SARS-CoV-2 Serological Tests for the Diagnosis of COVID-19 through the Evaluation of Three Immunoassays: Two Automated Immunoassays (Euroimmun and Abbott) and One Rapid Lateral Flow Immunoassay (NG Biotech). *J. Clin. Virol.* **2020**, *129*, 104511. [CrossRef]
24. European Centre for Disease Prevention and Control. COVID-19 Testing Strategies and Objectives. Available online: https://www.ecdc.europa.eu/en/publications-data/covid-19-testing-strategies-and-objectives (accessed on 23 May 2022).
25. Hasöksüz, M.; Kiliç, S.; Saraç, F. Coronaviruses and SARS-COV-2. *Turk. J. Med. Sci.* **2020**, *50*, 549–556. [CrossRef]
26. Gilbert, G.L. SARS, MERS and COVID-19—New Threats; Old Lessons. *Int. J. Epidemiol.* **2020**, *49*, 726–728. [CrossRef] [PubMed]
27. Kadam, S.B.; Sukhramani, G.S.; Bishnoi, P.; Pable, A.A.; Barvkar, V.T. SARS-CoV-2, the Pandemic Coronavirus: Molecular and Structural Insights. *J. Basic Microbiol.* **2021**, *61*, 180–202. [CrossRef] [PubMed]
28. Khailany, R.A.; Safdar, M.; Ozaslan, M. Genomic Characterization of a Novel SARS-CoV-2. *Gene Rep.* **2020**, *19*, 100682. [CrossRef] [PubMed]
29. Kim, D.; Lee, J.-Y.; Yang, J.-S.; Kim, J.W.; Kim, V.N.; Chang, H. The Architecture of SARS-CoV-2 Transcriptome. *Cell* **2020**, *181*, 914–921.e10. [CrossRef]
30. Bačenková, D.; Trebuňová, M.; Špakovská, T.; Schnitzer, M.; Bednarčíková, L.; Živčák, J. Comparison of Selected Characteristics of SARS-CoV-2, SARS-CoV, and HCoV-NL63. *Appl. Sci.* **2021**, *11*, 1497. [CrossRef]
31. Kirtipal, N.; Bharadwaj, S.; Kang, S.G. From SARS to SARS-CoV-2, Insights on Structure, Pathogenicity and Immunity Aspects of Pandemic Human Coronaviruses. *Infect. Genet. Evol.* **2020**, *85*, 104502. [CrossRef]
32. Greenhalgh, T.; Jimenez, J.L.; Prather, K.A.; Tufekci, Z.; Fisman, D.; Schooley, R. Ten Scientific Reasons in Support of Airborne Transmission of SARS-CoV-2. *Lancet* **2021**, *397*, 1603–1605. [CrossRef]
33. Jackson, C.B.; Farzan, M.; Chen, B.; Choe, H. Mechanisms of SARS-CoV-2 Entry into Cells. *Nat. Rev. Mol. Cell Biol.* **2021**, *23*, 3–20. [CrossRef]
34. Hoffmann, M.; Kleine-Weber, H.; Schroeder, S.; Krüger, N.; Herrler, T.; Erichsen, S.; Schiergens, T.S.; Herrler, G.; Wu, N.-H.; Nitsche, A.; et al. SARS-CoV-2 Cell Entry Depends on ACE2 and TMPRSS2 and Is Blocked by a Clinically Proven Protease Inhibitor. *Cell* **2020**, *181*, 271–280.e8. [CrossRef]
35. Papa, G.; Mallery, D.L.; Albecka, A.; Welch, L.G.; Cattin-Ortolá, J.; Luptak, J.; Paul, D.; McMahon, H.T.; Goodfellow, I.G.; Carter, A.; et al. Furin Cleavage of SARS-CoV-2 Spike Promotes but Is Not Essential for Infection and Cell-Cell Fusion. *PLoS Pathog.* **2021**, *17*, e1009246. [CrossRef] [PubMed]
36. Padmanabhan, P.; Desikan, R.; Dixit, N.M. Targeting TMPRSS2 and Cathepsin B/L Together May Be Synergistic against SARS-CoV-2 Infection. *PLoS Comput. Biol.* **2020**, *16*, e1008461. [CrossRef] [PubMed]
37. Prasad, K.; AlOmar, S.Y.; Almuqri, E.A.; Rudayni, H.A.; Kumar, V. Genomics-Guided Identification of Potential Modulators of SARS-CoV-2 Entry Proteases, TMPRSS2 and Cathepsins B/L. *PLoS ONE* **2021**, *16*, e0256141. [CrossRef] [PubMed]

38. Sungnak, W.; Huang, N.; Bécavin, C.; Berg, M.; Queen, R.; Litvinukova, M.; Talavera-López, C.; Maatz, H.; Reichart, D.; Sampaziotis, F.; et al. SARS-CoV-2 Entry Factors Are Highly Expressed in Nasal Epithelial Cells Together with Innate Immune Genes. *Nat. Med.* **2020**, *26*, 681–687. [CrossRef]
39. Lukassen, S.; Chua, R.L.; Trefzer, T.; Kahn, N.C.; Schneider, M.A.; Muley, T.; Winter, H.; Meister, M.; Veith, C.; Boots, A.W.; et al. SARS-CoV-2 Receptor ACE2 and TMPRSS2 Are Primarily Expressed in Bronchial Transient Secretory Cells. *EMBO J.* **2020**, *39*, e105114. [CrossRef] [PubMed]
40. Zhou, L.; Xu, Z.; Castiglione, G.M.; Soiberman, U.S.; Eberhart, C.G.; Duh, E.J. ACE2 and TMPRSS2 Are Expressed on the Human Ocular Surface, Suggesting Susceptibility to SARS-CoV-2 Infection. *Ocul. Surf.* **2020**, *18*, 537–544. [CrossRef]
41. Fodoulian, L.; Tuberosa, J.; Rossier, D.; Boillat, M.; Kan, C.; Pauli, V.; Egervari, K.; Lobrinus, J.A.; Landis, B.N.; Carleton, A.; et al. SARS-CoV-2 Receptors and Entry Genes Are Expressed in the Human Olfactory Neuroepithelium and Brain. *iScience* **2020**, *23*, 101839. [CrossRef]
42. World Health Organization. Tracking SARS-CoV-2 Variants. Available online: https://www.who.int/activities/tracking-SARS-CoV-2-variants (accessed on 23 May 2022).
43. Khandia, R.; Singhal, S.; Alqahtani, T.; Kamal, M.A.; El-Shall, N.A.; Nainu, F.; Desingu, P.A.; Dhama, K. Emergence of SARS-CoV-2 Omicron (B.1.1.529) Variant, Salient Features, High Global Health Concerns and Strategies to Counter It amid Ongoing COVID-19 Pandemic. *Environ. Res.* **2022**, *209*, 112816. [CrossRef]
44. Choi, J.Y.; Smith, D.M. SARS-CoV-2 Variants of Concern. *Yonsei Med. J.* **2021**, *62*, 961–968. [CrossRef]
45. Johansson, M.A.; Quandelacy, T.M.; Kada, S.; Prasad, P.V.; Steele, M.; Brooks, J.T.; Slayton, R.B.; Biggerstaff, M.; Butler, J.C. SARS-CoV-2 Transmission from People Without COVID-19 Symptoms. *JAMA Netw. Open* **2021**, *4*, e2035057. [CrossRef]
46. Diamond, M.S.; Kanneganti, T.-D. Innate Immunity: The First Line of Defense against SARS-CoV-2. *Nat. Immunol.* **2022**, *23*, 165–176. [CrossRef] [PubMed]
47. Boechat, J.L.; Chora, I.; Morais, A.; Delgado, L. The Immune Response to SARS-CoV-2 and COVID-19 Immunopathology—Current Perspectives. *Pulmonology* **2021**, *27*, 423–437. [CrossRef] [PubMed]
48. Thorne, L.G.; Reuschl, A.-K.; Zuliani-Alvarez, L.; Whelan, M.V.X.; Turner, J.; Noursadeghi, M.; Jolly, C.; Towers, G.J. SARS-CoV-2 Sensing by RIG-I and MDA5 Links Epithelial Infection to Macrophage Inflammation. *EMBO J.* **2021**, *40*, e107826. [CrossRef] [PubMed]
49. Severa, M.; Diotti, R.A.; Etna, M.P.; Rizzo, F.; Fiore, S.; Ricci, D.; Iannetta, M.; Sinigaglia, A.; Lodi, A.; Mancini, N.; et al. Differential Plasmacytoid Dendritic Cell Phenotype and Type I Interferon Response in Asymptomatic and Severe COVID-19 Infection. *PLOS Pathog.* **2021**, *17*, e1009878. [CrossRef]
50. Blanco-Melo, D.; Nilsson-Payant, B.E.; Liu, W.-C.; Uhl, S.; Hoagland, D.; Møller, R.; Jordan, T.X.; Oishi, K.; Panis, M.; Sachs, D.; et al. Imbalanced Host Response to SARS-CoV-2 Drives Development of COVID-19. *Cell* **2020**, *181*, 1036–1045.e9. [CrossRef]
51. Leisman, D.E.; Ronner, L.; Pinotti, R.; Taylor, M.D.; Sinha, P.; Calfee, C.S.; Hirayama, A.V.; Mastroiani, F.; Turtle, C.J.; Harhay, M.O.; et al. Cytokine Elevation in Severe and Critical COVID-19: A Rapid Systematic Review, Meta-Analysis, and Comparison with Other Inflammatory Syndromes. *Lancet Respir. Med.* **2020**, *8*, 1233–1244. [CrossRef]
52. García-Pérez, B.E.; González-Rojas, J.A.; Salazar, M.I.; Torres-Torres, C.; Castrejón-Jiménez, N.S. Taming the Autophagy as a Strategy for Treating COVID-19. *Cells* **2020**, *9*, 2679. [CrossRef]
53. Casadevall, A.; Joyner, M.J.; Pirofski, L.-A. SARS-CoV-2 Viral Load and Antibody Responses: The Case for Convalescent Plasma Therapy. *J. Clin. Invest.* **2020**, *130*, 5112–5114. [CrossRef]
54. Wang, H.; Yuan, Y.; Xiao, M.; Chen, L.; Zhao, Y.; Zhang, H.; Long, P.; Zhou, Y.; Xu, X.; Lei, Y.; et al. Dynamics of the SARS-CoV-2 Antibody Response up to 10 Months after Infection. *Cell Mol. Immunol.* **2021**, *18*, 1832–1834. [CrossRef]
55. Xu, L.; Li, D.; Ramadan, S.; Li, Y.; Klein, N. Facile Biosensors for Rapid Detection of COVID-19. *Biosens. Bioelectron.* **2020**, *170*, 112673. [CrossRef]
56. Yongchen, Z.; Shen, H.; Wang, X.; Shi, X.; Li, Y.; Yan, J.; Chen, Y.; Gu, B. Different Longitudinal Patterns of Nucleic Acid and Serology Testing Results Based on Disease Severity of COVID-19 Patients. *Emerg. Microbes Infect.* **2020**, *9*, 833–836. [CrossRef] [PubMed]
57. Herroelen, P.H.; Martens, G.A.; De Smet, D.; Swaerts, K.; Decavele, A.-S. Humoral Immune Response to SARS-CoV-2: Comparative Clinical Performance of Seven Commercial Serology Tests. *Am. J. Clin. Pathol.* **2020**, *154*, 610–619. [CrossRef] [PubMed]
58. Okba, N.M.A.; Müller, M.A.; Li, W.; Wang, C.; GeurtsvanKessel, C.H.; Corman, V.M.; Lamers, M.M.; Sikkema, R.S.; de Bruin, E.; Chandler, F.D.; et al. Severe Acute Respiratory Syndrome Coronavirus 2-Specific Antibody Responses in Coronavirus Disease Patients. *Emerg. Infect. Dis.* **2020**, *26*, 1478–1488. [CrossRef] [PubMed]
59. Long, Q.-X.; Liu, B.-Z.; Deng, H.-J.; Wu, G.-C.; Deng, K.; Chen, Y.-K.; Liao, P.; Qiu, J.-F.; Lin, Y.; Cai, X.-F.; et al. Antibody Responses to SARS-CoV-2 in Patients with COVID-19. *Nat. Med.* **2020**, *26*, 845–848. [CrossRef] [PubMed]
60. Loos, C.; Atyeo, C.; Fischinger, S.; Burke, J.; Slein, M.D.; Streeck, H.; Lauffenburger, D.; Ryan, E.T.; Charles, R.C.; Alter, G. Evolution of Early SARS-CoV-2 and Cross-Coronavirus Immunity. *mSphere* **2020**, *5*, e00622-20. [CrossRef]
61. Luo, H.; Jia, T.; Chen, J.; Zeng, S.; Qiu, Z.; Wu, S.; Li, X.; Lei, Y.; Wang, X.; Wu, W.; et al. The Characterization of Disease Severity Associated IgG Subclasses Response in COVID-19 Patients. *Front. Immunol.* **2021**, *12*, 632814. [CrossRef]
62. Kyei-Barffour, I.; Addo, S.A.; Aninagyei, E.; Ghartey-Kwansah, G.; Acheampong, D.O. Sterilizing Immunity against COVID-19: Developing Helper T Cells I and II Activating Vaccines Is Imperative. *Biomed. Pharmacother.* **2021**, *144*, 112282. [CrossRef]

63. Garcia-Beltran, W.F.; Lam, E.C.; St Denis, K.; Nitido, A.D.; Garcia, Z.H.; Hauser, B.M.; Feldman, J.; Pavlovic, M.N.; Gregory, D.J.; Poznansky, M.C.; et al. Multiple SARS-CoV-2 Variants Escape Neutralization by Vaccine-Induced Humoral Immunity. *Cell* **2021**, *184*, 2372–2383.e9. [CrossRef]
64. Planas, D.; Veyer, D.; Baidaliuk, A.; Staropoli, I.; Guivel-Benhassine, F.; Rajah, M.M.; Planchais, C.; Porrot, F.; Robillard, N.; Puech, J.; et al. Reduced Sensitivity of SARS-CoV-2 Variant Delta to Antibody Neutralization. *Nature* **2021**, *596*, 276–280. [CrossRef]
65. Sethuraman, N.; Jeremiah, S.S.; Ryo, A. Interpreting Diagnostic Tests for SARS-CoV-2. *JAMA* **2020**, *323*, 2249–2251. [CrossRef]
66. Caliendo, A.M.; Gilbert, D.N.; Ginocchio, C.C.; Hanson, K.E.; May, L.; Quinn, T.C.; Tenover, F.C.; Alland, D.; Blaschke, A.J.; Bonomo, R.A.; et al. Better Tests, Better Care: Improved Diagnostics for Infectious Diseases. *Clin. Infect. Dis.* **2013**, *57*, S139–S170. [CrossRef] [PubMed]
67. Kevadiya, B.D.; Machhi, J.; Herskovitz, J.; Oleynikov, M.D.; Blomberg, W.R.; Bajwa, N.; Soni, D.; Das, S.; Hasan, M.; Patel, M.; et al. Diagnostics for SARS-CoV-2 Infections. *Nat. Mater.* **2021**, *20*, 593–605. [CrossRef] [PubMed]
68. Corman, V.M.; Drosten, C. Authors' Response: SARS-CoV-2 Detection by Real-Time RT-PCR. *Eurosurveillance* **2020**, *25*, 2001035. [CrossRef] [PubMed]
69. Food and Drug Administration. *In Vitro Diagnostics EUAs—Antigen Diagnostic Tests for SARS-CoV-2*; FDA: Washington, DC, USA, 2022.
70. CDC. Clinical Laboratory Improvement Amendments (CLIA). Available online: https://www.cdc.gov/clia/index.html (accessed on 27 August 2022).
71. St John, A.; Price, C.P. Existing and Emerging Technologies for Point-of-Care Testing. *Clin. Biochem. Rev.* **2014**, *35*, 155–167.
72. Infectious Diseases Society of America. Antibody Testing. Available online: https://www.idsociety.org/covid-19-real-time-learning-network/diagnostics/antibody-testing/ (accessed on 24 May 2022).
73. European Commission. COVID-19 In Vitro Diagnostic Devices and Test Methods Database. Available online: https://covid-19-diagnostics.jrc.ec.europa.eu/ (accessed on 24 May 2022).
74. Van Elslande, J.; Houben, E.; Depypere, M.; Brackenier, A.; Desmet, S.; André, E.; Van Ranst, M.; Lagrou, K.; Vermeersch, P. Diagnostic Performance of Seven Rapid IgG/IgM Antibody Tests and the Euroimmun IgA/IgG ELISA in COVID-19 Patients. *Clin. Microbiol. Infect.* **2020**, *26*, 1082–1087. [CrossRef]
75. Sørensen, C.A.; Clemmensen, A.; Sparrewath, C.; Tetens, M.M.; Krogfelt, K.A. Children Naturally Evading COVID-19—Why Children Differ from Adults. *COVID* **2022**, *2*, 25. [CrossRef]
76. Scotta, M.C.; David CN, d.e.; Varela, F.H.; Sartor, I.T.S.; Polese-Bonatto, M.; Fernandes, I.R.; Zavaglia, G.O.; Ferreira, C.F.; Kern, L.B.; Santos, A.P.; et al. Low Performance of a SARS-CoV-2 Point-of-Care Lateral Flow Immunoassay in Symptomatic Children during the Pandemic. *J. Pediatr.* **2022**, *98*, 136–141. [CrossRef] [PubMed]
77. Fearon, E.; Buchan, I.E.; Das, R.; Davis, E.L.; Fyles, M.; Hall, I.; Hollingsworth, T.D.; House, T.; Jay, C.; Medley, G.F.; et al. SARS-CoV-2 Antigen Testing: Weighing the False Positives against the Costs of Failing to Control Transmission. *Lancet Respir. Med.* **2021**, *9*, 685–687. [CrossRef]
78. Andryukov, B.G. Six Decades of Lateral Flow Immunoassay: From Determining Metabolic Markers to Diagnosing COVID-19. *AIMS Microbiol.* **2020**, *6*, 280–304. [CrossRef]
79. Wen, T.; Huang, C.; Shi, F.-J.; Zeng, X.-Y.; Lu, T.; Ding, S.-N.; Jiao, Y.-J. Development of a Lateral Flow Immunoassay Strip for Rapid Detection of IgG Antibody against SARS-CoV-2 Virus. *Analyst* **2020**, *145*, 5345–5352. [CrossRef]
80. Mahmoudinobar, F.; Britton, D.; Montclare, J.K. Protein-Based Lateral Flow Assays for COVID-19 Detection. *Protein Eng. Des. Sel.* **2021**, *34*, gzab010. [CrossRef] [PubMed]
81. Exinger, J.; Hartard, C.; Lafferrière, F.; Fenninger, C.; Charbonnière, L.J.; Jeulin, H. Evaluation of a Lateral Flow Immunoassay COVIDTECH® SARS-CoV-2 IgM/IgG Antibody Rapid Test. *Jpn. J. Infect. Dis.* **2022**, *75*, 334–340. [CrossRef] [PubMed]
82. Koczula, K.M.; Gallotta, A. Lateral Flow Assays. *Essays Biochem.* **2016**, *60*, 111–120. [CrossRef] [PubMed]
83. Pieri, M.; Nicolai, E.; Nuccetelli, M.; Sarubbi, S.; Tomassetti, F.; Pelagalli, M.; Minieri, M.; Terrinoni, A.; Bernardini, S. Validation of a Quantitative Lateral Flow Immunoassay (LFIA)-Based Point-of-Care (POC) Rapid Test for SARS-CoV-2 Neutralizing Antibodies. *Arch. Virol.* **2022**, *167*, 1285–1291. [CrossRef] [PubMed]
84. Ward, H.; Whitaker, M.; Flower, B.; Tang, S.N.; Atchison, C.; Darzi, A.; Donnelly, C.A.; Cann, A.; Diggle, P.J.; Ashby, D.; et al. Population Antibody Responses Following COVID-19 Vaccination in 212,102 Individuals. *Nat. Commun.* **2022**, *13*, 907. [CrossRef] [PubMed]
85. Qi, H.; Liu, B.; Wang, X.; Zhang, L. The Humoral Response and Antibodies against SARS-CoV-2 Infection. *Nat. Immunol.* **2022**, *23*, 1008–1020. [CrossRef]
86. Nickel, O.; Rockstroh, A.; Borte, S.; Wolf, J. Evaluation of Simple Lateral Flow Immunoassays for Detection of SARS-CoV-2 Neutralizing Antibodies. *Vaccines* **2022**, *10*, 347. [CrossRef]
87. Tanne, J.H. Covid-19: FDA Approves Use of Convalescent Plasma to Treat Critically Ill Patients. *BMJ* **2020**, *368*, m1256. [CrossRef]
88. Duan, K.; Liu, B.; Li, C.; Zhang, H.; Yu, T.; Qu, J.; Zhou, M.; Chen, L.; Meng, S.; Hu, Y.; et al. Effectiveness of Convalescent Plasma Therapy in Severe COVID-19 Patients. *Proc. Natl. Acad. Sci. USA* **2020**, *117*, 9490–9496. [CrossRef]
89. Galipeau, Y.; Greig, M.; Liu, G.; Driedger, M.; Langlois, M.-A. Humoral Responses and Serological Assays in SARS-CoV-2 Infections. *Front. Immunol.* **2020**, *11*, 610688. [CrossRef]
90. Guo, L.; Ren, L.; Yang, S.; Xiao, M.; Chang, D.; Yang, F.; Dela Cruz, C.S.; Wang, Y.; Wu, C.; Xiao, Y.; et al. Profiling Early Humoral Response to Diagnose Novel Coronavirus Disease (COVID-19). *Clin. Infect. Dis.* **2020**, *71*, 778–785. [CrossRef] [PubMed]

91. Deeks, J.J.; Dinnes, J.; Takwoingi, Y.; Davenport, C.; Spijker, R.; Taylor-Phillips, S.; Adriano, A.; Beese, S.; Dretzke, J.; Ferrante di Ruffano, L.; et al. Antibody Tests for Identification of Current and Past Infection with SARS-CoV-2. *Cochrane Database Syst. Rev.* **2020**, *6*, CD013652. [CrossRef] [PubMed]
92. Shen, B.; Zheng, Y.; Zhang, X.; Zhang, W.; Wang, D.; Jin, J.; Lin, R.; Zhang, Y.; Zhu, G.; Zhu, H.; et al. Clinical Evaluation of a Rapid Colloidal Gold Immunochromatography Assay for SARS-Cov-2 IgM/IgG. *Am. J. Transl. Res.* **2020**, *12*, 1348–1354. [PubMed]
93. Novello, S.; Terzolo, M.; Paola, B.; Gianetta, M.; Bianco, V.; Arizio, F.; Brero, D.; Perini, A.M.E.; Boccuzzi, A.; Caramello, V.; et al. Humoral Immune Response to SARS-CoV-2 in Five Different Groups of Individuals at Different Environmental and Professional Risk of Infection. *Sci. Rep.* **2021**, *11*, 24503. [CrossRef]
94. Chen, P.-Y.; Ko, C.-H.; Wang, C.J.; Chen, C.-W.; Chiu, W.-H.; Hong, C.; Cheng, H.-M.; Wang, I.-J. The Early Detection of Immunoglobulins via Optical-Based Lateral Flow Immunoassay Platform in COVID-19 Pandemic. *PLoS ONE* **2021**, *16*, e0254486. [CrossRef]
95. Brochot, E.; Demey, B.; Touzé, A.; Belouzard, S.; Dubuisson, J.; Schmit, J.-L.; Duverlie, G.; Francois, C.; Castelain, S.; Helle, F. Anti-Spike, Anti-Nucleocapsid and Neutralizing Antibodies in SARS-CoV-2 Inpatients and Asymptomatic Individuals. *Front. Microbiol.* **2020**, *11*, 584251. [CrossRef]
96. van den Hoogen, L.L.; Smits, G.; van Hagen, C.C.E.; Wong, D.; Vos, E.R.A.; van Boven, M.; de Melker, H.E.; van Vliet, J.; Kuijer, M.; Woudstra, L.; et al. Seropositivity to Nucleoprotein to Detect Mild and Asymptomatic SARS-CoV-2 Infections: A Complementary Tool to Detect Breakthrough Infections after COVID-19 Vaccination? *Vaccine* **2022**, *40*, 2251–2257. [CrossRef]
97. Smits, V.A.J.; Hernández-Carralero, E.; Paz-Cabrera, M.C.; Cabrera, E.; Hernández-Reyes, Y.; Hernández-Fernaud, J.R.; Gillespie, D.A.; Salido, E.; Hernández-Porto, M.; Freire, R. The Nucleocapsid Protein Triggers the Main Humoral Immune Response in COVID-19 Patients. *Biochem. Biophys. Res. Commun.* **2021**, *543*, 45–49. [CrossRef]
98. Michel, M.; Bouam, A.; Edouard, S.; Fenollar, F.; Di Pinto, F.; Mège, J.-L.; Drancourt, M.; Vitte, J. Evaluating ELISA, Immunofluorescence, and Lateral Flow Assay for SARS-CoV-2 Serologic Assays. *Front. Microbiol.* **2020**, *11*, 597529. [CrossRef]
99. Ochola, L.; Ogongo, P.; Mungai, S.; Gitaka, J.; Suliman, S. Performance Evaluation of Lateral Flow Assays for Coronavirus Disease-19 Serology. *Clin. Lab. Med.* **2022**, *42*, 31–56. [CrossRef]
100. Tan, E.; Frew, E.; Cooper, J.; Humphrey, J.; Holden, M.; Mand, A.R.; Li, J.; Anderson, S.; Bi, M.; Hatler, J.; et al. Use of Lateral Flow Immunoassay to Characterize SARS-CoV-2 RBD-Specific Antibodies and Their Ability to React with the UK, SA and BR P.1 Variant RBDs. *Diagnostics* **2021**, *11*, 1190. [CrossRef] [PubMed]
101. Huang, R.-L.; Fu, Y.-C.; Wang, Y.-C.; Hong, C.; Yang, W.-C.; Wang, I.-J.; Sun, J.-R.; Chen, Y.; Shen, C.-F.; Cheng, C.-M. A Lateral Flow Immunoassay Coupled with a Spectrum-Based Reader for SARS-CoV-2 Neutralizing Antibody Detection. *Vaccines* **2022**, *10*, 271. [CrossRef] [PubMed]
102. Hung, K.-F.; Hung, C.-H.; Hong, C.; Chen, S.-C.; Sun, Y.-C.; Wen, J.-W.; Kuo, C.-H.; Ko, C.-H.; Cheng, C.-M. Quantitative Spectrochip-Coupled Lateral Flow Immunoassay Demonstrates Clinical Potential for Overcoming Coronavirus Disease 2019 Pandemic Screening Challenges. *Micromachines* **2021**, *12*, 321. [CrossRef] [PubMed]
103. Chen, S.; Meng, L.; Wang, L.; Huang, X.; Ali, S.; Chen, X.; Yu, M.; Yi, M.; Li, L.; Chen, X.; et al. SERS-Based Lateral Flow Immunoassay for Sensitive and Simultaneous Detection of Anti-SARS-CoV-2 IgM and IgG Antibodies by Using Gap-Enhanced Raman Nanotags. *Sens. Actuators B Chem.* **2021**, *348*, 130706. [CrossRef]
104. Shurrab, F.M.; Younes, N.; Al-Sadeq, D.W.; Liu, N.; Qotba, H.; Abu-Raddad, L.J.; Nasrallah, G.K. Performance Evaluation of Novel Fluorescent-Based Lateral Flow Immunoassay (LFIA) for Rapid Detection and Quantification of Total Anti-SARS-CoV-2 S-RBD Binding Antibodies in Infected Individuals. *Int. J. Infect. Dis.* **2022**, *118*, 132–137. [CrossRef]
105. Feng, M.; Chen, J.; Xun, J.; Dai, R.; Zhao, W.; Lu, H.; Xu, J.; Chen, L.; Sui, G.; Cheng, X. Development of a Sensitive Immunochromatographic Method Using Lanthanide Fluorescent Microsphere for Rapid Serodiagnosis of COVID-19. *ACS Sens.* **2020**, *5*, 2331–2337. [CrossRef]
106. Chen, Z.; Zhang, Z.; Zhai, X.; Li, Y.; Lin, L.; Zhao, H.; Bian, L.; Li, P.; Yu, L.; Wu, Y.; et al. Rapid and Sensitive Detection of Anti-SARS-CoV-2 IgG, Using Lanthanide-Doped Nanoparticles-Based Lateral Flow Immunoassay. *Anal. Chem.* **2020**, *92*, 7226–7231. [CrossRef]
107. Zhou, Y.; Chen, Y.; Liu, W.; Fang, H.; Li, X.; Hou, L.; Liu, Y.; Lai, W.; Huang, X.; Xiong, Y. Development of a Rapid and Sensitive Quantum Dot Nanobead-Based Double-Antigen Sandwich Lateral Flow Immunoassay and Its Clinical Performance for the Detection of SARS-CoV-2 Total Antibodies. *Sens. Actuators B Chem.* **2021**, *343*, 130139. [CrossRef]
108. Wang, P. Combination of Serological Total Antibody and RT-PCR Test for Detection of SARS-COV-2 Infections. *J. Virol. Methods* **2020**, *283*, 113919. [CrossRef]
109. Dinnes, J.; Deeks, J.J.; Berhane, S.; Taylor, M.; Adriano, A.; Davenport, C.; Dittrich, S.; Emperador, D.; Takwoingi, Y.; Cunningham, J.; et al. Rapid, Point-of-care Antigen Tests for Diagnosis of SARS-CoV-2 Infection. *Cochrane Database Syst. Rev.* **2021**, *2021*, CD013705. [CrossRef]
110. Mistry, D.A.; Wang, J.Y.; Moeser, M.-E.; Starkey, T.; Lee, L.Y.W. A Systematic Review of the Sensitivity and Specificity of Lateral Flow Devices in the Detection of SARS-CoV-2. *BMC Infect. Dis.* **2021**, *21*, 828. [CrossRef]
111. Tapari, A.; Braliou, G.G.; Papaefthimiou, M.; Mavriki, H.; Kontou, P.I.; Nikolopoulos, G.K.; Bagos, P.G. Performance of Antigen Detection Tests for SARS-CoV-2: A Systematic Review and Meta-Analysis. *Diagnostics* **2022**, *12*, 1388. [CrossRef] [PubMed]

112. Peto, T.; Affron, D.; Afrough, B.; Agasu, A.; Ainsworth, M.; Allanson, A.; Allen, K.; Allen, C.; Archer, L.; Ashbridge, N.; et al. COVID-19: Rapid Antigen Detection for SARS-CoV-2 by Lateral Flow Assay: A National Systematic Evaluation of Sensitivity and Specificity for Mass-Testing. *EClinicalMedicine* **2021**, *36*, 100924. [CrossRef] [PubMed]
113. Giberti, I.; Costa, E.; Domnich, A.; Ricucci, V.; De Pace, V.; Garzillo, G.; Guarona, G.; Icardi, G. High Diagnostic Accuracy of a Novel Lateral Flow Assay for the Point-of-Care Detection of SARS-CoV-2. *Biomedicines* **2022**, *10*, 1558. [CrossRef] [PubMed]
114. WHO. Antigen-Detection in the Diagnosis of SARS-CoV-2 Infection. Available online: https://www.who.int/publications-detail-redirect/antigen-detection-in-the-diagnosis-of-sars-cov-2infection-using-rapid-immunoassays (accessed on 23 August 2022).
115. De Marinis, Y.; Pesola, A.-K.; Söderlund Strand, A.; Norman, A.; Pernow, G.; Aldén, M.; Yang, R.; Rasmussen, M. Detection of SARS-CoV-2 by Rapid Antigen Tests on Saliva in Hospitalized Patients with COVID-19. *Infect. Ecol. Epidemiol.* **2021**, *11*, 1993535. [CrossRef]
116. Kivrane, A.; Igumnova, V.; Liepina, E.E.; Skrastina, D.; Leonciks, A.; Rudevica, Z.; Kistkins, S.; Reinis, A.; Zilde, A.; Kazaks, A.; et al. Development of Rapid Antigen Test Prototype for Detection of SARS-CoV-2 in Saliva Samples. *Upsala J. Med. Sci.* **2022**, *127*, e8207. [CrossRef]
117. Zhang, Y.; Liu, X.; Wang, L.; Yang, H.; Zhang, X.; Zhu, C.; Wang, W.; Yan, L.; Li, B. Improvement in Detection Limit for Lateral Flow Assay of Biomacromolecules by Test-Zone Pre-Enrichment. *Sci. Rep.* **2020**, *10*, 9604. [CrossRef]
118. Ardekani, L.S.; Thulstrup, P.W. Gold Nanoparticle-Mediated Lateral Flow Assays for Detection of Host Antibodies and COVID-19 Proteins. *Nanomaterials* **2022**, *12*, 1456. [CrossRef]
119. Peng, T.; Jiao, X.; Liang, Z.; Zhao, H.; Zhao, Y.; Xie, J.; Jiang, Y.; Yu, X.; Fang, X.; Dai, X. Lateral Flow Immunoassay Coupled with Copper Enhancement for Rapid and Sensitive SARS-CoV-2 Nucleocapsid Protein Detection. *Biosensors* **2022**, *12*, 13. [CrossRef]
120. Diao, B.; Wen, K.; Zhang, J.; Chen, J.; Han, C.; Chen, Y.; Wang, S.; Deng, G.; Zhou, H.; Wu, Y. Accuracy of a Nucleocapsid Protein Antigen Rapid Test in the Diagnosis of SARS-CoV-2 Infection. *Clin. Microbiol. Infect.* **2021**, *27*, 289.e1–289.e4. [CrossRef]
121. Kiro, V.V.; Gupta, A.; Singh, P.; Sharad, N.; Khurana, S.; Prakash, S.; Dar, L.; Malhotra, R.; Wig, N.; Kumar, A.; et al. Evaluation of COVID-19 Antigen Fluorescence Immunoassay Test for Rapid Detection of SARS-CoV-2. *J. Glob. Infect. Dis.* **2021**, *13*, 91. [CrossRef] [PubMed]
122. Wang, D.; He, S.; Wang, X.; Yan, Y.; Liu, J.; Wu, S.; Liu, S.; Lei, Y.; Chen, M.; Li, L.; et al. Rapid Lateral Flow Immunoassay for the Fluorescence Detection of SARS-CoV-2 RNA. *Nat. Biomed. Eng.* **2020**, *4*, 1150–1158. [CrossRef] [PubMed]
123. Wang, C.; Cheng, X.; Liu, L.; Zhang, X.; Yang, X.; Zheng, S.; Rong, Z.; Wang, S. Ultrasensitive and Simultaneous Detection of Two Specific SARS-CoV-2 Antigens in Human Specimens Using Direct/Enrichment Dual-Mode Fluorescence Lateral Flow Immunoassay. *ACS Appl. Mater. Interfaces* **2021**, *13*, 40342–40353. [CrossRef] [PubMed]
124. Zhu, Q.; Zhou, X. A Colorimetric Sandwich-Type Bioassay for SARS-CoV-2 Using a HACE2-Based Affinity Peptide Pair. *J. Hazard. Mater.* **2022**, *425*, 127923. [CrossRef]
125. Lee, J.-H.; Lee, Y.; Lee, S.K.; Kim, J.; Lee, C.-S.; Kim, N.H.; Kim, H.G. Versatile Role of ACE2-Based Biosensors for Detection of SARS-CoV-2 Variants and Neutralizing Antibodies. *Biosens. Bioelectron.* **2022**, *203*, 114034. [CrossRef]
126. Porras, J.; Bernuz, M.; Marfa, J.; Pallares-Rusiñol, A.; Martí, M.; Pividori, M.I. Comparative Study of Gold and Carbon Nanoparticles in Nucleic Acid Lateral Flow Assay. *Nanomaterials* **2021**, *11*, 741. [CrossRef]
127. FDA. *Mesa Biotech, Inc., Recalls Certain Accula SARS-CoV-2 Tests for Risk of False Positives Caused by Contamination*; FDA: Washington, DC, USA, 2022.
128. Agarwal, S.; Warmt, C.; Henkel, J.; Schrick, L.; Nitsche, A.; Bier, F.F. Lateral Flow–Based Nucleic Acid Detection of SARS-CoV-2 Using Enzymatic Incorporation of Biotin-Labeled DUTP for POCT Use. *Anal. Bioanal. Chem.* **2022**, *414*, 3177–3186. [CrossRef]
129. Zheng, C.; Wang, K.; Zheng, W.; Cheng, Y.; Li, T.; Cao, B.; Jin, Q.; Cui, D. Rapid Developments in Lateral Flow Immunoassay for Nucleic Acid Detection. *Analyst* **2021**, *146*, 1514–1528. [CrossRef]
130. Rahman, M.M. Progress in Electrochemical Biosensing of SARS-CoV-2 Virus for COVID-19 Management. *Chemosensors* **2022**, *10*, 287. [CrossRef]

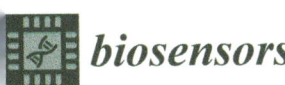

Review

A Framework for Biosensors Assisted by Multiphoton Effects and Machine Learning

Jose Alberto Arano-Martinez [1], Claudia Lizbeth Martínez-González [1], Ma Isabel Salazar [2] and Carlos Torres-Torres [1,*]

[1] Sección de Estudios de Posgrado e Investigación, Escuela Superior de Ingeniería Mecánica y Eléctrica, Unidad Zacatenco, Instituto Politécnico Nacional, Mexico City 07738, Mexico

[2] Departamento de Microbiología, Escuela Nacional de Ciencias Biológicas, Instituto Politécnico Nacional, Mexico City 11340, Mexico

* Correspondence: ctorrest@ipn.mx

Abstract: The ability to interpret information through automatic sensors is one of the most important pillars of modern technology. In particular, the potential of biosensors has been used to evaluate biological information of living organisms, and to detect danger or predict urgent situations in a battlefield, as in the invasion of SARS-CoV-2 in this era. This work is devoted to describing a panoramic overview of optical biosensors that can be improved by the assistance of nonlinear optics and machine learning methods. Optical biosensors have demonstrated their effectiveness in detecting a diverse range of viruses. Specifically, the SARS-CoV-2 virus has generated disturbance all over the world, and biosensors have emerged as a key for providing an analysis based on physical and chemical phenomena. In this perspective, we highlight how multiphoton interactions can be responsible for an enhancement in sensibility exhibited by biosensors. The nonlinear optical effects open up a series of options to expand the applications of optical biosensors. Nonlinearities together with computer tools are suitable for the identification of complex low-dimensional agents. Machine learning methods can approximate functions to reveal patterns in the detection of dynamic objects in the human body and determine viruses, harmful entities, or strange kinetics in cells.

Keywords: optical biosensors; photonics; machine learning; nonlinear optics; SARS-CoV-2

1. Introduction

The field of biosensors is highly dynamic, with scientific research advances that have mainly flourished in the last decades. Numerous biosensors have been developed for nanotechnology, engineering, molecular biology, computer, and optics [1]. In general, there are three types of biosensors: electrochemical, optical, and piezoelectric; each kind has its own method for transducing signals [2]. Nanoscale functions have been shown to be attractive for manufacturing biosensors [3].

A biosensor is a tool with the ability to detect and determine biological expressions in an environment [4]. This involves a biorecognition fragment for a detailed union and specifies the target molecules (enzymes, antibodies, proteins, cell receptors, toxins, DNA, pharmacists, etc.) [5]. Due to the powerful optical characteristics of semiconductors, they have provided great sensitivity and repeatability for integrated photonic biosensors based on silicon [6]. The performance of the optical sensors in semiconductor platforms may be impacted by two-photon absorption and free carrier dispersion, even if silicon offers optical advantages [7]. Therefore, different scientific groups have oriented their work to design other low-cost materials with advanced characteristics for developing optical biosensors [8].

Optical biosensors outperform standard analytical techniques by allowing real-time, label-free detection of biological and chemical compounds in a highly sensitive, selective, and cost-effective way [9]. Optical biosensors have been developed for detecting optical signals related to analytes via biocatalytic or bio-affinitive processes [10]. They are categorized according to the mechanism for biosensing, which can be refraction, reflection, Raman scattering, infrared emission, fluorescence, chemiluminescence, absorption, dispersion, or phosphorescence [11].

Optical biosensors can be assisted by plasmonic effects in order to easily identify a virus confirmed by molecules in exhaled air, or droplets such as those represented by nasopharyngeal swabs and saliva [12]. In essence, plasmonic detection techniques act as a viral pre-screening tool to enable the detection of infected individuals [13]. Biosensors have demonstrated their ability to detect viruses in human blood: an example is dengue [14] or chikungunya [15].

Surface plasmon resonance (SPR) has become the most sensitive label-free technique for the detection of various molecular species in solution, and it is of great significance in drug, food safety, and biological reaction studies [16]. SPR excitations are the result of free electron density oscillations and the interaction of electromagnetic waves between dielectric and metal film surfaces; the collective electronic excitations are the fundamental mechanism behind SPR experiments [1]. The reflected light in SPR systems is significantly reduced when the evanescent wave and the surface plasma wave produced by light resonate.

SPR technology has been utilized to produce biosensors for a variety of uses, including plasmonic detectors, optical polarization encoding, sensing technologies, and bio-photonic sensors [17]. SPR has been employed in several biosensor applications because it is highly sensitive to the refractive index of materials nearby [18]. The oscillation of free electrons in the conducting band of the metal is known as surface plasmons. They can only be excited by a polarized wave that is orthogonal to the plane of incidence and the direction of propagation of the surface plasmons [19]. Additionally, remarkable discoveries have been reported for biosensors based on the Raman effect, which is an inflexible shift in radiation frequency caused by optical light in vibrating molecules [20].

Plasmon-based technologies, such as SPR biosensors, have outstanding performance and versatility, and they are one kind of biosensor that is able to detect COVID-19 [21]. An SPR biosensor is capable of completing a reliable COVID-19 test in a matter of minutes compared to other long PCR or antigen tests that patients must perform in medical centers or hospitals [22]. Therefore, SPR-based techniques attract attention for developing biosensors. The detailed processing in SPR simply involves excitation of the coupled-resonator optical-waveguide at a fixed wavelength and imaging of coupled-resonator optical-out-of-plane waveguide's elastic light-scattering huge factor [23]. The method can make use of a discontinuous transition of the coupled-resonator optical waveguide (CROW) eigenstate excited at a fixed laser wavelength in response to a slight change inside the coating refractive index [24].

Single protein detection has been achieved using several label-free optical techniques, including two with imaging capabilities. One involves heating a protein solution with a laser in an indirect manner while the change in the solvent's refractive index is recorded. Interferometric scattering is the base of another technique [25]. The typical method for detecting the scattering light of plasmonic nanoparticles is based on scanning the spectra of nanoparticles using dark-field microscopy, which is time-consuming, laborious, and the small capacity of the sample regularly acts as a limitation [26]. On the other hand, surface-enhanced Raman scattering (SERS) methods are also assisted by SPR effects provided by specific metal nanoparticles such as their main component [20]. The double recognition biosensor SERS is an effective way to measure a variety of biological agents in the laboratory [27].

Biosensors based on bimetallic nanostructures have demonstrated high sensitivity in the detection of different substances, acting as an alternative for use [28]. In addition to their portability and high detection efficiency, some biosensors based on SERS can be reused more than three times when replacing the thread of the DNA substrate and washing the microfluidic device again [29]. Recently, several SERS substrates have been developed for biosensor applications with a high signal improvement for superimposed plasmonic fields. SERS is very attractive as an alternative method for detecting quantitative and co-multiplexed DNA because it can generate specific molecular oscillation spectra [30].

SERS-based methods have had a high impact on biomolecular analysis due to several factors, such as the fingerprint signal from the SERS nanotag and the stability [31]. As a rule, when a laser illuminates nanoparticles immobilized with the Raman reporter molecule, a local hotspot is initiated, and the Raman signal intensity of the reporter molecule is amplified by several orders of magnitude [32]. So far, research papers have been published demonstrating the potential of SERS-based methods for detecting sensitive and multiplexed biomarkers [33]. The dispersion of the cross-section spectrum shows a peak whose position also depends on the thickness of the biomolecular layer of the nanoparticles. The dependence of the cross-section spectra and the corresponding maximum changes in the thickness of the biomolecular layer are presented by a dispersing effect. Compared with the peaks of the absorption and dispersion spectra, the position of the peak of the dispersion spectrum is more sensitive to changes in the thickness of the biomolecule layer. The peak dispersion change can be about 8 nm, while the saturable absorption can be 2.5 nm [34]. In previous investigations, it has been pointed out that the optical characteristics of cadmium telluride nanorods have a better property under laser excitation with the absorption coefficient of two-photon absorption of 12.0×10^{-10} m/W at 100 µJ. Applications of cadmium telluride nanorods seems to be promising for the next-generation nonenzymatic biosensors and memory devices [35]. However, nonlinear optical (NLO) properties of semiconductors are limited by power level requirements. Nonlinear semiconductors are designed to exhibit high nonlinearity in refraction without effects associated with two-photon absorption; this method allows waveguides to operate at low power levels. For example, it has been indicated that silicon photon waveguide biosensors can detect variations in the transmission spectrum at 1550 nm of the urine glucose concentration with the evaluation of the refractive index [36].

It must be highlighted that NLO processes have opened up a variety of options for improving biosensors. There are many important factors to consider when designing nonlinear biosensors, including the refractive index of the optical media being used [37]. In particular, optical biosensors based on photonic crystals have been reported for detecting the concentration of the SARS-CoV-2 pathogen in water [38].

Moreover, in view of the need to overcome these issues, two branches of artificial intelligence (AI): machine learning (ML) and soft computing, have achieved a notable improvement in several research fields by providing agility and efficiency in different applications. Soft computing is an approach that incorporates the uncertainty and imprecision inherent to real world, inspired by systems in nature, mostly the human brain. Thus, a main process in these techniques is learning; machine learning, then, is related to the capability of a machine to infer an approximate solution from past data or to discover patterns and rules from unknown data.

In view of all these points, we analyzed different panoramic opportunities for optical biosensors based on NLOs for the detection of SARS-CoV-2. In this direction, we highlight how different NLO applications assisted by ML have increased their efficiency and speed to carry out tasks assigned to advanced algorithms with a potential for their use in sensing performance.

2. SARS-CoV-2 Biosensors

Compared to SARS-CoV and Middle East respiratory syndrome coronavirus, SARS-CoV-2 has been shown to be far more contagious [39]. The virus, also known as SARS-CoV-2, has had a significant negative impact on the environment and mankind, increasing mortality rates and causing significant economic losses around the globe [40]. In the years 2002 to 2003, the severe acute respiratory syndrome (SARS) was spread by SARS-CoV-2, a single-stranded RNA virus from the genus Beta coronavirus [41]. In 2021, RNA SARS-CoV-

2 was frequently detected on surfaces in the medical environment, even in adaptive and unrelated sewage [42].

Coronavirus disease (COVID-19) outbreaks in several communities have compelled governments worldwide to enact stringent controls such as blockades, border closures, and widespread screening [43]. The SARS-CoV-2 virus is compatible with the coronavirus family with single-stranded gene RNA and surface proteins such as membranes, envelopes, nucleocapsids, and spikes [44]. Cryo-electron microscopy was utilized to establish the structure of the SARS-CoV-2 spike glycoprotein, which was then used for the creation of cell-specific vaccinations [45].

The symptoms of being infected by the SARS-CoV-2 virus can be varied; some symptoms are coughing, discomfort, and fever [46]. Several techniques are available for rapid measurement of antigen levels from both nasopharyngeal secretions and saliva, providing fairly satisfactory duplication of molecular assay results [47]. When performing the standard diagnosis, RNA extraction of the nasopharyngeal swab is required, followed by quantitative reverse transcription PCR (RT-QPCR) [48]. In recent years, some of the investigations have been focused on the design of optical biosensors for the efficient and rapid detection of the SARS-CoV-2 virus. The recognition elements of optical biosensors can be divided into aptamers, molecular imprint polymers (MIPs), and antibodies [49]. Wenjuan and his colleagues created the first unique microfluidic biosensor using Fresnel reflection for the detection of SARS-CoV-2 without a label that is quick, simple, and sensitive [50].

In order to identify the SARS-CoV-2 virus, optical biosensors can generate several wavelengths and collect data on heart rate, nitric oxide levels, pulse oximetry, and kidney function [51]. Courtney and colleagues created a successful biosensor with the ability to detect nucleic acids and with the option to improve with high convergence and mismatch [52]. Silicon nitride low-loss photonic wires have been used in the optical transmission waveguide devices to develop a complementary metal-oxide semiconductor compatible with the plasma-enhanced chemical vapor deposition process [53]. Ebola, HIV, and norovirus viruses have been detected by optical biosensors based on resonators, optical biosensors based on the waveguides, photonic biosensors based on crystals, and fiber-based optical biosensors [54]. In the latest investigations, the possibility of detecting the COVID-19 virus with a low 0.22 pm detection limit has been reported and the difference between SARS-CoV of the SARS-CoV-2 was distinguished by a plasmonic sensor [55].

One of the most intriguing and extensively researched devices is one made by utilizing surface nanopatterning technology. Nanopattern subwavelength characteristics promote actions such as guided mode resonance [56], SERS [56], or localized SPR [57]. Those structures make it possible to identify light interactions with certain biological analytes at the sensor surface effectively.

In order to increase the sensibility of sensing materials, photonic crystals have been proposed as periodic arrangements of dielectric materials built in an area of incoming radiation [58]. Similar to the bandgap in semiconductors, they have a photonic bandgap where it is forbidden for some wavelengths to pass through their structure [59].

In the past two decades, integrated photonic biosensors have become the focus of significant study because they can be miniaturized and can effectively detect relatively low concentrations of analytes in real time [60]. According to Srivastava and colleagues, the magnified changes caused by the conversion to photonics are sensitive to changes in the refraction index of the sensing medium; this makes the nanostructures an excellent choice for a biosensor [61]. Most of the photonic integrated sensors employ the concept of evanescent field detection, where the analyte adheres to a bioreaction layer on the surface of the wave guide and interacts with the evanescent field of the guided wave [62]. The initial displacement in particular biosensors may be increased by about four orders of magnitude by utilizing preselection to choose the polarization and postselection to create destructive interference [63]. This signal enhancement approach can simplify the optical components and lower the cost of the sensor device in addition to measuring the spin-dependent splitting in biosensors [64]. Furthermore, due to its distinct optical characteristics, the photonic spin Hall effect has generated a lot of study in recent years [62]. On-chip resonant or interferometric devices are used to translate changes in the optical phase, which cannot be detected directly, into changes in the optical power [63].

SPR biosensors are particularly effective in detecting bacterial viruses and pathogens among various biodetection methodologies [65]. By using this method, slow PCR and ELISA techniques are avoided. The first investigation by Wrapp and colleagues focused on the high affinity of the SARS-CoV-2 protein with ACE2 [66]. More recently, a unique localized SPR biosensor with the twin capabilities of plasmonic photothermal and sensing transduction was presented [67].

A very efficient technique for rapid detection is worth mentioning. It is without labels and is precise for a variety of pathogens and viruses that have been based on SPR [68]. In the past, it was asserted that an SPR-based biosensor could recognize the feline calicivirus in about 15 min [69]. In the same way, a very similar discovery was obtained for human enterovirus 71 (EV71) [70]. Research has found different forms of rapid and precise detection of COVID-19, and nanophotonic biosensors have been developed [67]. An SPR optical biosensor with a gold nanoparticle coating was successfully developed by researchers as a COVID-19 detection device [71]. For the potential detection of coronavirus illness, different optical biosensors with localized SPR have been presented [72].

It is possible to improve SPR platforms of localized SPR devices for the identification of COVID-19 [73]. Ren-min and Oulton's study demonstrated the use of the nanolaser method as a biological optical detector [74]. For monitoring small chemical molecules, photonic glass fiber biosensors have been integrated by using porous silicon structures [75]. In order to find comparative chemical compounds, photonic crystal fiber biosensors based on a porous silicon have also been described [76]. Typically, the SPR biosensor is employed to identify biological or chemical materials [77]. Previous experiments demonstrated the potential of SPR biosensors for viral detection without real-time labels [78]. An overview of representative works in this area is shown in Table 1.

Table 1. Representative optical biosensors papers for the detection of SARS-CoV-2.

Journal	Detection Limit	Analyte Types	Optical Effect	Year	Reference
Biosensors and Bioelectronics	2 µL	The genes of S, N, and Orf1ab	Evanescent wave fluorescence	2021	[79]
Talanta	1.0 mg/mL	Immunoglobulins (G, M, and A)	Colorimetric	2021	[80]
Talanta	12.5 ng/mL	IgG antibody	Evanescent wave fluorescence	2021	[81]
Sensors and Actuators B: Chemical	1 and 0.033 ng/mL	Spike 1 protein	Fluorescent bifunctional	2022	[82]
Chemical Engineering Journal	43.70 aM	RNA-dependent RNA polymerase gene	Electrochemiluminescence	2022	[83]
Environmental Science: Nano	32.80 aM	RNA-dependent RNA polymerase gene	Electrochemiluminescence	2022	[84]
Biosensors and Bioelectronics	2.75 fM	Spike protein, matrix protein, envelope protein, and nucleocapsid	Colorimetry G-quadruplex	2020	[85]
Virology	-	Nucleocapsid protein	Luminescence	2021	[86]
Talanta	59 aM	Nucleic acid	Electrochemiluminescence	2022	[87]
Chemical Engineering Journal	7.8 aM	RNA-dependent RNA polymerase gene	Electrochemiluminescence	2022	[88]
Viruses	50 µg/mL	Angiotensin-converting enzyme 2	Bioluminescent	2021	[89]
Cold Spring Harbor Laboratory	50 µg/mL	Angiotensin-converting enzyme 2	Bioluminescent	2020	[90]
Physica Scripta	1020 nm/refractive index unit (RIU)	Pathogens of SARS-CoV-2	Refractive index	2022	[38]

Table 1. Cont.

Journal	Detection Limit	Analyte Types	Optical Effect	Year	Reference
Sensors and Actuators B: Chemical	-	Spike protein	Optical interferometry	2021	[91]
SSRN Electronic Journal	833.33 nm/RIU	Spike glycoprotein	Refractive index	2022	[92]
Talanta	514 aM	spike protein, nucleocapsid protein, the RNA-dependent RNA polymerase gene	Electrochemiluminescence	2022	[93]
Sensors	0.1 fM	Open reading frames 1ab gene	Electrochemiluminescence	2022	[94]
Talanta	0.22 pM	Spike protein	Refractive index	2021	[55]
Analytica Chimica Acta	48 ng/mL	SARS-CoV-2 spike antigen	Colorimetric	2021	[95]
Analytica Chimica Acta	1.0×10^{-6} RIU	Spike protein receptor-binding domain	Fresnel reflection	2021	[96]
2021 IEEE 15th International Conference on Nano/Molecular Medicine & Engineering (NANOMED)	114.07 nm RIU^{-1}	COVID-19 virus detection by delivering quick, dependable results	Refractive index	2021	[22]
Scilight	~106 virions/mL	SARS-CoV-2 proteins (membrane, envelope, and spike)	Colorimetric	2021	[97]
Biosensors and Bioelectronics	17 aM	SARS-CoV-2 RNAs with single molecule sensitivity	Electro-optofluidic	2021	[98]
Biosensors and Bioelectronics	-	Nucleic-acid-based testing	Colorimetric	2021	[99]
Journal of the American Chemical Society	-	Spike antigen and cultured virus	Luminescent	2022	[100]
Biosensors and Bioelectronics	370 vp/mL	SARS-CoV-2 virus particles in one step	Nanoplasmonic resonance	2021	[101]
ACS Applied Materials & Interfaces	0.21 fM	RNA-dependent RNA polymerase gene	Electrochemiluminescence	2021	[102]
In vitro models	1 µg/mL	S protein of SARS-CoV-2	Colorimetric	2022	[103]
Biosensors and Bioelectronics	3 copies/µL	Two regions in nucleocapsid gene (N1 and N2 genes)	Fluorescence polarization	2021	[104]
Biosensors and Bioelectronics	1 mg/mL	Immunoglobulins G and M	Optical/chemiluminescence	2021	[105]
Viruses	100 pM	Spike proteins, nucleocapsid proteins	Fluorescent	2022	[106]
Microchimica Acta	4.98 ng/mL^{-1}	Angiotensin-converting enzyme 2	Colorimetric	2021	[107]

From Table 1, we can observe different optical and photonic biosensors that perform the function of detecting SARS-CoV-2. The advantage of using optical biosensors is the ease of use. The optics tools have demonstrated with some applications the ability to improve the resolution, speed, and efficiency of biosensors. Moreover, biosensors based on nonlinear absorption, Raman dispersion, or SPR can present advantages in biosensing regarding the potential for multiphoton effects. Table 2 presents these characteristics for detection of SARS-CoV-2. Table 1 describes biosensors assisted by optical effects, while Table 2 mentions biosensors that are related to multiphoton effects.

Table 2. Representative multiphoton biosensors papers for the detection of SARS-CoV-2.

Journal	Detection Limit	Analyte Types	Optical Effect	Year	Reference
IEEE Sensors Journal	2.5 ng/mL	Nucleocapsid protein	Plasmonic fiber optic absorbance	2021	[108]
Biosensors	0.047 µg/mL	SARS-CoV-2 pseudovirus	Surface plasmon resonance	2022	[109]
Biosensors and Bioelectronics	0.77 fg/mL^{-1}	Spike protein	Raman scattering	2021	[110]
Sensors and Actuators B: Chemical	50 and 10 pfu/mL	Angiotensin-converting enzyme 2	Raman scattering	2022	[111]
ECS Meeting Abstracts	-	Antibodies to SARS-CoV-2	Surface plasmon resonance	2021	[112]
Analytical Chemistry	45.6 to 86 ng mL^{-1}	Nucleocapsid protein	Plasmonics	2022	[21]
Biosensors and Bioelectronics	2 ng/spot	spike S1, spike S1 S2, and the nucleocapsid protein	Fluorescent plasmonics	2021	[113]
Sensors	4.2 µg/mL	Spike protein	Photonics	2021	[114]
Analyst	12 fg mL^{-1}	Spike S1 protein	Surface plasmon resonance	2022	[115]
Biomedical Vibrational Spectroscopy 2022: Advances in Research and Industry	-	Spike protein	Raman spectroscopy	2022	[116]
Plasmonics	152°/RIU	Spike proteins, membrane proteins, envelop proteins, and nucleoprotein	Surface plasmon resonance	2022	[117]
Sensors	250 µg/mL	Spike (S1 and S2) proteins	Surface plasmon resonance	2021	[118]
IEEE SENSORS 2021	8.34 ng/mL	Spike protein	Surface plasmon resonance	2021	[119]
Biosensors and Bioelectronics	1 µg/mL	Nucleocapsid antibody	Surface plasmon resonance	2022	[120]
AIP Advances	54.04 RIU^{-1}	Spike glycoprotein	Surface plasmon resonance	2021	[67]
Analytical Chemistry	-	Spike surface glycoprotein	Surface-enhanced infrared absorption	2021	[13]
Matter	10 PFU/mL	Spike glycoprotein and membrane protein	Raman scattering	2022	[121]
ACS Applied Nano Materials	200 PFU/mL	Spike proteins	Raman scattering	2022	[122]
ACS Nano	0.22 pM	RNA-dependent RNA polymerase	Localized surface plasmon resonance	2020	[123]
Analytical Chemistry	-	Angiotensin-converting enzyme 2	Surface plasmon resonance	2020	[124]
Biosensors and Bioelectronics	150 ng/ml	Detect SARS-CoV-2 nucleocapsid proteins	Localized surface Plasmon resonance	2022	[125]
Analytical Methods	200 µL	Spike and nucleocapsid proteins	Surface plasmon resonance	2021	[126]
Sensors & Diagnostics	10 RU	Spike protein	Surface plasmon resonance	2022	[127]
Biosensors and Bioelectronics	2×10^{11} particles/mL	Nucleocapsid phosphoprotein gene	Raman scattering	2022	[128]
BioChip Journal	1.02 pM	Antibodies against nucleoprotein	Surface plasmon resonance	2020	[129]
Nanoscale Advances	4.5 fg/mL^{-1}	SARS-CoV-2 spike protein	Raman scattering	2022	[130]

Table 2. Cont.

Journal	Detection Limit	Analyte Types	Optical Effect	Year	Reference
Biosensors and Bioelectronics	0.08 ng/mL	SARS-CoV-2 spike protein	Localized surface plasmon resonance	2020	[131]
Analytical Chemistry	4 mg/mL	SARS-CoV-2 spike protein	Surface plasmon resonance	2021	[132]
Plasmonics	1×10^{13} per m^2	Thiol-tethered DNA of SARS-CoV-2	Surface plasmon resonance	2021	[133]
Talanta	0.046 ng/mL	SARS-CoV-2 spike protein	Raman scattering	2022	[134]
Talanta	100 pg/mL^{-1}	Measurement of SARS-CoV-2 antibody	Photonic resonator absorption	2021	[135]
Talanta	37 nM	SARS-CoV-2 spike glycoprotein	Surface plasmon resonance	2021	[136]

3. Biosensors Assisted by Machine Learning

As was mentioned before, ML is a subfield of artificial intelligence (AI) that provides another way to gain insight into complex data [137]. ML uses computational systems to simulate human learning and gives the algorithm the ability to recognize and acquire knowledge of the environment to improve performance [138]. Complex biological systems are naturally compatible with ML methods that can effectively detect hidden patterns [139]. Predictive information multiplexed can be obtained by increasing analysis of responses in a sequence [140].

ML-assisted biosensors can be used in complex environments and without having the characteristics of a laboratory study [141]. A typical process is shown in Figure 1. Raw data acquired by a biosensor are preprocessed (data filtering, missing values, segmentation; normalization is also carried out early in this step to homogenize scales or data types) according to the nature of the data. Features or characteristics are then extracted to represent the differences in the data and also to reduce the amount of data. This features set X is called features space. Dimensionality reduction of X is carried out to select the most significant variables and decrease complexity. It is worth mentioning that the quality of data is relevant. ML learns from the sample; if there is noise or the sample is not significant, overfitting will occur and the performance of the algorithm will be poor.

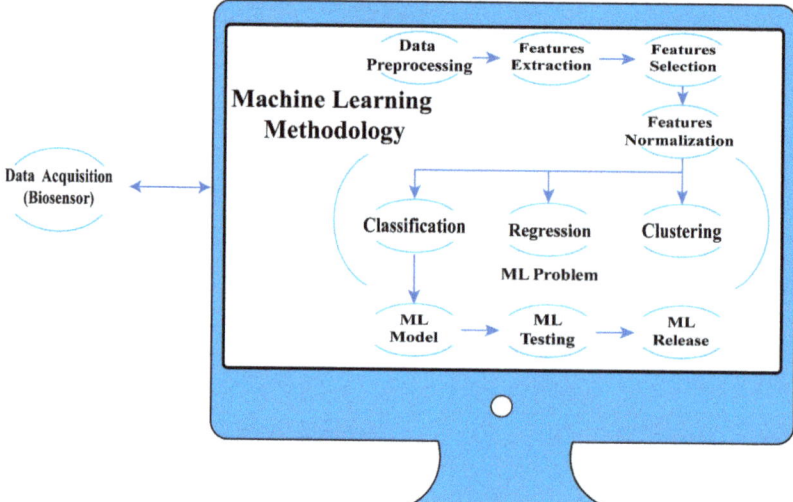

Figure 1. Biosensors assisted by ML.

In general, three types of problems can be approximated with ML: classification, regression, and clustering problems. Dimensionality reduction by itself is also considered a type of problem solved by ML, and clustering is commonly a previous step in a classification problem.

According to the nature of X, the learning process in ML is divided into two main categories: supervised and unsupervised learning (Figure 2). When the inputs X are known or labeled, the learning process is called supervised. The objective in a problem of classification or prediction (regression) is to approximate a function $f(X) = Y + \varepsilon$, to approximate the output or labels Y with an error ε. In this learning process, ML methods use a subset of X to train a model. Once the model has been trained, it is tested with the rest of the available data. This step is repeated until the approximate function reaches an error goal; then, the model is released to classify or predict new unknown data. A balance among two types of error should be taken into account: bias, which is the result of the assumptions of data behavior in learning the objective function, and variance, which indicates how different the function approach will be according to the training dataset used. Different algorithms are used for these learning processes; some of them are usually applied to data analysis, such as linear regression. Other algorithms categorized in ML are logistic regression, support vector machines (SVM), naïve Bayes, decision trees, and k-nearest neighbors (KNN). On the other hand, the learning process is called unsupervised when X is not labeled; here, the objective is to discover the patterns in the data to generate clusters with similar features. The most popular algorithm for this learning process is k-means.

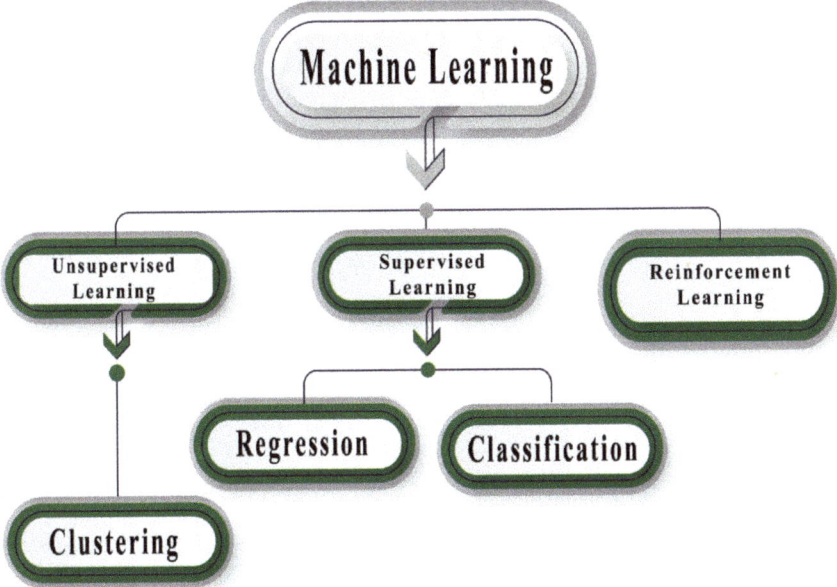

Figure 2. ML categories according to the nature of the features space.

Soft computing algorithms are those strictly inspired by nature, for instance, artificial neural networks (ANNs), fuzzy systems, genetic algorithms, swarm algorithms, and ant colony optimization algorithms. Soft computing methods are especially useful for optimization problems; in this sense, ANNs and other ML algorithms optimize the error of the objective function.

The acquisition of information can be enhanced by automatic learning tools [142]; in this direction, optical biosensors have made a great contribution to medicine by being non-invasive and ultrafast. On the other hand, ML can improve these results, simplifying the analysis of the raw data from the biosensors output, to approximate a solution to different problems. For instance, (a) classification, for detection or diagnosis and treatment decisions support; (b) regression, to predict and prevent non-desirable events; and (c) clustering, to find groups of data that share features, such as symptoms, characteristics of a disease, or a strange behavior in different scales (e.g., enzymes, hormones, cells, organs, systems, and the whole body). The signals provided by the optical biosensor can be monitored in real time to outflow tract constructions that are useful in ML methods [143].

For instance, a supervised automatic learning method with optimized characteristics has been implemented to consider the effects of decreased enzymatic activity [144] or glucose in a sample [145]. ML regression statistical models have been applied to estimate the current response of a second-generation amperometry glucose oxidase biosensor [146].

Neural Networks in Biosensors

An artificial neural network (ANN) consists of a node layer that has an input layer, one or additional hidden layers, and an output layer [147]. Every node or artificial nerve cell connects to a different node and has acceptable weights and thresholds [148]. Once a private node output exceeds a threshold, that node is activated and sends data to a consequent layer within the network [149], as illustrated in Figure 3.

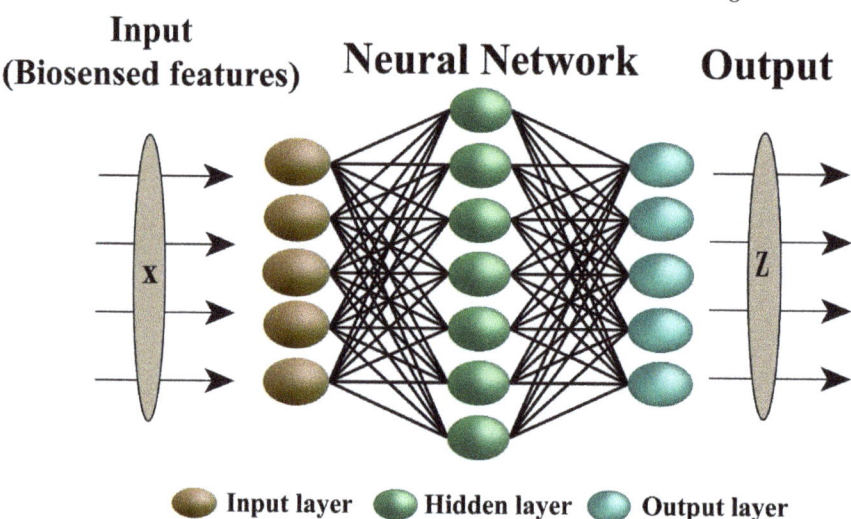

Figure 3. ANN common structure.

There is research demonstrating the improvement in the use of neural networks (NNs) in the enhancement of signal processing. In fact, it has been found that the combination of spectrum in spectrograms is an effective way to classify strong signs of biosensors [150]. In biosensors, pathogen agents and neurons associated with the disease have an important value. In recognition of the excellent classification capacity of the convolutional neuronal network model, it is also possible to perform the classification of a disease using biosensors [151]. An example of this is Mennel and colleagues, who conducted an image detection study applying an ANN [152].

In recent years, optical biosensors have received attention from the scientific community due to their advantages, such as detection with high sensitivity [153]. Different fluorescent materials such as quantum dots [154] and fluorescent microspheres have been used [155]. A technique to measure the fluorescent signal is excitation using a sensitive fluorometer; this determines the concentration of the bacteria. Instead of determining the target bacteria concentration, fluorescent bacteria can also be counted directly. NNs algorithms fulfill the function of processing the images obtained from fluorescent bacteria.

NNs processing manages to calculate the amount of fluorescent points faster to determine the target bacteria [156].

4. NLO Processes Analyzed with ML

Prediction of nanoscale functions in multiphoton experiments is attractive for describing different NLO effects [157]. Analysis of third-order NLO techniques by ML has conjointly progressed throughout the last decade [158], considering all-optical functions for sensing and signal processing by ML [159]. There has been growing interest in generating pulses with repetitive frequencies on the order of gigacycle per second with the assistance of deep learning [160]. Measurements of ultrafast optical pulses for sensing represent challenges for scientific research in ML methods [161].

A roadmap of representative research on NLO applying ML methods is shown in Figure 4. ML for studying chaotic nonlinear dynamics [162], self-tuning for mode-locked lasers [163], laser optimization [164], and the measurement of extremely short pulses; it should be noted that their duration is much shorter than the response times of most photodetectors [165]. Ultrashort pulses are widely used to monitor chemical reactions, control THz radiation, cipher pulses for communication, and form optical pulses [166]. ML has been used to measure time unit pulse duration using time unit detectors [167].

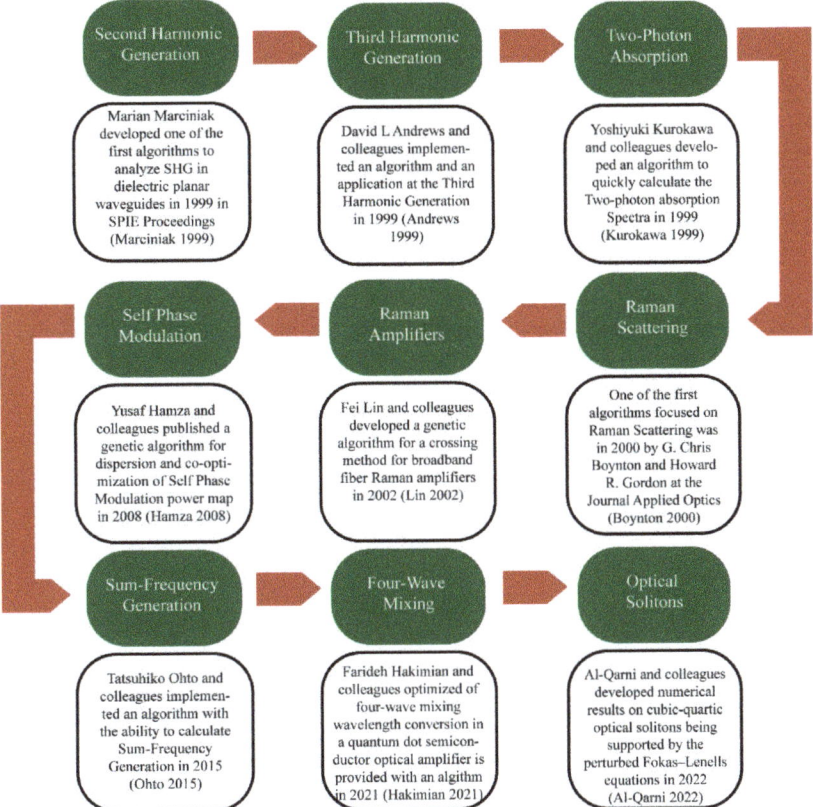

Figure 4. Roadmap of investigations based on NLO processes assisted by ML and soft computing [168–176].

The most promising methodology to atone for nonlinearities in single channel systems is the digital backpropagation algorithm, which works by digitally modeling the fiber channel [177]. The disadvantages of this method are the high procedure complexity of the time period application and also the impossibility of accurately modeling the channel because of the looks of random parameters [178]. For these reasons, analysis on nonlinear compensation is currently centered on computing techniques [179]. Extraordinarily short pulses are troublesome to explain due to the massive variety of the parameters concerned [180]. With such systems, small changes in state variables will cause changes in momentum dynamics, which is particularly necessary with ML-based algorithms [168–176] (Roadmap).

4.1. Second-Harmonic Generation

The second-order NLO process in which photons that interact with a nonlinear material "combine" effectively is known as second-harmonic generation (SHG) [181]. SHG, which depends on a second-order NLO difference system, permits specialists to perform non-checking and non-horrendous imaging of tissue structures at the cell level [182]. Currently, when relevant areas in SHG images are detected, further medical actions can be proposed [183]. However, no simplifying assumptions or analytic solutions have been found to obtain SHG's accurate spatial phase distribution [184]. The core measures employed in SHG simulation continue to be numerical techniques such as the split-step method and the Fourier-space algorithm [185].

The variation that uses SHG is simple for frequency-resolved optical gating (FROG). In fact, the pulse-shaping community frequently employs SHG FROG in nonlinear spectroscopy and coherent anti-Stokes Raman diffusing to discover potential extremely complex beats [186]. Furthermore, due to well-known trivial ambiguities, it has been mathematically demonstrated that all pulses may be uniquely predicted by SHG FROG [187]. More recently, a nonlinear time-domain finite difference method was developed by modifying Yee's algorithm into a potent modeling technique that can take nonlinear phenomena such as second- or third-harmonic generation into consideration [188]. Intrinsic signals can be viewed as label-free using a nonlinear mode of multiphoton excitation called SHG [189]. Qun and colleagues have applied the SHG effect with the help of ML methods to develop images of the samples of thick heart tissue [190].

Since the discovery of quartz's piezoelectricity more than a century ago, the need for effective materials for novel piezoelectric and NLO applications has steadily increased. Although piezoelectric materials are supposed to have the highest electromechanical coefficients, excellent SHG characteristics are crucial for NLO applications [191]. ANNs speed up optimization of genetic algorithms and store sample information that can be easily generalized to other samples with minimal additional training [192]. Hall and colleagues developed an impartial and efficient algorithm to quantify the images of SHG in tissues [193].

The continuous wave laser radiation in the UV range is often realized due to nonlinear effects such as four-wavelength mixing or SHG [194]. ANNs speed up optimization of genetic algorithms and store sample information that can be easily generalized to other samples with minimal additional training [195]. Deep-ultraviolet NLO crystals for current and upcoming basic research and technology requirements, a succinct SHG output wavelength, and a frequency conversion ratio are crucial [196]. SHG coefficients are shown to be inversely related to the band gap via the sum-over-states formula [197].

By using second-order NLO differential elements in SHG imaging, specialists can conduct label-free, non-destructive studies of tissue architecture [198]. Up to the current date, there is no published study that suggests using ML to instruct users about adjustable NLO vulnerability and exchanging behavior for sensing [199].

4.2. Nonlinear Optical Absorption

The optical absorption coefficient of a material that depends on irradiance is known as nonlinear optical absorption [200]. The absorption coefficient disappears at the dissipation intensity. In other cases, absorption is observed at low intensities, but the absorption coefficient increases or decreases at high intensities [201]. In order to address nonlinear tomographic absorption spectroscopy issues, Deng et al. looked deeper into how well other complicated deep ANNs, such as deep belief networks and recurrent ANNs, performed [202]. It is advantageous for photonic computing applications because of its straightforward design, very quick operation, and high NLO coefficient [203]. However, only basic investigations of direct absorption-spectroscopy-based deep learning algorithms for nonlinear tomography issues have been performed [204]. Only temperature or particle concentration may be reconstructed using the deep learning network provided [202].

4.3. Optical Kerr Effect

The Kerr nonlinearity has an NLO impact when light induces a change in the refractive index by different physical mechanisms such as electronic polarization or molecular orientation. It can be portrayed as an induced birefringence caused by optical irradiance and is dependent on the square of the electric field that can be supervised by ML [205].

The Kerr law of nonlinearity emerges when a light wave in an optical fiber meets nonlinear responses because of nonharmonic mobility of electrons trapped in molecules produced by an external electric field [206]. Solli and colleagues observed for the first time the rogue waves in one-dimensional settings in the field of optics [207]. Chalcogenide glass, which has a very strong Kerr effect and reacts right away to electrical stimulation, was employed by Gopalakrishnan and colleagues to obtain experimentally meaningful values for the above described [208]. Jhangeer and his colleagues developed an algorithm capable of obtaining wave solutions of exact paths of complex nonlinear partial differential equations [209]. This is achieved by improving the perturbative nonlinear Schrödinger equation with the nonlinear Kerr effect, which is an important equation for soliton testing in optical communication networks.

4.4. Sum Frequency Generation

A second-order NLO mechanism called sum frequency generation (SFG) works by annihilating two input photons with each frequency ω_1 and ω_2 while simultaneously generating one photon with frequency ω_3 [210]. When imaging self-assembled thiol monolayers on gold using the SFG spectroscopic method, ANNs are utilized as a substitute for chemical identification [211]. ANNs are also particularly helpful for solving issues when it is difficult or impossible to provide realistic physical or mathematical models [212].

4.5. Self-Phase Modulation

An NLO result for the interaction between matter and the vectorial nature of light is self-phase modulation (SPM). Due to the optical Kerr effect, a medium's refractive index changes when an ultrashort light pulse passes across it [213]. Since NN can adaptively correct for distortion, NN-based digital signal processing has been researched to account for nonlinear effects in wireless communication systems [214]. Only intensity-modulated direct detection transmission methods have been analyzed for nonlinear distortion correction in optical communication systems. In order to correct for the distorted multilevel optical signal caused by SPM, Shotaro and colleagues suggested a novel nonlinear equalization technique employing NN [215]. Caballero and colleagues developed a method with the ability to estimate signal-to-noise linear ratio and nonlinear ratio considering SPM assisted with an NN [216].

4.6. Raman Amplifiers

The reasonable choice of pump powers and wavelengths is a key element in accomplishing a wanted Raman pick-up profile. This is often a challenging assignment as the relationship between power profile versus pump powers and wavelengths is nonlinear and requires broad numerical reenactments to anticipate [217]. Raman amplifiers have lately attracted fresh interest as a result of their ability to amplify broadband signals by the assistance of ML when used in a multi-pump laser arrangement [218]. In addition, they have reduced noise when using distributed amplifiers and ML [219]. The Raman amplifiers' capacity to arbitrarily set the gain by varying the pump power and wavelength is another distinctive quality improved by ML [220]. This gives optical amplifiers and optical communication systems unprecedented flexibility and capacity for dynamic adaptation by using deep learning techniques [221]. An example is distributed Raman amplifier (DRA), which is an important amplification method in optical communication systems due to its low noise figure and flexible wideband gain obtained by using ML [222]. Raman gain design and analysis have benefited greatly from the successful use of ML in other domains of optical communication in recent years [223].

Optimizing the pump design to obtain the appropriate gain spectrum at the amplifier output is the key research goal of the Raman amplifier [218]. This challenging optimization issue calls for the solution of a set of nonlinear differential equations. Many algorithms have been developed [224], as well as ANN [225] or ML [226] to find a solution to the conflict between the pump setting and the intended spectral gain setting. Currently, an ML strategy has been proposed for single-mode fibers [227] and few-mode fibers [225]. A dataset of hundreds of advantage bends made with erratic pump powers and wavelengths is used to train an NN to consider the relationship between the pump parameters [228].

4.7. Surface-Enhanced Raman Scattering

Molecular polarizability can be used to explain Raman scattering [229]. Electrons and nuclei are shifted when a molecule is put in an electric field [230]. An electric dipole moment is produced in the molecule because of the separation of charged species, and the molecule is said to be polarized [231]. A molecule scatters irradiant light from a source laser in the Raman method, which is a light scattering technique [232]. Most of the scattered light is of the same wavelength as the laser source and hence useless, but a tiny quantity of light is dispersed at various wavelengths and so is beneficial [233].

The molecules can be coherently driven to a state of breath and can then generate signals that are usually of a stronger magnitude than the spontaneous Raman dispersion [234]. This happens when there is a difference between the pump field and the Stokes field in the coincidence in active vibrations of the molecules in the sample [235]. By analyzing NLO effects, a quick and efficient response is required; an example is the impact of amplified spontaneous emission and nonlinear interference reported by Margareth and colleagues [236].

Raman microscopy is another option for label-free imaging; however, because of the poor effectiveness of Raman scattering, neuron imaging with ordinary spontaneous Raman scattering needs a considerable exposure period [237]. Plasmonic materials have been employed to boost the Raman technique's sensitivity. Pengju and colleagues utilized a calculation based on ML to classify the ordinary and extracellular cancer vesicles and parties [238].

SERS, which has sensitivity down to the level of a single molecule, is perfect for multichannel detection [239]. Based on this idea, SERS physiology was very recently developed in order to offer speculative details about nearby cellular metabolites [240] by accumulating time-based SERS spectra constantly. The way the data were processed also had limitations in the original photophysiological trials for SERS. An ML method that is adaptable was proposed by Leong and colleagues [241].

4.8. Summary of Representative Nonlinear Optical Effects Assisted by ML Algorithms

The progress and development of new research in ML has opened up the opportunity to advance new techniques for the collection and interpretation of information in applications in different sciences. By joining the different optical processes to the interpretation of ML data, it opens up a variety of options and applications. The development of biosensors based on optical processes has provided the ability to detect biological agents in different organisms, facilitating their analysis. The study of the NLO processes assisted by ML involves the extraction of the properties that can represent fundamental information for sensitive classifying and segmentation.

NLO processes have been developed for the use of detection of different materials that can be used for improving biosensors. The most used multiphoton process for the detection of the SARS-CoV-2 virus has been Raman scattering; this is due to its advantages in the field of optics. Table 3 shows different NLO processes that are assisted by computer systems.

Table 3. NLO processes assisted by computational methods.

Journal or Conference Event	Application	Optical Effect	Year	Reference
Sensors	Optical biosensors supported by algorithms for rigorous monitoring and control in the identification of bacteria	Light Diffraction	2020	[242]
PLOS ONE	Comparison between Marquardt Algorithm vs. Newton Iteration Algorithm for biomolecular interaction process between antigen and antibodies or receptors	Optical Surface Plasmon Resonance	2015	[243]
Scientific Reports	Improves the image difference between normal tissues and tumors	SHG	2021	[244]
BMC Cancer	An independent predictive measure of metastasis-free survival in patients with invasive ductal cancer	SHG	2020	[245]
SPIE LASE	Enhanced Pulse Extraction Algorithm FROG used for geometry	SHG	2019	[246]
Atmospheric Measurement Techniques	Measures the error between CO and CO_2 by nonlinear absorption and fluctuations in interference coefficients	Nonlinear Absorption	2013	[240]
Journal of Lightwave Technology	A scheme allowing the soliton comb to be determined under a specific pump scan, with an error of <8%, verified by experimental measurements	Optical Kerr Effect	2020	[247]
SSRN Electronic Journal	Tackling the effects of the intra-polarization self-phase modulation and inter-polarization cross-phase modulation	SFM	2022	[248]
Optics Express	Optimizes the pump wavelength	Raman Amplifiers	2020	[249]
Optical Fiber Communication Conference (OFC) 2020	Gains improvements for a few mode fiber amplifiers	Raman Amplifiers	2020	[250]
Spectrochimica Acta Part A: Molecular and Biomolecular Spectroscopy	Detection of quantity of chlorpyrifos in rice.	Raman Scattering	2021	[251]
Food Chemistry	Quantifies the systemic fungicide residues of Benzimidazole (Thiabendazole) in apples	Raman Scattering	2021	[252]
ACS Nano	Performs the measurement simultaneously from gradients, at least eight in vitro metabolites along with different cell lines	Raman Scattering	2019	[253]
2021 IEEE International Conference on Big Data (Big Data)	Improves rapidity in the inspection of the techniques of images of cellular and tissue pathology	Raman Scattering	2021	[254]
2018 Cross Strait Quad-Regional Radio Science and Wireless Technology Conference (CSQRWC)	Sorts different varieties of honey	Raman Scattering	2018	[255]
In Proceedings of the 2021 IEEE 21st International Conference on Nanotechnology	Label-free method for detection of protective anthrax antigens based on SERS	Raman Scattering	2021	[256]

Table 4 shows different applications that improve the analysis of the processes of the NLOs assisted by computer systems. Figure 5 shows the different nonlinear optical effects mentioned in this work, with a sample of SARS-CoV-2 as an example.

Table 4. Publications about NLO processes assisted by ML.

Journal	Application	Algorithm	Nonlinear Optical	Year	Reference
Journal of Lightwave Technology	A standard for optical quality	A new approach to direct-learning-based pre-distortion using ANN	High throughput coherent optical	2020	[257]
2017 International Conference on Orange Technologies (ICOT)	Using a Computer-Aided Diagnosis (CAD) system, stem cells in the stratum basale are studied	Convolutional ANN	Third-harmonic generation	2017	[258]
Optical and Quantum Electronics	Optimizing the wavelength conversion for four-wave mixing in a quantum dot semiconductor optical amplifier	A fresh method based on ANN and genetic algorithms	Four-wave mixing	2021	[176]
IEEE Photonics Journal	Extrapolates helpful characteristics and details from the SERS signal	A novel approach to enhance SERS signals using principal component analysis as an ML approach	Raman scattering	2020	[259]
Applied Optics	Encryption scheme	A fresh nonlinear picture encryption method using the Fresnel transform domain's Gerchberg–Saxton phase retrieval algorithm	Fresnel transform domain	2014	[260]
Micromachines	In optical micro-resonators, achieves high-fidelity harmonic production	Algorithm Broyden Fletcher Goldfarb Shanno	High-fidelity harmonic	2020	[261]
APL Photonics	A unique method for eliminating Cross-Phase Modulation (XPM) coherent artifacts in ultrafast pumping	XPMnet algorithm	Cross-phase modulation	2021	[262]
IEEE Photonics Journal	Showcases an optical phase conjugation photoelectric nonlinear compensation method	Complex-valued deep NN	Optical phase conjugation	2021	[263]
Optics Express	The deep residual network is used to forecast the Raman spectra of ice and water to detect the ice-water contact as an identification challenge	Deep-learning-based component identification for mixed Raman spectra	Raman scattering	2019	[264]
Environmental Science and Pollution Research	Examines the impact of the fungicide difenoconazole on the quality of rat sperm	Compare the effectiveness of three categorization algorithms	Raman scattering	2019	[265]
IEICE Communications Express	Improved performance in terms of bit error rate and error vector magnitude by effectively compensating for the nonlinear distortion brought on by cross-phase modulation	A cutting-edge digital signal processing method based on ANN for cross-phase modulation correction	Cross-phase modulation	2018	[266]
Optics Communications	Creates empirical physical formulations based on experimental evidence for the light-scattering amplitude response functions of nematic liquid crystals, which are intrinsically nonlinear	Layered feedforward ANN	Light-scattering	2011	[267]
IEICE Communications Express	Compensates nonlinear distortion in optical communication systems	A three-layer ANN	Self-phase modulation	2017	[268]
Scientific Reports	SHG coefficients of NLO crystals with different diamond-like features are being studied	Random forests regression	Second-harmonic generation	2020	[269]
IEEE Journal of Selected Topics in Quantum Electronics	A nonlinear activation function in a feed forward optical NN	Optical ANN	Electro-optic	2019	[270]

Table 4. Cont.

Journal	Application	Algorithm	Nonlinear Optical	Year	Reference
2019 9th International Conference on Cloud Computing	Provides scenarios that demonstrate the relationship between quantum computers and a light of light in the NLO	Algorithm assisting photonic operations	Four-wave mixing and cross-phase	2019	[271]
Chemical Communications	Ratiometric analysis is used to provide a model for the prediction of the depth of two "flavors" of SERS active nanotags buried inside pig tissue	A proof-of-concept approach for the prediction	Raman scattering	2022	[272]
International Journal of Optics	Inference abilities for the task of classifying images	The deep NN with all-optical diffraction	Nonlinear diffraction	2021	[273]
Advanced Photonics	Enhancement of the third-harmonic generation in optimized metasurfaces and contributes to improving the amplitude of optomechanical vibrations	Deep learning techniques for the inverse design of nanophotonics	Third-harmonic generation	2020	[274]
Conference on Lasers and Electro-Optics	Performs image and audio classification	A universal algorithm for backpropagating	Second-harmonic generation	2021	[275]
Optical Materials Express	Activation functions for fully connected ANN, emulated in tensor flow	Photonic ANN	Induced transparency and reverse saturated absorption	2018	[276]
Optik	Encryption security has been improved to the greatest extent possible to fend off attempts	Modified Gerchberg Saxton Iterative Algorithm	Optical nonlinear cryptosystem	2021	[277]
Optics and Lasers in Engineering	Checks the security of a dual random-phase-coding-based nonlinear optical cryptosystem	chosen-plaintext attack algorithm and known-plaintext attack algorithm modifications	Based on double random phase encoding, the NLO cryptosystem	2021	[278]

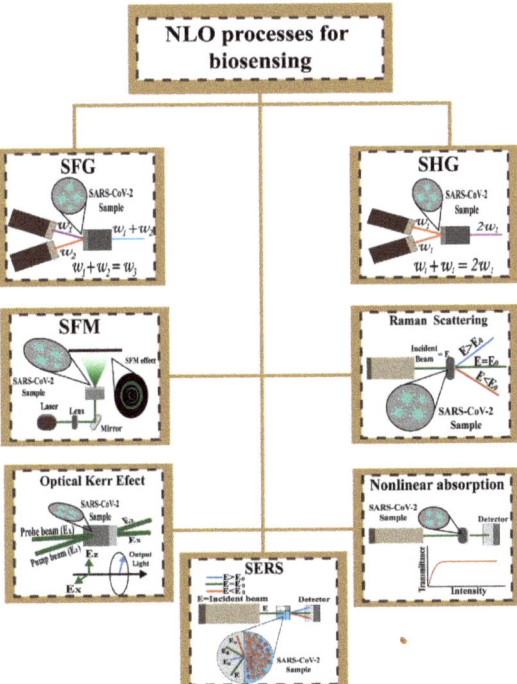

Figure 5. NLO effect schemes proposed for biosensing.

5. Perspectives

Optical biosensors have evolved to visualize biological functions as a microscope has evolved to identify effects of energy. Some optical biosensors can focus the impact of optical and multiphoton nonlinearities to detect the SARS-CoV-2 virus. The optical effect of fluorescence has been used to identify the SARS-CoV-2 virus as well as bacteria, cancer cells, and other viruses. The signature of optics in biosensors has taken advantage of the collection of more information for the detection of biological agents as a non-invasive tool.

Due to the frequency and phase-changing capabilities of the laser light that interacts with NLO materials, they rank among the most intelligent materials of our time [264]. A cutting-edge topic of study for the theoretical and experimental community is the creation of NLO documents [279]. Organic materials must have relatively nonlinear properties due to electrons moving to orbits $\pi - \pi$ [280]. This expectation explains the extensive research on NLO materials for developing biocrystals.

The use of organic crystals as NLO materials has been increasingly promoted by the easy manipulation of these crystals, allowing control of the NLO properties of the material. Compounds exhibiting strong nonlinearity are of great interest to the field of nonlinear optics, as they are used to fabricate devices operating at high speeds [281]. Researchers have been able to produce silicon-organic hybrid waveguides with bandwidths as high as 100 Gbit per second using organic NLO materials [282].

Optical biosensors can be applied to acquire information from remote sensing and one of the tools used for the interpretation of information can be based on ML. The function of the use of ML in biosensors allows automating the device to perform an action depending on the information collected. The diverse forms of emission and optical absorption in nonlinear biosensors are fascinating and are unexplored in several conditions that can be addressed by ML techniques for describing biological functions.

The disadvantage of AI derivatives is that there is a paucity of existing information on studies with NLO effects and nanomaterials, but this opens up an opportunity for new discoveries.

In the collection of information, different algorithms were found that analyze NLO effects. In Table 4, some algorithms are observed in different applications; NLO processes are unexplored for designing platforms related to biosensing performance, but they have promising potential.

6. Conclusions

ML has the potential to fundamentally change the practice of data analysis. Optical biosensors are well positioned to take advantage of ML, which leads to greater efficiency and precision. By combining the ML analysis tools and multiphotonic effects for the increase in applications in optical biosensors, it is clear that there is potential for a better interpretation of biological agents. In this work, a perspective for optical biosensors in virus detection is described.

The processing and classification of large amounts of data allowed by ML lead to extraordinary interpretations and unique predictions in the study with optical biosensors. In this work, optical biosensors assisted by ML for virus detection are proposed, specifically for SARS-CoV-2. By applying different NLO phenomena, the use of ML can optimize the biosensing performance due to its ability to handle large amounts of information. It was pointed out that there is still a vast field of research regarding the party effect of ML on nonlinear optical biosensors.

In this work, it is observed that ML can be useful for estimating different NLO interactions, although the current limited evidence does not support the superiority of ML and automation over study analysis in NLO processes. However, the handling and classification of large amounts of data allow envisioning that ML can play a crucial role in predictions of NLO-based biosensors. In this work, various studies that can be envisioned for the classification and organization of information in experiments with AI are proposed.

Author Contributions: Investigation, J.A.A.-M., C.L.M.-G., M.I.S. and C.T.-T.; Writing—original draft, J.A.A.-M.; Writing—review and editing, J.A.A.-M., C.L.M.-G., M.I.S. and C.T.-T.; Conceptualization, C.T.-T. All the authors contributed equally to the proposal and development of this research. The manuscript was written with the contribution of all authors. All authors have read and agreed to the published version of the manuscript.

Funding: This research was funded by Instituto Politécnico Nacional (SIP-2022) and Consejo Nacional de Ciencia y Tecnología (CONACyT).

Institutional Review Board Statement: Not applicable.

Informed Consent Statement: Not applicable.

Data Availability Statement: Data and materials are available upon reasonable request to C. Torres-Torres (ctorrest@ipn.mx).

Acknowledgments: The authors kindly acknowledge the financial support from the Instituto Politécnico Nacional and Consejo Nacional de Ciencia y Tecnología.

Conflicts of Interest: The authors declare no conflict of interest.

References

1. Lei, Z.-L.; Guo, B. 2D Material-Based Optical Biosensor: Status and Prospect. *Adv. Sci.* **2022**, *9*, 2102924. [CrossRef] [PubMed]
2. Khalil, I.; Julkapli, N.; Yehye, W.; Basirun, W.; Bhargava, S. Graphene–Gold Nanoparticles Hybrid—Synthesis, Functionalization, and Application in a Electrochemical and Surface-Enhanced Raman Scattering Biosensor. *Materials* **2016**, *9*, 406. [CrossRef] [PubMed]
3. Malhotra, B.D.; Ali, M.A. Nanomaterials in Biosensors. In *Nanomaterials for Biosensors*; Elsevier: Amsterdam, The Netherlands, 2018; pp. 1–74.
4. Shumeiko, V.; Malach, E.; Helman, Y.; Paltiel, Y.; Bisker, G.; Hayouka, Z.; Shoseyov, O. A Nanoscale Optical Biosensor Based on Peptide Encapsulated SWCNTs for Detection of Acetic Acid in the Gaseous Phase. *Sens. Actuators B Chem.* **2021**, *327*, 128832. [CrossRef]
5. Samani, S.S.; Khojastehnezhad, A.; Ramezani, M.; Alibolandi, M.; Yazdi, F.T.; Mortazavi, S.A.; Khoshbin, Z.; Abnous, K.; Taghdisi, S.M. Ultrasensitive Detection of Micrococcal Nuclease Activity and Staphylococcus Aureus Contamination Using Optical Biosensor Technology-A Review. *Talanta* **2021**, *226*, 122168. [CrossRef]
6. Portes, A.V.R.; Martins, A.J.L.; Guerrero, J.A.; Carvalho, M.M.; Amaya-Fernandez, F.O.; Saito, L.A.M.; Ramirez, J.C. Electro-Optical Biosensor Based on Embedded Double-Monolayer of Graphene Capacitor in Polymer Technology. *Polymers* **2021**, *13*, 3564. [CrossRef]
7. Aldaya, I.; Gil-Molina, A.; Pita, J.L.; Gabrielli, L.H.; Fragnito, H.L.; Dainese, P. Nonlinear Carrier Dynamics in Silicon Nano-Waveguides. *Optica* **2017**, *4*, 1219. [CrossRef]
8. Ramirez, J.C.; Lechuga, L.M.; Gabrielli, L.H.; Hernandez-Figueroa, H.E. Study of a Low-Cost Trimodal Polymer Waveguide for Interferometric Optical Biosensors. *Opt. Express* **2015**, *23*, 11985. [CrossRef]
9. Singh, P. Surface Plasmon Resonance: A Boon for Viral Diagnostics. In *Reference Module in Life Sciences*; Elsevier: Amsterdam, The Netherlands, 2017; ISBN 978-0-12-809633-8.
10. Su, Y.; Xia, S.; Wang, R.; Xiao, L. Phytohormonal Quantification Based on Biological Principles. In *Hormone Metabolism and Signaling in Plants*; Li, J., Li, C., Smith, S.M., Eds.; Elsevier: Amsterdam, The Netherlands, 2017; pp. 431–470. ISBN 978-0-12-811562-6.
11. Cajigas, S.; Soto, D.; Orozco, J. Biosensors: Biosensors With Signal Amplification. In *Reference Module in Biomedical Sciences*; Elsevier: Amsterdam, The Netherlands, 2021; ISBN 978-0-12-801238-3.
12. Shrivastav, A.M.; Cvelbar, U.; Abdulhalim, I. A Comprehensive Review on Plasmonic-Based Biosensors Used in Viral Diagnostics. *Commun. Biol.* **2021**, *4*, 70. [CrossRef] [PubMed]
13. Li, D.; Zhou, H.; Hui, X.; He, X.; Mu, X. Plasmonic Biosensor Augmented by a Genetic Algorithm for Ultra-Rapid, Label-Free, and Multi-Functional Detection of COVID-19. *Anal. Chem.* **2021**, *93*, 9437–9444. [CrossRef]
14. Sharma, S.; Kumar, A. Design of a Biosensor for the Detection of Dengue Virus Using 1D Photonic Crystals. *Plasmonics* **2022**, *17*, 675–680. [CrossRef]
15. Sharma, S.; Kumar, A.; Singh, K.S.; Tyagi, H.K. 2D Photonic Crystal Based Biosensor for the Detection of Chikungunya Virus. *Optik* **2021**, *237*, 166575. [CrossRef]
16. Zhou, J.; Yang, T.; Chen, J.; Wang, C.; Zhang, H.; Shao, Y. Two-Dimensional Nanomaterial-Based Plasmonic Sensing Applications: Advances and Challenges. *Coord. Chem. Rev.* **2020**, *410*, 213218. [CrossRef]
17. Meradi, K.A.; Tayeboun, F.; Guerinik, A.; Zaky, Z.A.; Aly, A.H. Optical Biosensor Based on Enhanced Surface Plasmon Resonance: Theoretical Optimization. *Opt. Quantum Electron.* **2022**, *54*, 124. [CrossRef]
18. Lertvachirapaiboon, C.; Baba, A.; Ekgasit, S.; Shinbo, K.; Kato, K.; Kaneko, F. Transmission Surface Plasmon Resonance Techniques and Their Potential Biosensor Applications. *Biosens. Bioelectron.* **2018**, *99*, 399–415. [CrossRef]

19. Kushwaha, A.S.; Kumar, A.; Kumar, R.; Srivastava, S.K. A Study of Surface Plasmon Resonance (SPR) Based Biosensor with Improved Sensitivity. *Photonics Nanostruct.-Fundam. Appl.* **2018**, *31*, 99–106. [CrossRef]
20. Lu, Y.; Tan, Y.; Xiao, Y.; Li, Z.; Sheng, E.; Dai, Z. A Silver@gold Nanoparticle Tetrahedron Biosensor for Multiple Pesticides Detection Based on Surface-Enhanced Raman Scattering. *Talanta* **2021**, *234*, 122585. [CrossRef] [PubMed]
21. Calvo-Lozano, O.; Sierra, M.; Soler, M.; Estévez, M.C.; Chiscano-Camón, L.; Ruiz-Sanmartin, A.; Ruiz-Rodriguez, J.C.; Ferrer, R.; González-López, J.J.; Esperalba, J.; et al. Label-Free Plasmonic Biosensor for Rapid, Quantitative, and Highly Sensitive COVID-19 Serology: Implementation and Clinical Validation. *Anal. Chem.* **2022**, *94*, 975–984. [CrossRef]
22. Sidhu, R.; Zheng, R.; Rasheed, A.; Khan, M.A. The Development of Point-of-Care Plasmonic-Based Biosensor for Early Detection of COVID-19 Virus. In Proceedings of the 2021 IEEE 15th International Conference on Nano/Molecular Medicine & Engineering (NANOMED), Taipei, Taiwan, 15–17 November 2021; IEEE: Manhattan, NY, USA, 2021; pp. 23–27.
23. Wang, J.; Yao, Z.; Lei, T.; Poon, A.W. Silicon Coupled-Resonator Optical-Waveguide-Based Biosensors Using Light-Scattering Pattern Recognition with Pixelized Mode-Field-Intensity Distributions. *Sci. Rep.* **2015**, *4*, 7528. [CrossRef]
24. Wang, J.; Yao, Z.; Poon, A.W. Silicon-Nitride-Based Integrated Optofluidic Biochemical Sensors Using a Coupled-Resonator Optical Waveguide. *Front. Mater.* **2015**, *2*, 34. [CrossRef]
25. Zhang, P.; Ma, G.; Dong, W.; Wan, Z.; Wang, S.; Tao, N. Plasmonic Scattering Imaging of Single Proteins and Binding Kinetics. *Nat. Methods* **2020**, *17*, 1010–1017. [CrossRef]
26. Song, M.K.; Chen, S.X.; Hu, P.P.; Huang, C.Z.; Zhou, J. Automated Plasmonic Resonance Scattering Imaging Analysis via Deep Learning. *Anal. Chem.* **2021**, *93*, 2619–2626. [CrossRef] [PubMed]
27. Pang, Y.; Wan, N.; Shi, L.; Wang, C.; Sun, Z.; Xiao, R.; Wang, S. Dual-Recognition Surface-Enhanced Raman Scattering(SERS)Biosensor for Pathogenic Bacteria Detection by Using Vancomycin-SERS Tags and Aptamer-Fe_3O_4@Au. *Anal. Chim. Acta* **2019**, *1077*, 288–296. [CrossRef] [PubMed]
28. Mao, K.; Zhou, Z.; Han, S.; Zhou, X.; Hu, J.; Li, X.; Yang, Z. A Novel Biosensor Based on Au@Ag Core-Shell Nanoparticles for Sensitive Detection of Methylamphetamine with Surface Enhanced Raman Scattering. *Talanta* **2018**, *190*, 263–268. [CrossRef] [PubMed]
29. He, X.; Zhou, X.; Liu, Y.; Wang, X. Ultrasensitive, Recyclable and Portable Microfluidic Surface-Enhanced Raman Scattering (SERS) Biosensor for Uranyl Ions Detection. *Sens. Actuators B Chem.* **2020**, *311*, 127676. [CrossRef]
30. Khalil, I.; Yehye, W.A.; Muhd Julkapli, N.; Ibn Sina, A.A.; Islam Chowdhury, F.; Khandaker, M.U.; Hsiao, V.K.S.; Basirun, W.J. Simultaneous Detection of Dual Food Adulterants Using Graphene Oxide and Gold Nanoparticle Based Surface Enhanced Raman Scattering Duplex DNA Biosensor. *Vib. Spectrosc.* **2021**, *116*, 103293. [CrossRef]
31. Vendrell, M.; Maiti, K.K.; Dhaliwal, K.; Chang, Y.-T. Surface-Enhanced Raman Scattering in Cancer Detection and Imaging. *Trends Biotechnol.* **2013**, *31*, 249–257. [CrossRef]
32. Dey, S.; Ahmed, E.; Somvanshi, P.S.; Sina, A.A.I.; Wuethrich, A.; Trau, M. An Electrochemical and Raman Scattering Dual Detection Biosensor for Rapid Screening and Biomolecular Profiling of Cancer Biomarkers. *Chemosensors* **2022**, *10*, 93. [CrossRef]
33. Granger, J.H.; Granger, M.C.; Firpo, M.A.; Mulvihill, S.J.; Porter, M.D. Toward Development of a Surface-Enhanced Raman Scattering (SERS)-Based Cancer Diagnostic Immunoassay Panel. *Analyst* **2013**, *138*, 410–416. [CrossRef]
34. Lopatynskyi, A.M.; Lopatynska, O.G.; Guo, L.J.; Chegel, V.I. Localized Surface Plasmon Resonance Biosensor—Part I: Theoretical Study of Sensitivity—Extended Mie Approach. *IEEE Sens. J.* **2011**, *11*, 361–369. [CrossRef]
35. Manikandan, M.; Revathi, C.; Senthilkumar, P.; Amreetha, S.; Dhanuskodi, S.; Rajendra Kumar, R.T. CdTe Nanorods for Nonenzymatic Hydrogen Peroxide Biosensor and Optical Limiting Applications. *Ionics* **2020**, *26*, 2003–2010. [CrossRef]
36. Prasanna Kumaar, S.; Sivasubramanian, A. Optimization of the Transverse Electric Photonic Strip Waveguide Biosensor for Detecting Diabetes Mellitus from Bulk Sensitivity. *J. Healthc. Eng.* **2021**, *2021*, 6081570. [CrossRef]
37. Panda, A.; Puspa Devi, P. Photonic Crystal Biosensor for Refractive Index Based Cancerous Cell Detection. *Opt. Fiber Technol.* **2020**, *54*, 102123. [CrossRef]
38. Efimov, I.M.; Vanyushkin, N.A.; Gevorgyan, A.H.; Golik, S.S. Optical Biosensor Based on a Photonic Crystal with a Defective Layer Designed to Determine the Concentration of SARS-CoV-2 in Water. *Phys. Scr.* **2022**, *97*, 055506. [CrossRef]
39. Abrego-Martinez, J.C.; Jafari, M.; Chergui, S.; Pavel, C.; Che, D.; Siaj, M. Aptamer-Based Electrochemical Biosensor for Rapid Detection of SARS-CoV-2: Nanoscale Electrode-Aptamer-SARS-CoV-2 Imaging by Photo-Induced Force Microscopy. *Biosens. Bioelectron.* **2022**, *195*, 113595. [CrossRef]
40. Ranjan, A.K.; Patra, A.K.; Gorai, A.K. Effect of Lockdown Due to SARS COVID-19 on Aerosol Optical Depth (AOD) over Urban and Mining Regions in India. *Sci. Total Environ.* **2020**, *745*, 141024. [CrossRef]
41. Cennamo, N.; D'Agostino, G.; Perri, C.; Arcadio, F.; Chiaretti, G.; Parisio, E.M.; Camarlinghi, G.; Vettori, C.; Di Marzo, F.; Cennamo, R.; et al. Proof of Concept for a Quick and Highly Sensitive On-Site Detection of SARS-CoV-2 by Plasmonic Optical Fibers and Molecularly Imprinted Polymers. *Sensors* **2021**, *21*, 1681. [CrossRef]
42. Liu, Y.-N.; Lv, Z.-T.; Yang, S.-Y.; Liu, X.-W. Optical Tracking of the Interfacial Dynamics of Single SARS-CoV-2 Pseudoviruses. *Environ. Sci. Technol.* **2021**, *55*, 4115–4122. [CrossRef]
43. Gomez-Gonzalez, E.; Barriga-Rivera, A.; Fernandez-Muñoz, B.; Navas-Garcia, J.M.; Fernandez-Lizaranzu, I.; Munoz-Gonzalez, F.J.; Parrilla-Giraldez, R.; Requena-Lancharro, D.; Gil-Gamboa, P.; Rosell-Valle, C.; et al. Optical Imaging Spectroscopy for Rapid, Primary Screening of SARS-CoV-2: A Proof of Concept. *Sci. Rep.* **2022**, *12*, 2356. [CrossRef]

44. Daoudi, K.; Ramachandran, K.; Alawadhi, H.; Boukherroub, R.; Dogheche, E.; El Khakani, M.A.; Gaidi, M. Ultra-Sensitive and Fast Optical Detection of the Spike Protein of the SARS-CoV-2 Using AgNPs/SiNWs Nanohybrid Based Sensors. *Surf. Interfaces* **2021**, *27*, 101454. [CrossRef]
45. Li, Z.; Hirst, J.D. Computed Optical Spectra of SARS-CoV-2 Proteins. *Chem. Phys. Lett.* **2020**, *758*, 137935. [CrossRef]
46. Rabiee, N.; Fatahi, Y.; Ahmadi, S.; Abbariki, N.; Ojaghi, A.; Rabiee, M.; Radmanesh, F.; Dinarvand, R.; Bagherzadeh, M.; Mostafavi, E.; et al. Bioactive Hybrid Metal-Organic Framework (MOF)-Based Nanosensors for Optical Detection of Recombinant SARS-CoV-2 Spike Antigen. *Sci. Total Environ.* **2022**, *825*, 153902. [CrossRef] [PubMed]
47. Minopoli, A.; Scardapane, E.; Acunzo, A.; Campanile, R.; Della Ventura, B.; Velotta, R. Analysis of the Optical Response of a SARS-CoV-2-Directed Colorimetric Immunosensor. *AIP Adv.* **2021**, *11*, 065319. [CrossRef]
48. Diaz, L.M.; Johnson, B.E.; Jenkins, D.M. Real-Time Optical Analysis of a Colorimetric LAMP Assay for SARS-CoV-2 in Saliva with a Handheld Instrument Improves Accuracy Compared with Endpoint Assessment. *J. Biomol. Tech.* **2021**, *32*, 158–171. [CrossRef] [PubMed]
49. Tao, Y.; Bian, S.; Wang, P.; Zhang, H.; Bi, W.; Zhu, P.; Sawan, M. Rapid Optical Biosensing of SARS-CoV-2 Spike Proteins in Artificial Samples. *Sensors* **2022**, *22*, 3768. [CrossRef]
50. Xu, W.; Liu, J.; Song, D.; Li, C.; Zhu, A.; Long, F. Rapid, Label-Free, and Sensitive Point-of-Care Testing of Anti-SARS-CoV-2 IgM/IgG Using All-Fiber Fresnel Reflection Microfluidic Biosensor. *Microchim. Acta* **2021**, *188*, 261. [CrossRef]
51. Doulou, S.; Leventogiannis, K.; Tsilika, M.; Rodencal, M.; Katrini, K.; Antonakos, N.; Kyprianou, M.; Karofylakis, E.; Karageorgos, A.; Koufargyris, P.; et al. A Novel Optical Biosensor for the Early Diagnosis of Sepsis and Severe Covid-19: The PROUD Study. *BMC Infect. Dis.* **2020**, *20*, 860. [CrossRef]
52. Courtney, S.; Stromberg, Z.; Myers y Gutiérrez, A.; Jacobsen, D.; Stromberg, L.; Lenz, K.; Theiler, J.; Foley, B.; Gans, J.; Yusim, K.; et al. Optical Biosensor Platforms Display Varying Sensitivity for the Direct Detection of Influenza RNA. *Biosensors* **2021**, *11*, 367. [CrossRef]
53. Schotter, J.; Schrittwieser, S.; Muellner, P.; Melnik, E.; Hainberger, R.; Koppitsch, G.; Schrank, F.; Soulantika, K.; Lentijo-Mozo, S.; Pelaz, B.; et al. Optical Biosensor Technologies for Molecular Diagnostics at the Point-of-Care. *Proc. SPIE* **2015**, *9490*, 94900B. [CrossRef]
54. El-Sherif, D.M.; Abouzid, M.; Gaballah, M.S.; Ahmed, A.A.; Adeel, M.; Sheta, S.M. New Approach in SARS-CoV-2 Surveillance Using Biosensor Technology: A Review. *Environ. Sci. Pollut. Res.* **2022**, *29*, 1677–1695. [CrossRef]
55. Lee, S.-L.; Kim, J.; Choi, S.; Han, J.; Seo, G.; Lee, Y.W. Fiber-Optic Label-Free Biosensor for SARS-CoV-2 Spike Protein Detection Using Biofunctionalized Long-Period Fiber Grating. *Talanta* **2021**, *235*, 122801. [CrossRef]
56. Sun, Y.; Shi, L.; Mi, L.; Guo, R.; Li, T. Recent Progress of SERS Optical Nanosensors for MiRNA Analysis. *J. Mater. Chem. B* **2020**, *8*, 5178–5183. [CrossRef] [PubMed]
57. Yildirim, D.U.; Ghobadi, A.; Ozbay, E. Nanosensors Based on Localized Surface Plasmon Resonance. In *Plasmonic Sensors and Their Applications*; Wiley Online Books; Wiley: Hoboken, NJ, USA, 2021; pp. 23–54, ISBN 9783527830343.
58. Dziekan, Z.; Pituła, E.; Kwietniewski, N.; Stonio, B.; Janik, M.; Śmiarowski, T.; Koba, M.; Parzuchowski, P.; Niedziółka-Jönsson, J.; Śmietana, M. Performance of Nanoimprinted and Nanocoated Optical Label-Free Biosensor-Nanocoating Properties Perspective. *Opt. Lasers Eng.* **2022**, *153*, 107009. [CrossRef]
59. Threm, D.; Nazirizadeh, Y.; Gerken, M. Photonic Crystal Biosensors towards On-Chip Integration. *J. Biophotonics* **2012**, *5*, 601–616. [CrossRef]
60. Fernández Gavela, A.; Grajales García, D.; Ramirez, J.; Lechuga, L. Last Advances in Silicon-Based Optical Biosensors. *Sensors* **2016**, *16*, 285. [CrossRef] [PubMed]
61. Srivastava, A.; Sharma, A.K.; Kumar Prajapati, Y. On the Sensitivity-Enhancement in Plasmonic Biosensor with Photonic Spin Hall Effect at Visible Wavelength. *Chem. Phys. Lett.* **2021**, *774*, 138613. [CrossRef]
62. Li, N.; Tang, T.; Li, J.; Luo, L.; Li, C.; Shen, J.; Yao, J. Highly Sensitive Biosensor with Graphene-MoS$_2$ Heterostructure Based on Photonic Spin Hall Effect. *J. Magn. Magn. Mater.* **2019**, *484*, 445–450. [CrossRef]
63. Leuermann, J.; Stamenkovic, V.; Ramirez-Priego, P.; Sánchez-Postigo, A.; Fernández-Gavela, A.; Chapman, C.A.; Bailey, R.C.; Lechuga, L.M.; Perez-Inestrosa, E.; Collado, D.; et al. Coherent Silicon Photonic Interferometric Biosensor with an Inexpensive Laser Source for Sensitive Label-Free Immunoassays. *Opt. Lett.* **2020**, *45*, 6595. [CrossRef]
64. Xie, L.; Zhang, Z.; Du, J. The Photonic Spin Hall Effect Sensor. In *Applied Optical Metrology II*; Novak, E., Trolinger, J.D., Eds.; SPIE: Bellingham, WA, USA, 2017; Volume 10373, p. 10.
65. Mavrikou, S.; Moschopoulou, G.; Tsekouras, V.; Kintzios, S. Development of a Portable, Ultra-Rapid and Ultra-Sensitive Cell-Based Biosensor for the Direct Detection of the SARS-CoV-2 S1 Spike Protein Antigen. *Sensors* **2020**, *20*, 3121. [CrossRef]
66. Wrapp, D.; Wang, N.; Corbett, K.S.; Goldsmith, J.A.; Hsieh, C.-L.; Abiona, O.; Graham, B.S.; McLellan, J.S. Cryo-EM Structure of the 2019-NCoV Spike in the Prefusion Conformation. *Science* **2020**, *367*, 1260–1263. [CrossRef]
67. Ruiz-Vega, G.; Soler, M.; Lechuga, L.M. Nanophotonic Biosensors for Point-of-Care COVID-19 Diagnostics and Coronavirus Surveillance. *J. Phys. Photonics* **2021**, *3*, 011002. [CrossRef]
68. Moznuzzaman, M.; Khan, I.; Islam, M.R. Nano-Layered Surface Plasmon Resonance-Based Highly Sensitive Biosensor for Virus Detection: A Theoretical Approach to Detect SARS-CoV-2. *AIP Adv.* **2021**, *11*, 065023. [CrossRef] [PubMed]
69. Bai, H.; Wang, R.; Hargis, B.; Lu, H.; Li, Y. A SPR Aptasensor for Detection of Avian Influenza Virus H5N1. *Sensors* **2012**, *12*, 12506–12518. [CrossRef] [PubMed]

70. Prabowo, B.A.; Wang, R.Y.L.; Secario, M.K.; Ou, P.-T.; Alom, A.; Liu, J.-J.; Liu, K.-C. Rapid Detection and Quantification of Enterovirus 71 by a Portable Surface Plasmon Resonance Biosensor. *Biosens. Bioelectron.* **2017**, *92*, 186–191. [CrossRef]
71. Murugan, D.; Bhatia, H.; Sai, V.V.R.; Satija, J. P-FAB: A Fiber-Optic Biosensor Device for Rapid Detection of COVID-19. *Trans. Indian Natl. Acad. Eng.* **2020**, *5*, 211–215. [CrossRef]
72. Alathari, M.J.A.; Al Mashhadany, Y.; Mokhtar, M.H.H.; Burham, N.; Bin Zan, M.S.D.; A Bakar, A.A.; Arsad, N. Human Body Performance with COVID-19 Affectation According to Virus Specification Based on Biosensor Techniques. *Sensors* **2021**, *21*, 8362. [CrossRef]
73. Taha, B.A.; Al Mashhadany, Y.; Hafiz Mokhtar, M.H.; Dzulkefly Bin Zan, M.S.; Arsad, N. An Analysis Review of Detection Coronavirus Disease 2019 (COVID-19) Based on Biosensor Application. *Sensors* **2020**, *20*, 6764. [CrossRef] [PubMed]
74. Ma, R.-M.; Oulton, R.F. Applications of Nanolasers. *Nat. Nanotechnol.* **2019**, *14*, 12–22. [CrossRef]
75. Rodriguez, G.A.; Markov, P.; Cartwright, A.P.; Choudhury, M.H.; Afzal, F.O.; Cao, T.; Halimi, S.I.; Retterer, S.T.; Kravchenko, I.I.; Weiss, S.M. Photonic Crystal Nanobeam Biosensors Based on Porous Silicon. *Opt. Express* **2019**, *27*, 9536. [CrossRef]
76. Kim, H.; Hwang, J.; Kim, J.H.; Lee, S.; Kang, M. Sensitive Detection of Multiple Fluoresence Probes Based on Surface-Enhanced Raman Scattering (SERS) for MERS-CoV. In Proceedings of the 2019 IEEE 14th International Conference on Nano/Micro Engineered and Molecular Systems (NEMS), Bangkok, Thailand, 11–14 April 2019; IEEE: Manhattan, NY, USA, 2019; pp. 498–501.
77. Kumar, A.; Kumar, A.; Kushwaha, A.S.; Dubey, S.K.; Srivastava, S.K. A Comparative Study of Different Types of Sandwiched Structures of SPR Biosensor for Sensitive Detection of SsDNA. *Photonics Nanostruct.-Fundam. Appl.* **2022**, *48*, 100984. [CrossRef]
78. Syed Nor, S.N.; Rasanang, N.S.; Karman, S.; Zaman, W.S.W.K.; Harun, S.W.; Arof, H. A Review: Surface Plasmon Resonance-Based Biosensor for Early Screening of SARS-CoV2 Infection. *IEEE Access* **2022**, *10*, 1228–1244. [CrossRef]
79. Yang, Y.; Liu, J.; Zhou, X. A CRISPR-Based and Post-Amplification Coupled SARS-CoV-2 Detection with a Portable Evanescent Wave Biosensor. *Biosens. Bioelectron.* **2021**, *190*, 113418. [CrossRef] [PubMed]
80. Cavalera, S.; Colitti, B.; Rosati, S.; Ferrara, G.; Bertolotti, L.; Nogarol, C.; Guiotto, C.; Cagnazzo, C.; Denina, M.; Fagioli, F.; et al. A Multi-Target Lateral Flow Immunoassay Enabling the Specific and Sensitive Detection of Total Antibodies to SARS CoV-2. *Talanta* **2021**, *223*, 121737. [CrossRef] [PubMed]
81. Song, D.; Liu, J.; Xu, W.; Han, X.; Wang, H.; Cheng, Y.; Zhuo, Y.; Long, F. Rapid and Quantitative Detection of SARS-CoV-2 IgG Antibody in Serum Using Optofluidic Point-of-Care Testing Fluorescence Biosensor. *Talanta* **2021**, *235*, 122800. [CrossRef]
82. Han, H.; Wang, C.; Yang, X.; Zheng, S.; Cheng, X.; Liu, Z.; Zhao, B.; Xiao, R. Rapid Field Determination of SARS-CoV-2 by a Colorimetric and Fluorescent Dual-Functional Lateral Flow Immunoassay Biosensor. *Sens. Actuators B Chem.* **2022**, *351*, 130897. [CrossRef]
83. Zhang, K.; Fan, Z.; Ding, Y.; Xie, M. A PH-Engineering Regenerative DNA Tetrahedron ECL Biosensor for the Assay of SARS-CoV-2 RdRp Gene Based on CRISPR/Cas12a Trans-Activity. *Chem. Eng. J.* **2022**, *429*, 132472. [CrossRef]
84. Zhang, K.; Fan, Z.; Ding, Y.; Zhu, S.; Xie, M.; Hao, N. Exploring the Entropy-Driven Amplification Reaction and Trans -Cleavage Activity of CRISPR-Cas12a for the Development of an Electrochemiluminescence Biosensor for the Detection of the SARS-CoV-2 RdRp Gene in Real Samples and Environmental Surveillance. *Environ. Sci. Nano* **2022**, *9*, 162–172. [CrossRef]
85. Xi, H.; Juhas, M.; Zhang, Y. G-Quadruplex Based Biosensor: A Potential Tool for SARS-CoV-2 Detection. *Biosens. Bioelectron.* **2020**, *167*, 112494. [CrossRef]
86. O'Brien, A.; Chen, D.-Y.; Hackbart, M.; Close, B.J.; O'Brien, T.E.; Saeed, M.; Baker, S.C. Detecting SARS-CoV-2 3CLpro Expression and Activity Using a Polyclonal Antiserum and a Luciferase-Based Biosensor. *Virology* **2021**, *556*, 73–78. [CrossRef]
87. Zhang, K.; Fan, Z.; Huang, Y.; Ding, Y.; Xie, M.; Wang, M. Hybridization Chain Reaction Circuit-Based Electrochemiluminescent Biosensor for SARS-Cov-2 RdRp Gene Assay. *Talanta* **2022**, *240*, 123207. [CrossRef] [PubMed]
88. Fan, Z.; Yao, B.; Ding, Y.; Xu, D.; Zhao, J.; Zhang, K. Rational Engineering the DNA Tetrahedrons of Dual Wavelength Ratiometric Electrochemiluminescence Biosensor for High Efficient Detection of SARS-CoV-2 RdRp Gene by Using Entropy-Driven and Bipedal DNA Walker Amplification Strategy. *Chem. Eng. J.* **2022**, *427*, 131686. [CrossRef]
89. Yang, X.; Liu, L.; Hao, Y.; So, E.; Emami, S.S.; Zhang, D.; Gong, Y.; Sheth, P.M.; Wang, Y. A Bioluminescent Biosensor for Quantifying the Interaction of SARS-CoV-2 and Its Receptor ACE2 in Cells and In Vitro. *Viruses* **2021**, *13*, 1055. [CrossRef] [PubMed]
90. Yang, X.; Liu, L.; Hao, Y.; So, Y.W.; Emami, S.S.; Zhang, D.; Gong, Y.; Sheth, P.M.; Wang, Y.T. An Ultrasensitive Biosensor for Quantifying the Interaction of SARS-CoV-2 and Its Receptor ACE2 in Cells and In Vitro. *bioRxiv* **2020**, 424698. [CrossRef]
91. Murillo, A.M.M.; Tomé-Amat, J.; Ramírez, Y.; Garrido-Arandia, M.; Valle, L.G.; Hernández-Ramírez, G.; Tramarin, L.; Herreros, P.; Santamaría, B.; Díaz-Perales, A.; et al. Developing an Optical Interferometric Detection Method Based Biosensor for Detecting Specific SARS-CoV-2 Immunoglobulins in Serum and Saliva, and Their Corresponding ELISA Correlation. *Sens. Actuators B Chem.* **2021**, *345*, 130394. [CrossRef]
92. Liu, N.; Wang, S.; Wang, J.; Lv, J.; Cheng, Q.; Ma, W.; Lu, Y. Promising Refractive Index and Temperature Biosensor Based on Hybrid Gmr/Fp System Employed for the Detection of SARS-CoV-2. *SSRN Electron. J.* **2022**. [CrossRef]
93. Gutiérrez-Gálvez, L.; del Caño, R.; Menéndez-Luque, I.; García-Nieto, D.; Rodríguez-Peña, M.; Luna, M.; Pineda, T.; Pariente, F.; García-Mendiola, T.; Lorenzo, E. Electrochemiluminescent Nanostructured DNA Biosensor for SARS-CoV-2 Detection. *Talanta* **2022**, *240*, 123203. [CrossRef] [PubMed]
94. Jiang, C.; Mu, X.; Liu, S.; Liu, Z.; Du, B.; Wang, J.; Xu, J. A Study of the Detection of SARS-CoV-2 ORF1ab Gene by the Use of Electrochemiluminescent Biosensor Based on Dual-Probe Hybridization. *Sensors* **2022**, *22*, 2402. [CrossRef]

95. Karakuş, E.; Erdemir, E.; Demirbilek, N.; Liv, L. Colorimetric and Electrochemical Detection of SARS-CoV-2 Spike Antigen with a Gold Nanoparticle-Based Biosensor. *Anal. Chim. Acta* **2021**, *1182*, 338939. [CrossRef]
96. Xu, W.; Zhuo, Y.; Song, D.; Han, X.; Xu, J.; Long, F. Development of a Novel Label-Free All-Fiber Optofluidic Biosensor Based on Fresnel Reflection and Its Applications. *Anal. Chim. Acta* **2021**, *1181*, 338910. [CrossRef] [PubMed]
97. Kim, M. Detecting SARS-CoV-2 with a Rapid, Cost-Effective Colorimetric Biosensor. *Scilight* **2021**, *2021*, 251103. [CrossRef]
98. Sampad, M.J.N.; Zhang, H.; Yuzvinsky, T.D.; Stott, M.A.; Hawkins, A.R.; Schmidt, H. Optical Trapping Assisted Label-Free and Amplification-Free Detection of SARS-CoV-2 RNAs with an Optofluidic Nanopore Sensor. *Biosens. Bioelectron.* **2021**, *194*, 113588. [CrossRef]
99. Ahmad, M.; Sharma, P.; Kamai, A.; Agrawal, A.; Faruq, M.; Kulshreshtha, A. HRPZyme Assisted Recognition of SARS-CoV-2 Infection by Optical Measurement (HARIOM). *Biosens. Bioelectron.* **2021**, *187*, 113280. [CrossRef]
100. Ravalin, M.; Roh, H.; Suryawanshi, R.; Kumar, G.R.; Pak, J.E.; Ott, M.; Ting, A.Y. A Single-Component Luminescent Biosensor for the SARS-CoV-2 Spike Protein. *J. Am. Chem. Soc.* **2022**, *144*, 13663–13672. [CrossRef]
101. Huang, L.; Ding, L.; Zhou, J.; Chen, S.; Chen, F.; Zhao, C.; Xu, J.; Hu, W.; Ji, J.; Xu, H.; et al. One-Step Rapid Quantification of SARS-CoV-2 Virus Particles via Low-Cost Nanoplasmonic Sensors in Generic Microplate Reader and Point-of-Care Device. *Biosens. Bioelectron.* **2021**, *171*, 112685. [CrossRef] [PubMed]
102. Yao, B.; Zhang, J.; Fan, Z.; Ding, Y.; Zhou, B.; Yang, R.; Zhao, J.; Zhang, K. Rational Engineering of the DNA Walker Amplification Strategy by Using a Au@Ti$_3$C$_2$@PEI-Ru(Dcbpy)32+ Nanocomposite Biosensor for Detection of the SARS-CoV-2 RdRp Gene. *ACS Appl. Mater. Interfaces* **2021**, *13*, 19816–19824. [CrossRef]
103. Bhattacharjee, A.; Sabino, R.M.; Gangwish, J.; Manivasagam, V.K.; James, S.; Popat, K.C.; Reynolds, M.; Li, Y.V. A Novel Colorimetric Biosensor for Detecting SARS-CoV-2 by Utilizing the Interaction between Nucleocapsid Antibody and Spike Proteins. *Vitr. Model.* **2022**, *1*, 241–247. [CrossRef]
104. Lee, C.Y.; Degani, I.; Cheong, J.; Lee, J.-H.; Choi, H.-J.; Cheon, J.; Lee, H. Fluorescence Polarization System for Rapid COVID-19 Diagnosis. *Biosens. Bioelectron.* **2021**, *178*, 113049. [CrossRef] [PubMed]
105. Roda, A.; Cavalera, S.; Di Nardo, F.; Calabria, D.; Rosati, S.; Simoni, P.; Colitti, B.; Baggiani, C.; Roda, M.; Anfossi, L. Dual Lateral Flow Optical/Chemiluminescence Immunosensors for the Rapid Detection of Salivary and Serum IgA in Patients with COVID-19 Disease. *Biosens. Bioelectron.* **2021**, *172*, 112765. [CrossRef] [PubMed]
106. Zheng, Y.; Song, K.; Cai, K.; Liu, L.; Tang, D.; Long, W.; Zhai, B.; Chen, J.; Tao, Y.; Zhao, Y.; et al. B-Cell-Epitope-Based Fluorescent Quantum Dot Biosensors for SARS-CoV-2 Enable Highly Sensitive COVID-19 Antibody Detection. *Viruses* **2022**, *14*, 1031. [CrossRef]
107. Büyüksünetçi, Y.T.; Çitil, B.E.; Tapan, U.; Anık, Ü. Development and Application of a SARS-CoV-2 Colorimetric Biosensor Based on the Peroxidase-Mimic Activity of γ-Fe$_2$O$_3$ Nanoparticles. *Microchim. Acta* **2021**, *188*, 335. [CrossRef]
108. Divagar, M.; Gayathri, R.; Rasool, R.; Shamlee, J.K.; Bhatia, H.; Satija, J.; Sai, V.V.R. Plasmonic Fiberoptic Absorbance Biosensor (P-FAB) for Rapid Detection of SARS-CoV-2 Nucleocapsid Protein. *IEEE Sens. J.* **2021**, *21*, 22758–22766. [CrossRef]
109. Zheng, Y.; Bian, S.; Sun, J.; Wen, L.; Rong, G.; Sawan, M. Label-Free LSPR-Vertical Microcavity Biosensor for On-Site SARS-CoV-2 Detection. *Biosensors* **2022**, *12*, 151. [CrossRef] [PubMed]
110. Zhang, M.; Li, X.; Pan, J.; Zhang, Y.; Zhang, L.; Wang, C.; Yan, X.; Liu, X.; Lu, G. Ultrasensitive Detection of SARS-CoV-2 Spike Protein in Untreated Saliva Using SERS-Based Biosensor. *Biosens. Bioelectron.* **2021**, *190*, 113421. [CrossRef] [PubMed]
111. Li, Y.; Lin, C.; Peng, Y.; He, J.; Yang, Y. High-Sensitivity and Point-of-Care Detection of SARS-CoV-2 from Nasal and Throat Swabs by Magnetic SERS Biosensor. *Sens. Actuators B Chem.* **2022**, *365*, 131974. [CrossRef]
112. Hojjat Jodaylami, M.; Djaileb, A.; Live, L.S.; Boudreau, D.; Pelletier, J.; Masson, J.-F. Rapid Quantification of SARS-CoV-2 Antibodies with a Portable Surface Plasmon Resonance Biosensor. *ECS Meet. Abstr.* **2021**, *MA2021-01*, 2026. [CrossRef]
113. Cady, N.C.; Tokranova, N.; Minor, A.; Nikvand, N.; Strle, K.; Lee, W.T.; Page, W.; Guignon, E.; Pilar, A.; Gibson, G.N. Multiplexed Detection and Quantification of Human Antibody Response to COVID-19 Infection Using a Plasmon Enhanced Biosensor Platform. *Biosens. Bioelectron.* **2021**, *171*, 112679. [CrossRef] [PubMed]
114. Cognetti, J.S.; Miller, B.L. Monitoring Serum Spike Protein with Disposable Photonic Biosensors Following SARS-CoV-2 Vaccination. *Sensors* **2021**, *21*, 5857. [CrossRef] [PubMed]
115. Wu, Q.; Wu, W.; Chen, F.; Ren, P. Highly Sensitive and Selective Surface Plasmon Resonance Biosensor for the Detection of SARS-CoV-2 Spike S1 Protein. *Analyst* **2022**, *147*, 2809–2818. [CrossRef]
116. Ebrem Bilgin, B.; Torun, H.; Ilgü, M.; Yanik, C.; Batur, S.N.; Çelik, S.; Öztürk, H.; Dogan, Ö.; Ergönül, Ö.; Solaroglu, I.; et al. Clinical Validation of SERS Metasurface SARS-CoV-2 Biosensor. In *Biomedical Vibrational Spectroscopy 2022: Advances in Research and Industry*; Huang, Z., Ed.; SPIE: Bellingham, WA, USA, 2022; Volume 11957, p. 36.
117. Kumar, A.; Kumar, A.; Srivastava, S.K. Silicon Nitride-BP-Based Surface Plasmon Resonance Highly Sensitive Biosensor for Virus SARS-CoV-2 Detection. *Plasmonics* **2022**, *17*, 1065–1077. [CrossRef]
118. Akib, T.B.A.; Mou, S.F.; Rahman, M.M.; Rana, M.M.; Islam, M.R.; Mehedi, I.M.; Mahmud, M.A.P.; Kouzani, A.Z. Design and Numerical Analysis of a Graphene-Coated SPR Biosensor for Rapid Detection of the Novel Coronavirus. *Sensors* **2021**, *21*, 3491. [CrossRef]
119. Anshori, I.; Nugroho, A.E.; Jessika, A.S.; Yusuf, M.; Hartati, Y.W.; Sari, S.P.; Tohari, T.R.; Yuliarto, B.; Gumilar, G.; Nuraviana, L.; et al. Single-Chained Fragment Variable (ScFv) Recombinant as a Potential Receptor for SARS-CoV-2 Biosensor Based on Surface Plasmon Resonance (SPR). In *2021 IEEE Sensors*; IEEE: Piscataway, NJ, USA, 2021; p. 21487738.

120. Dai, Z.; Xu, X.; Wang, Y.; Li, M.; Zhou, K.; Zhang, L.; Tan, Y. Surface Plasmon Resonance Biosensor with Laser Heterodyne Feedback for Highly-Sensitive and Rapid Detection of COVID-19 Spike Antigen. *Biosens. Bioelectron.* **2022**, *206*, 114163. [CrossRef]
121. Peng, Y.; Lin, C.; Li, Y.; Gao, Y.; Wang, J.; He, J.; Huang, Z.; Liu, J.; Luo, X.; Yang, Y. Identifying Infectiousness of SARS-CoV-2 by Ultra-Sensitive SnS_2 SERS Biosensors with Capillary Effect. *Matter* **2022**, *5*, 694–709. [CrossRef] [PubMed]
122. Lee, W.-I.; Subramanian, A.; Mueller, S.; Levon, K.; Nam, C.-Y.; Rafailovich, M.H. Potentiometric Biosensors Based on Molecular-Imprinted Self-Assembled Monolayer Films for Rapid Detection of Influenza A Virus and SARS-CoV-2 Spike Protein. *ACS Appl. Nano Mater.* **2022**, *5*, 5045–5055. [CrossRef] [PubMed]
123. Qiu, G.; Gai, Z.; Tao, Y.; Schmitt, J.; Kullak-Ublick, G.A.; Wang, J. Dual-Functional Plasmonic Photothermal Biosensors for Highly Accurate Severe Acute Respiratory Syndrome Coronavirus 2 Detection. *ACS Nano* **2020**, *14*, 5268–5277. [CrossRef] [PubMed]
124. Forssén, P.; Samuelsson, J.; Lacki, K.; Fornstedt, T. Advanced Analysis of Biosensor Data for SARS-CoV-2 RBD and ACE2 Interactions. *Anal. Chem.* **2020**, *92*, 11520–11524. [CrossRef]
125. Behrouzi, K.; Lin, L. Gold Nanoparticle Based Plasmonic Sensing for the Detection of SARS-CoV-2 Nucleocapsid Proteins. *Biosens. Bioelectron.* **2022**, *195*, 113669. [CrossRef]
126. Basso, C.R.; Malossi, C.D.; Haisi, A.; de Albuquerque Pedrosa, V.; Barbosa, A.N.; Grotto, R.T.; Araujo Junior, J.P. Fast and Reliable Detection of SARS-CoV-2 Antibodies Based on Surface Plasmon Resonance. *Anal. Methods* **2021**, *13*, 3297–3306. [CrossRef]
127. Saada, H.; Pagneux, Q.; Wei, J.; Live, L.; Roussel, A.; Dogliani, A.; Die Morini, L.; Engelmann, I.; Alidjinou, E.K.; Rolland, A.S.; et al. Sensing of COVID-19 Spike Protein in Nasopharyngeal Samples Using a Portable Surface Plasmon Resonance Diagnostic System. *Sens. Diagn.* **2022**. [CrossRef]
128. Moitra, P.; Chaichi, A.; Abid Hasan, S.M.; Dighe, K.; Alafeef, M.; Prasad, A.; Gartia, M.R.; Pan, D. Probing the Mutation Independent Interaction of DNA Probes with SARS-CoV-2 Variants through a Combination of Surface-Enhanced Raman Scattering and Machine Learning. *Biosens. Bioelectron.* **2022**, *208*, 114200. [CrossRef]
129. Bong, J.-H.; Kim, T.-H.; Jung, J.; Lee, S.J.; Sung, J.S.; Lee, C.K.; Kang, M.-J.; Kim, H.O.; Pyun, J.-C. Pig Sera-Derived Anti-SARS-CoV-2 Antibodies in Surface Plasmon Resonance Biosensors. *BioChip J.* **2020**, *14*, 358–368. [CrossRef]
130. Achadu, O.J.; Nwaji, N.; Lee, D.; Lee, J.; Akinoglu, E.M.; Giersig, M.; Park, E.Y. 3D Hierarchically Porous Magnetic Molybdenum Trioxide@gold Nanospheres as a Nanogap-Enhanced Raman Scattering Biosensor for SARS-CoV-2. *Nanoscale Adv.* **2022**, *4*, 871–883. [CrossRef]
131. Funari, R.; Chu, K.-Y.; Shen, A.Q. Detection of Antibodies against SARS-CoV-2 Spike Protein by Gold Nanospikes in an Opto-Microfluidic Chip. *Biosens. Bioelectron.* **2020**, *169*, 112578. [CrossRef] [PubMed]
132. Gutgsell, A.R.; Gunnarsson, A.; Forssén, P.; Gordon, E.; Fornstedt, T.; Geschwindner, S. Biosensor-Enabled Deconvolution of the Avidity-Induced Affinity Enhancement for the SARS-CoV-2 Spike Protein and ACE2 Interaction. *Anal. Chem.* **2022**, *94*, 1187–1194. [CrossRef] [PubMed]
133. Saad, Y.; Gazzah, M.H.; Mougin, K.; Selmi, M.; Belmabrouk, H. Sensitive Detection of SARS-CoV-2 Using a Novel Plasmonic Fiber Optic Biosensor Design. *Plasmonics* **2022**. [CrossRef]
134. Bistaffa, M.J.; Camacho, S.A.; Pazin, W.M.; Constantino, C.J.L.; Oliveira, O.N.; Aoki, P.H.B. Immunoassay Platform with Surface-Enhanced Resonance Raman Scattering for Detecting Trace Levels of SARS-CoV-2 Spike Protein. *Talanta* **2022**, *244*, 123381. [CrossRef] [PubMed]
135. Zhao, B.; Che, C.; Wang, W.; Li, N.; Cunningham, B.T. Single-Step, Wash-Free Digital Immunoassay for Rapid Quantitative Analysis of Serological Antibody against SARS-CoV-2 by Photonic Resonator Absorption Microscopy. *Talanta* **2021**, *225*, 122004. [CrossRef] [PubMed]
136. Cennamo, N.; Pasquardini, L.; Arcadio, F.; Lunelli, L.; Vanzetti, L.; Carafa, V.; Altucci, L.; Zeni, L. SARS-CoV-2 Spike Protein Detection through a Plasmonic D-Shaped Plastic Optical Fiber Aptasensor. *Talanta* **2021**, *233*, 122532. [CrossRef] [PubMed]
137. Zhang, Z.-Y.; Liu, X.; Shen, L.; Chen, L.; Fang, W.-H. Machine Learning with Multilevel Descriptors for Screening of Inorganic Nonlinear Optical Crystals. *J. Phys. Chem. C* **2021**, *125*, 25175–25188. [CrossRef]
138. Wang, X.; Wang, H.; Zhou, W.; Zhang, T.; Huang, H.; Song, Y.; Li, Y.; Liu, Y.; Kang, Z. Carbon Dots with Tunable Third-Order Nonlinear Coefficient Instructed by Machine Learning. *J. Photochem. Photobiol. A Chem.* **2022**, *426*, 113729. [CrossRef]
139. Fairbairn, C.E.; Kang, D.; Bosch, N. Using Machine Learning for Real-Time BAC Estimation from a New-Generation Transdermal Biosensor in the Laboratory. *Drug Alcohol Depend.* **2020**, *216*, 108205. [CrossRef]
140. Robison, H.M.; Chapman, C.A.; Zhou, H.; Erskine, C.L.; Theel, E.; Peikert, T.; Lindestam Arlehamn, C.S.; Sette, A.; Bushell, C.; Welge, M.; et al. Risk Assessment of Latent Tuberculosis Infection through a Multiplexed Cytokine Biosensor Assay and Machine Learning Feature Selection. *Sci. Rep.* **2021**, *11*, 20544. [CrossRef]
141. Kim, H.; Seong, W.; Rha, E.; Lee, H.; Kim, S.K.; Kwon, K.K.; Park, K.-H.; Lee, D.-H.; Lee, S.-G. Machine Learning Linked Evolutionary Biosensor Array for Highly Sensitive and Specific Molecular Identification. *Biosens. Bioelectron.* **2020**, *170*, 112670. [CrossRef] [PubMed]
142. Pennacchio, A.; Giampaolo, F.; Piccialli, F.; Cuomo, S.; Notomista, E.; Spinelli, M.; Amoresano, A.; Piscitelli, A.; Giardina, P. A Machine Learning-Enhanced Biosensor for Mercury Detection Based on an Hydrophobin Chimera. *Biosens. Bioelectron.* **2022**, *196*, 113696. [CrossRef] [PubMed]
143. Green, E.M.; van Mourik, R.; Wolfus, C.; Heitner, S.B.; Dur, O.; Semigran, M.J. Machine Learning Detection of Obstructive Hypertrophic Cardiomyopathy Using a Wearable Biosensor. *Npj Digit. Med.* **2019**, *2*, 57. [CrossRef]

144. Vakilian, K.A. A Nitrate Enzymatic Biosensor Based on Optimized Machine Learning Techniques. In *2022 9th Iranian Joint Congress on Fuzzy and Intelligent Systems (CFIS)*; IEEE: Piscataway, NJ, USA, 2022; p. 21758368.
145. Khor, S.M.; Choi, J.; Won, P.; Ko, S.H. Challenges and Strategies in Developing an Enzymatic Wearable Sweat Glucose Biosensor as a Practical Point-Of-Care Monitoring Tool for Type II Diabetes. *Nanomaterials* **2022**, *12*, 221. [CrossRef] [PubMed]
146. Gonzalez-Navarro, F.; Stilianova-Stoytcheva, M.; Renteria-Gutierrez, L.; Belanche-Muñoz, L.; Flores-Rios, B.; Ibarra-Esquer, J. Glucose Oxidase Biosensor Modeling and Predictors Optimization by Machine Learning Methods. *Sensors* **2016**, *16*, 1483. [CrossRef] [PubMed]
147. Boscolo, S.; Finot, C. Artificial Neural Networks for Nonlinear Pulse Shaping in Optical Fibers. *Opt. Laser Technol.* **2020**, *131*, 106439. [CrossRef]
148. Chicea, D.; Rei, S.M. A Fast Artificial Neural Network Approach for Dynamic Light Scattering Time Series Processing. *Meas. Sci. Technol.* **2018**, *29*, 105201. [CrossRef]
149. Talebi-Moghaddam, S.; Bauer, F.J.; Huber, F.J.T.; Will, S.; Daun, K.J. Inferring Soot Morphology through Multi-Angle Light Scattering Using an Artificial Neural Network. *J. Quant. Spectrosc. Radiat. Transf.* **2020**, *251*, 106957. [CrossRef]
150. Pelenis, D.; Barauskas, D.; Vanagas, G.; Dzikaras, M.; Viržonis, D. CMUT-Based Biosensor with Convolutional Neural Network Signal Processing. *Ultrasonics* **2019**, *99*, 105956. [CrossRef]
151. Byun, S.-J.; Kim, D.-G.; Park, K.-D.; Choi, Y.-J.; Kumar, P.; Ali, I.; Kim, D.-G.; Yoo, J.-M.; Huh, H.-K.; Jung, Y.-J.; et al. A Low-Power Analog Processor-in-Memory-Based Convolutional Neural Network for Biosensor Applications. *Sensors* **2022**, *22*, 4555. [CrossRef]
152. Mennel, L.; Symonowicz, J.; Wachter, S.; Polyushkin, D.K.; Molina-Mendoza, A.J.; Mueller, T. Ultrafast Machine Vision with 2D Material Neural Network Image Sensors. *Nature* **2020**, *579*, 62–66. [CrossRef] [PubMed]
153. Chen, C.; Wang, J. Optical Biosensors: An Exhaustive and Comprehensive Review. *Analyst* **2020**, *145*, 1605–1628. [CrossRef] [PubMed]
154. Yan, Y.; Gong, J.; Chen, J.; Zeng, Z.; Huang, W.; Pu, K.; Liu, J.; Chen, P. Recent Advances on Graphene Quantum Dots: From Chemistry and Physics to Applications. *Adv. Mater.* **2019**, *31*, 1808283. [CrossRef]
155. Zhao, Y.; Li, Y.; Zhang, P.; Yan, Z.; Zhou, Y.; Du, Y.; Qu, C.; Song, Y.; Zhou, D.; Qu, S.; et al. Cell-Based Fluorescent Microsphere Incorporated with Carbon Dots as a Sensitive Immunosensor for the Rapid Detection of Escherichia Coli O157 in Milk. *Biosens. Bioelectron.* **2021**, *179*, 113057. [CrossRef]
156. Hu, Q.; Wang, S.; Duan, H.; Liu, Y. A Fluorescent Biosensor for Sensitive Detection of Salmonella Typhimurium Using Low-Gradient Magnetic Field and Deep Learning via Faster Region-Based Convolutional Neural Network. *Biosensors* **2021**, *11*, 447. [CrossRef] [PubMed]
157. Zhu, X.; Liu, P.; Xue, T.; Ge, Y.; Ai, S.; Sheng, Y.; Wu, R.; Xu, L.; Tang, K.; Wen, Y. A Novel Graphene-like Titanium Carbide MXene/Au–Ag Nanoshuttles Bifunctional Nanosensor for Electrochemical and SERS Intelligent Analysis of Ultra-Trace Carbendazim Coupled with Machine Learning. *Ceram. Int.* **2021**, *47*, 173–184. [CrossRef]
158. Chen, G.; Du, J.; Sun, L.; Zhang, W.; Xu, K.; Chen, X.; Reed, G.T.; He, Z. Nonlinear Distortion Mitigation by Machine Learning of SVM Classification for PAM-4 and PAM-8 Modulated Optical Interconnection. *J. Light. Technol.* **2018**, *36*, 650–657. [CrossRef]
159. Lin, J.; Shen, G.; Zhai, Z.; Zheng, D.; Li, Y.; Chang, Z.; Zong, L.; Deng, N.; Chang, T. Delivering Distributed Machine Learning Services in All-Optical Datacenter Networks with Torus Topology. In *Asia Communications and Photonics Conference 2021*; Chang-Hasnain Willner, A., Shieh, W., Shum, P., Su, Y., Li, G., Eggleton, B., Essiambre, R., Dai, D., Ma, D.C., Eds.; Optica Publishing Group: Washington, DC, USA, 2021; p. W3C.5.
160. McConnon, A. Deep Learning Characterizes Optical Pulses Using Speckle Patterns at the End of Multimode Fibers. *Scilight* **2020**, *2020*, 381102. [CrossRef]
161. Noble, J.; Zhou, C.; Murray, W.T.; Liu, Z. Convolutional Neural Network Reconstruction of Ultrashort Optical Pulses. *Ultrafast Nonlinear Imaging Spectrosc. VIII* **2020**, *11497*, 20. [CrossRef]
162. Närhi, M.; Salmela, L.; Toivonen, J.; Billet, C.; Dudley, J.M.; Genty, G. Machine Learning Analysis of Extreme Events in Optical Fibre Modulation Instability. *Nat. Commun.* **2018**, *9*, 4923. [CrossRef]
163. Kokhanovskiy, A.; Kuprikov, E.; Bednyakova, A.; Popkov, I.; Smirnov, S.; Turitsyn, S. Inverse Design of Mode-Locked Fiber Laser by Particle Swarm Optimization Algorithm. *Sci. Rep.* **2021**, *11*, 13555. [CrossRef] [PubMed]
164. Woodward, R.I.; Kelleher, E.J.R. Towards 'Smart Lasers': Self-Optimisation of an Ultrafast Pulse Source Using a Genetic Algorithm. *Sci. Rep.* **2016**, *6*, 37616. [CrossRef] [PubMed]
165. Zahavy, T.; Dikopoltsev, A.; Moss, D.; Haham, G.I.; Cohen, O.; Mannor, S.; Segev, M. Deep Learning Reconstruction of Ultrashort Pulses. *Optica* **2018**, *5*, 666. [CrossRef]
166. Underwood, K.J.; Jones, A.M.; Gopinath, J.T. Synthesis of Coherent Optical Pulses Using a Field-Programmable Gate Array (FPGA)-Based Gradient Descent Phase-Locking Algorithm with Three Semiconductor Lasers. In *CLEO: 2015*; OSA: Washington, DC, USA, 2015; p. 15380458.
167. Wang, D.; Zhang, M.; Cai, Z.; Cui, Y.; Li, Z.; Han, H.; Fu, M.; Luo, B. Combatting Nonlinear Phase Noise in Coherent Optical Systems with an Optimized Decision Processor Based on Machine Learning. *Opt. Commun.* **2016**, *369*, 199–208. [CrossRef]
168. Marciniak, M. Two-Beam-Propagation Method Algorithm for Second-Harmonic Generation in Dielectric Planar Waveguides. In *Proceedings of SPIE*; Tuchin, V.V., Ryabukho, V.P., Zimnyakov, D.A., Eds.; SPIE: Bellingham, WA, USA, 1999; Volume 3726, p. 32.
169. Andrews, D.L.; Romero, L.C.D.; Meath, W.J. An Algorithm for the Nonlinear Optical Susceptibilities of Dipolar Molecules, and an Application to Third Harmonic Generation. *J. Phys. B At. Mol. Opt. Phys.* **1999**, *32*, 1. [CrossRef]

170. Kurokawa, Y.; Nomura, S.; Takemori, T.; Aoyagi, Y. Fast Algorithm for Calculating Two-Photon Absorption Spectra. *Phys. Rev. E* **1999**, *59*, 3694–3697. [CrossRef]
171. Boynton, G.C.; Gordon, H.R. Irradiance Inversion Algorithm for Estimating the Absorption and Backscattering Coefficients of Natural Waters: Raman-Scattering Effects. *Appl. Opt.* **2000**, *39*, 3012–3022. [CrossRef]
172. Lin, F.; Gong, Y.; Shum, P. Optimization Design By Genetic Algorithm With A New Crossover Method For Broadband Fiber Raman Amplifiers. In *Optical Communications and Networks*; World Scientific: Singapore, 2002; pp. 249–252, ISBN 978-981-238-232-0.
173. Hamza, M.Y.; Tariq, S.; Awais, M.M.; Yang, S. Mitigation of the Effects of Self Phase Modulation and Group-Velocity Dispersion in Fiber Optic Communications: Dispersion- and Power-Map Cooptimization Using the Genetic Algorithm. *Opt. Eng.* **2008**, *47*, 1–12. [CrossRef]
174. Ohto, T.; Usui, K.; Hasegawa, T.; Bonn, M.; Nagata, Y. Toward Ab Initio Molecular Dynamics Modeling for Sum-Frequency Generation Spectra; an Efficient Algorithm Based on Surface-Specific Velocity-Velocity Correlation Function. *J. Chem. Phys.* **2015**, *143*, 124702. [CrossRef]
175. Hakimian, F.; Shayesteh, M.R.; Moslemi, M.R. Optimization of Four-Wave Mixing Wavelength Conversion in a Quantum-Dot Semiconductor Optical Amplifier Based on the Genetic Algorithm. *Opt. Quantum Electron.* **2021**, *53*, 140. [CrossRef]
176. Al-Qarni, A.A.; Bakodah, H.O.; Alshaery, A.A.; Biswas, A.; Yıldırım, Y.; Moraru, L.; Moldovanu, S. Numerical Simulation of Cubic-Quartic Optical Solitons with Perturbed Fokas–Lenells Equation Using Improved Adomian Decomposition Algorithm. *Mathematics* **2022**, *10*, 138. [CrossRef]
177. Moreno-Larios, J.A.; Ramírez-Guerra, C.; Contreras-Martínez, R.; Rosete-Aguilar, M.; Garduño-Mejía, J. Algorithm to Filter the Noise in the Spectral Intensity of Ultrashort Laser Pulses. *Appl. Opt.* **2020**, *59*, 7233–7241. [CrossRef] [PubMed]
178. Fan, Q.; Zhou, G.; Gui, T.; Lu, C.; Lau, A.P.T. Advancing Theoretical Understanding and Practical Performance of Signal Processing for Nonlinear Optical Communications through Machine Learning. *Nat. Commun.* **2020**, *11*, 3694. [CrossRef] [PubMed]
179. Smolyaninov, I.I. Nonlinear Optics of Photonic Hyper-Crystals: Optical Limiting and Hyper-Computing. *J. Opt. Soc. Am. B* **2019**, *36*, 1629–1636. [CrossRef]
180. Dikopoltsev, A.; Zahavy, T.; Ziv, R.; Rubinstein, I.; Sidorenko, P.; Mannor, S.; Cohen, O.; Segev, M. Reconstruction of Ultrashort Pulses Using Deep Neural Networks. In *2018 2nd URSI Atlantic Radio Science Meeting (AT-RASC)*; IEEE: Piscataway, NJ, USA, 2018; p. 18144568.
181. Wang, Q.; Liu, W.; Chen, X.; Wang, X.; Chen, G.; Zhu, X. Quantification of Scar Collagen Texture and Prediction of Scar Development via Second Harmonic Generation Images and a Generative Adversarial Network. *Biomed. Opt. Express* **2021**, *12*, 5305–5319. [CrossRef] [PubMed]
182. Wang, G.; Sun, Y.; Jiang, S.; Wu, G.; Liao, W.; Chen, Y.; Lin, Z.; Liu, Z.; Zhuo, S. Machine Learning-Based Rapid Diagnosis of Human Borderline Ovarian Cancer on Second-Harmonic Generation Images. *Biomed. Opt. Express* **2021**, *12*, 5658–5669. [CrossRef]
183. Wu, B.; Judd, N.B.; Smith, J.T.; Icaza, M.; Mukherjee, S.; Jain, M.; Gallagher, R.M.; Szeligowski, R.V. A Pilot Study for Distinguishing Chromophobe Renal Cell Carcinoma and Oncocytoma Using Second Harmonic Generation Imaging and Convolutional Neural Network Analysis of Collagen Fibrillar Structure. In *Optical Biopsy XVI: Toward Real-Time Spectroscopic Imaging and Diagnosis*; Alfano, R.R., Demos, S.G., Eds.; SPIE: Bellingham, WA, USA, 2018; Volume 10489, p. 44.
184. Vidal-Codina, F.; Nguyen, N.-C.; Ciracì, C.; Oh, S.-H.; Peraire, J. A Nested Hybridizable Discontinuous Galerkin Method for Computing Second-Harmonic Generation in Three-Dimensional Metallic Nanostructures. *J. Comput. Phys.* **2021**, *429*, 110000. [CrossRef]
185. Xu, Z.; Wang, P.; Zhao, M.; Yang, M.; Zhao, W.; Hu, K.; Dong, L.; Wang, S.; Li, X.; Yang, P.; et al. Prediction of Second-Harmonic Generation Wave-Front Distribution by Extreme Learning Machine. *IEEE Photonics Technol. Lett.* **2020**, *32*, 693–696. [CrossRef]
186. Jafari, R.; Jones, T.; Trebino, R. 100% Reliable Algorithm for Second-Harmonic-Generation Frequency-Resolved Optical Gating. *Opt. Express* **2019**, *27*, 2112–2124. [CrossRef]
187. Jafari, R.; Jones, T.; Trebino, R. 100% Reliable Frequency-Resolved-Optical-Gating Pulse Retrieval Algorithmic Approach. In *Frontiers in Optics + Laser Science APS/DLS*; OSA: Washington, DC, USA, 2019; p. JW3A.33.
188. Saito, K.; Tanabe, T.; Oyama, Y. Numerical Analysis of Second Harmonic Generation for THz-Wave in a Photonic Crystal Waveguide Using a Nonlinear FDTD Algorithm. *Opt. Commun.* **2016**, *365*, 164–167. [CrossRef]
189. Schneidereit, D.; Nübler, S.; Prölß, G.; Reischl, B.; Schürmann, S.; Müller, O.J.; Friedrich, O. Optical Prediction of Single Muscle Fiber Force Production Using a Combined Biomechatronics and Second Harmonic Generation Imaging Approach. *Light Sci. Appl.* **2018**, *7*, 79. [CrossRef] [PubMed]
190. Liu, Q.; Mukhopadhyay, S.; Bastidas Rodriguez, M.X.; Fu, X.; Sahu, S.; Burk, D.; Gartia, M. A One-Shot Learning Framework for Assessment of Fibrillar Collagen from Second Harmonic Generation Images of an Infarcted Myocardium. In *2020 IEEE 17th International Symposium on Biomedical Imaging (ISBI)*; IEEE: Piscataway, NJ, USA, 2020; pp. 839–843.
191. Diatta, A.; Rouquette, J.; Armand, P.; Hermet, P. Density Functional Theory Prediction of the Second Harmonic Generation and Linear Pockels Effect in Trigonal $BaZnO_2$. *J. Phys. Chem. C* **2018**, *122*, 21277–21283. [CrossRef]
192. Comin, A.; Hartschuh, A. Efficient Optimization of SHG Hotspot Switching in Plasmonic Nanoantennas Using Phase-Shaped Laser Pulses Controlled by Neural Networks. *Opt. Express* **2018**, *26*, 33678–33686. [CrossRef] [PubMed]
193. Hall, G.; Liang, W.; Li, X. Efficient and Unbiased Fit-Free Algorithm for Quantification of Collagen Fiber Alignment for SHG Imaging Applications. In *Biomedical Optics 2016*; OSA: Washington, DC, USA, 2016.

194. Preißler, D.; Kiefer, D.; Führer, T.; Walther, T. Evolutionary Algorithm-Assisted Design of a UV SHG Cavity with Elliptical Focusing to Avoid Crystal Degradation. *Appl. Phys. B* **2019**, *125*, 220. [CrossRef]
195. Hall, G.; Liang, W.; Li, X. Fitting-Free Algorithm for Efficient Quantification of Collagen Fiber Alignment in SHG Imaging Applications. *Biomed. Opt. Express* **2017**, *8*, 4609–4620. [CrossRef]
196. Kang, L.; Liang, F.; Gong, P.; Lin, Z.; Liu, F.; Huang, B. Two Novel Deep-Ultraviolet Nonlinear Optical Crystals with Shorter Phase-Matching Second Harmonic Generation than KBe2BO3F2: A First-Principles Prediction. *Phys. Status Solidi–Rapid Res. Lett.* **2018**, *12*, 1800276. [CrossRef]
197. Zhang, B.; Tikhonov, E.; Xie, C.; Yang, Z.; Pan, S. Prediction of Fluorooxoborates with Colossal Second Harmonic Generation (SHG) Coefficients and Extremely Wide Band Gaps: Towards Modulating Properties by Tuning the BO_3/BO_3F Ratio in Layers. *Angew. Chem.* **2019**, *131*, 11852–11856. [CrossRef]
198. McLean, J.; DiMarzio, C. A Linear Algorithm for Quantitative Measure of Corneal Collagen Fiber Orientation Using Second Harmonic Generation Microscopy. *Proc. SPIE* **2016**, *9713*, 971317. [CrossRef]
199. Kumar, A.; Yadav, M.P.S. Computational Studies of Third-Order Nonlinear Optical Properties of Pyridine Derivative 2-Aminopyridinium p-Toluenesulphonate Crystal. *Pramana* **2017**, *89*, 7. [CrossRef]
200. Salem, M.A.; Twelves, I.; Brown, A. Prediction of Two-Photon Absorption Enhancement in Red Fluorescent Protein Chromophores Made from Non-Canonical Amino Acids. *Phys. Chem. Chem. Phys.* **2016**, *18*, 24408–24416. [CrossRef]
201. Eybposh, M.H.; Caira, N.W.; Atisa, M.; Chakravarthula, P.; Pégard, N.C. Enhanced Two-Photon Absorption with Deep Learning-Based Computer Generated Holography. In *Frontiers in Optics/Laser Science*; Lee Mazzali, C., Corwin, K., Jason Jones, R.B., Eds.; OSA: Washington, DC, USA, 2020.
202. Deng, A.; Huang, J.; Liu, H.; Cai, W. Deep Learning Algorithms for Temperature Field Reconstruction of Nonlinear Tomographic Absorption Spectroscopy. *Meas. Sens.* **2020**, *10–12*, 100024. [CrossRef]
203. Yadav, C.; Roy, S. Ultrafast Nonlinear Absorption in Hemoprotein Cytochrome-c and Its Application to Computing. *Opt. Quantum Electron.* **2016**, *48*, 377. [CrossRef]
204. Wang, Z.; Zhu, N.; Wang, W.; Chao, X. Y-Net: A Dual-Branch Deep Learning Network for Nonlinear Absorption Tomography with Wavelength Modulation Spectroscopy. *Opt. Express* **2022**, *30*, 2156–2172. [CrossRef] [PubMed]
205. Neskorniuk, V.; Freire, P.J.; Napoli, A.; Spinnler, B.; Schairer, W.; Prilepsky, J.E.; Costa, N.; Turitsyn, S.K. Simplifying the Supervised Learning of Kerr Nonlinearity Compensation Algorithms by Data Augmentation. In *2020 European Conference on Optical Communications (ECOC)*; IEEE: Piscataway, NJ, USA, 2020; pp. 1–4.
206. Yıldırım, Y.; Çelik, N.; Yaşar, E. Nonlinear Schrödinger Equations with Spatio-Temporal Dispersion in Kerr, Parabolic, Power and Dual Power Law Media: A Novel Extended Kudryashov's Algorithm and Soliton Solutions. *Results Phys.* **2017**, *7*, 3116–3123. [CrossRef]
207. Solli, D.R.; Ropers, C.; Koonath, P.; Jalali, B. Optical Rogue Waves. *Nature* **2007**, *450*, 1054–1057. [CrossRef]
208. Gopalakrishnan, S.S.; Panajotov, K.; Taki, M.; Tlidi, M. Dissipative Light Bullets in Kerr Cavities: Multistability, Clustering, and Rogue Waves. *Phys. Rev. Lett.* **2021**, *126*, 153902. [CrossRef]
209. Jhangeer, A.; Faridi, W.A.; Asjad, M.I.; Akgül, A. Analytical Study of Soliton Solutions for an Improved Perturbed Schrödinger Equation with Kerr Law Non-Linearity in Non-Linear Optics by an Expansion Algorithm. *Partial Differ. Equ. Appl. Math.* **2021**, *4*, 100102. [CrossRef]
210. Chase, H.M.; Rudshteyn, B.; Psciuk, B.T.; Upshur, M.A.; Strick, B.F.; Thomson, R.J.; Batista, V.S.; Geiger, F.M. Assessment of DFT for Computing Sum Frequency Generation Spectra of an Epoxydiol and a Deuterated Isotopologue at Fused Silica/Vapor Interfaces. *J. Phys. Chem. B* **2016**, *120*, 1919–1927. [CrossRef]
211. Shah, S.A.; Pikalov, A.A.; Baldelli, S. ChemSpecNet: A Neural Network for Chemical Analysis of Sum Frequency Generation Spectroscopic Imaging. *Opt. Commun.* **2022**, *507*, 127691. [CrossRef]
212. Jackson, W.; Zishan, W.; Xiong, W. Imaging Orientation of a Single Molecular Hierarchical Self-Assembled Sheet: The Combined Power of a Vibrational Sum Frequency Generation Microscopy and Neural Network. *ChemRxiv* **2022**. [CrossRef]
213. Cai, M.; Zhuge, Q.; Lun, H.; Fu, M.; Yi, L.; Hu, W. Pilot-Aided Self-Phase Modulation Noise Monitoring Based on Artificial Neural Network. In *Asia Communications and Photonics Conference (ACPC) 2019*; Optica Publishing Group: Chengdu, China, 2019; p. M4A.9.
214. Fumumoto, Y.; Owaki, S.; Nakamura, M. Effect of Number of Neurons of a Neural-Network on Compensation Performance of SPM Non-Linear Waveform Distortion. In *2017 Opto-Electronics and Communications Conference (OECC) and Photonics Global Conference (PGC)*; IEEE: Piscataway, NJ, USA, 2017; pp. 1–2.
215. Owaki, S.; Nakamura, M. Simultaneous Compensation of Waveform Distortion Caused by Chromatic Dispersion and SPM Using a Three-Layer Neural-Network. In *2017 Opto-Electronics and Communications Conference (OECC) and Photonics Global Conference (PGC)*; IEEE: Piscataway, NJ, USA, 2017; p. 17373621.
216. Caballero, F.J.V.; Ives, D.J.; Laperle, C.; Charlton, D.; Zhuge, Q.; O'Sullivan, M.; Savory, S.J. Machine Learning Based Linear and Nonlinear Noise Estimation. *J. Opt. Commun. Netw.* **2018**, *10*, 42–51. [CrossRef]
217. Brusin, A.M.R.; de Moura, U.C.; Curri, V.; Zibar, D.; Carena, A. Introducing Load Aware Neural Networks for Accurate Predictions of Raman Amplifiers. *J. Light. Technol.* **2020**, *38*, 6481–6491. [CrossRef]
218. Soltani, M.; Da Ros, F.; Carena, A.; Zibar, D. Spectral and Spatial Power Evolution Design With Machine Learning-Enabled Raman Amplification. *J. Light. Technol.* **2022**, *40*, 3546–3556. [CrossRef]

219. Soltani, M.; Da Ros, F.; Carena, A.; Zibar, D. Distance and Spectral Power Profile Shaping Using Machine Learning Enabled Raman Amplifiers. In *2021 IEEE Photonics Society Summer Topicals Meeting Series (SUM)*; IEEE: Piscataway, NJ, USA, 2021; p. 21048928.
220. de Moura, U.C.; Da Ros, F.; Zibar, D.; Rosa Brusin, A.M.; Carena, A. Optimization of Raman Amplifiers Using Machine Learning. In *2021 IEEE Photonics Society Summer Topicals Meeting Series (SUM)*; IEEE: Piscataway, NJ, USA, 2021; p. 21048937.
221. Marcon, G.; Galtarossa, A.; Palmieri, L.; Santagiustina, M. Model-Aware Deep Learning Method for Raman Amplification in Few-Mode Fibers. *J. Light. Technol.* **2021**, *39*, 1371–1380. [CrossRef]
222. Huang, Y.; Du, J.; Chen, Y.; Xu, K.; He, Z. Machine Learning Assisted Inverse Design for Ultrafine, Dynamic and Arbitrary Gain Spectrum Shaping of Raman Amplification. *Photonics* **2021**, *8*, 260. [CrossRef]
223. Ionescu, M.; Ghazisaeidi, A.; Renaudier, J. Machine Learning Assisted Hybrid EDFA-Raman Amplifier Design for C+L Bands. In *Proceedings of the 2020 European Conference on Optical Communications (ECOC)*, Virtual Event, 6–10 December 2020; IEEE: Piscataway, NJ, USA, 2020; p. 20349557.
224. Marcon, G.; Galtarossa, A.; Palmieri, L.; Santagiustina, M. C+L Band Gain Design in Few-Mode Fibers Using Raman Amplification and Machine Learning. In *2020 Italian Conference on Optics and Photonics (ICOP)*; IEEE: Piscataway, NJ, USA, 2020; p. 20264995.
225. Soltani, M.; Da Ros, F.; Carena, A.; Zibar, D. Inverse Design of a Raman Amplifier in Frequency and Distance Domains Using Convolutional Neural Networks. *Opt. Lett.* **2021**, *46*, 2650–2653. [CrossRef]
226. Zibar, D.; de Moura, U.C.; Rosa Brusin, A.M.; Carena, A.; Da Ros, F. Machine Learning Enabled Raman Amplifiers. In Proceedings of the 2021 Conference on Lasers and Electro-Optics Europe and European Quantum Electronics Conference, Virtual Event, 21–25 June 2021; Optica Publishing Group: Munich, Germany, 2021; p. ci_1_3.
227. Marcon, G.; Galtarossa, A.; Palmieri, L.; Santagiustina, M. Gain Design of Few-Mode Fiber Raman Amplifiers Using an Autoencoder-Based Machine Learning Approach. In *2020 European Conference on Optical Communications (ECOC)*; IEEE: Piscataway, NJ, USA, 2020; p. 20349595.
228. Gong, J.; Liu, F.; Wu, Y.; Zhang, Y.; Lei, S.; Zhu, Z. Raman Fiber Amplifier Design Scheme Based on Back Propagation Neural Network Algorithm. *Opt. Eng.* **2021**, *60*, 37103. [CrossRef]
229. Hunter, R.A.; Asare-Werehene, M.; Mandour, A.; Tsang, B.K.; Anis, H. Determination of Chemoresistance in Ovarian Cancer by Simultaneous Quantification of Exosomes and Exosomal Cisplatin with Surface Enhanced Raman Scattering. *Sens. Actuators B Chem.* **2022**, *354*, 131237. [CrossRef]
230. Chen, T.; Cheng, Q.; Lee, H.J. Machine-Learning-Mediated Single-Cell Classification by Hyperspectral Stimulated Raman Scattering Imaging. *Opt. Heal. Care Biomed. Opt. XI* **2021**, *11900*, 30. [CrossRef]
231. Viljoen, R.; Neethling, P.; Spangenberg, D.; Heidt, A.; Frey, H.-M.; Feurer, T.; Rohwer, E. Implementation of Temporal Ptychography Algorithm, I2PIE, for Improved Single-Beam Coherent Anti-Stokes Raman Scattering Measurements. *J. Opt. Soc. Am. B* **2020**, *37*, A259–A265. [CrossRef]
232. Melnikov, G.; Ignatenko, N.; Petrova, L.; Manzhos, O.; Gromkov, A. On the Influence of Clustering Processes in the Liquid Structure on Raman Scattering. *MATEC Web Conf.* **2021**, *344*, 01010. [CrossRef]
233. Fang, X.; Zeng, Q.; Yan, X.; Zhao, Z.; Chen, N.; Deng, Q.; Zhu, M.; Zhang, Y.; Li, S. Fast Discrimination of Tumor and Blood Cells by Label-Free Surface-Enhanced Raman Scattering Spectra and Deep Learning. *J. Appl. Phys.* **2021**, *129*, 123103. [CrossRef]
234. Weng, S.; Xu, X.; Li, J.; Wong, S.T.C. Combining Deep Learning and Coherent Anti-Stokes Raman Scattering Imaging for Automated Differential Diagnosis of Lung Cancer. *J. Biomed. Opt.* **2017**, *22*, 106017. [CrossRef] [PubMed]
235. Yamato, N.; Matsuya, M.; Niioka, H.; Miyake, J.; Hashimoto, M. Nerve Segmentation with Deep Learning from Label-Free Endoscopic Images Obtained Using Coherent Anti-Stokes Raman Scattering. *Biomolecules* **2020**, *10*, 1012. [CrossRef] [PubMed]
236. Brusin, A.M.R.; Zefreh, M.R.; Poggiolini, P.; Piciaccia, S.; Forghieri, F.; Carena, A. Machine Learning for Power Profiles Prediction in Presence of Inter-Channel Stimulated Raman Scattering. In *2021 European Conference on Optical Communication (ECOC)*; IEEE: Piscataway, NJ, USA, 2021; p. 21549326.
237. Yamato, N.; Niioka, H.; Miyake, J.; Hashimoto, M. Improvement of Nerve Imaging Speed with Coherent Anti-Stokes Raman Scattering Rigid Endoscope Using Deep-Learning Noise Reduction. *Sci. Rep.* **2020**, *10*, 15212. [CrossRef]
238. Yin, P.; Li, G.; Zhang, B.; Farjana, H.; Zhao, L.; Qin, H.; Hu, B.; Ou, J.; Tian, J. Facile PEG-Based Isolation and Classification of Cancer Extracellular Vesicles and Particles with Label-Free Surface-Enhanced Raman Scattering and Pattern Recognition Algorithm. *Analyst* **2021**, *146*, 1949–1955. [CrossRef]
239. Shi, H.; Wang, H.; Meng, X.; Chen, R.; Zhang, Y.; Su, Y.; He, Y. Setting Up a Surface-Enhanced Raman Scattering Database for Artificial-Intelligence-Based Label-Free Discrimination of Tumor Suppressor Genes. *Anal. Chem.* **2018**, *90*, 14216–14221. [CrossRef]
240. Sun, Y.W.; Liu, C.; Chan, K.L.; Xie, P.H.; Liu, W.Q.; Zeng, Y.; Wang, S.M.; Huang, S.H.; Chen, J.; Wang, Y.P.; et al. Stack Emission Monitoring Using Non-Dispersive Infrared Spectroscopy with an Optimized Nonlinear Absorption Cross Interference Correction Algorithm. *Atmos. Meas. Tech.* **2013**, *6*, 1993–2005. [CrossRef]
241. Leong, Y.X.; Lee, Y.H.; Koh, C.S.L.; Phan-Quang, G.C.; Han, X.; Phang, I.Y.; Ling, X.Y. Surface-Enhanced Raman Scattering (SERS) Taster: A Machine-Learning-Driven Multireceptor Platform for Multiplex Profiling of Wine Flavors. *Nano Lett.* **2021**, *21*, 2642–2649. [CrossRef]
242. Buzalewicz, I.; Suchwałko, A.; Karwańska, M.; Wieliczko, A.; Podbielska, H. Development of the Correction Algorithm to Limit the Deformation of Bacterial Colonies Diffraction Patterns Caused by Misalignment and Its Impact on the Bacteria Identification in the Proposed Optical Biosensor. *Sensors* **2020**, *20*, 5797. [CrossRef]

243. Hu, J.; Ma, L.; Wang, S.; Yang, J.; Chang, K.; Hu, X.; Sun, X.; Chen, R.; Jiang, M.; Zhu, J.; et al. Biomolecular Interaction Analysis Using an Optical Surface Plasmon Resonance Biosensor: The Marquardt Algorithm vs Newton Iteration Algorithm. *PLoS ONE* **2015**, *10*, e0132098. [CrossRef] [PubMed]
244. Mirsanaye, K.; Uribe Castaño, L.; Kamaliddin, Y.; Golaraei, A.; Augulis, R.; Kontenis, L.; Done, S.J.; Žurauskas, E.; Stambolic, V.; Wilson, B.C.; et al. Machine Learning-Enabled Cancer Diagnostics with Widefield Polarimetric Second-Harmonic Generation Microscopy. *Sci. Rep.* **2022**, *12*, 10290. [CrossRef] [PubMed]
245. Desa, D.E.; Strawderman, R.L.; Wu, W.; Hill, R.L.; Smid, M.; Martens, J.W.M.; Turner, B.M.; Brown, E.B. Intratumoral Heterogeneity of Second-Harmonic Generation Scattering from Tumor Collagen and Its Effects on Metastatic Risk Prediction. *BMC Cancer* **2020**, *20*, 1217. [CrossRef]
246. Jafari, R.; Jones, T.; Trebino, R. 100% Robust and Fast Algorithm for Second-Harmonic-Generation Frequency-Resolved Optical Gating. *Real-Time Meas. Rogue Phenom. Single-Shot Appl. IV SPIE LASE* **2019**, *10903*, 22. [CrossRef]
247. Tan, T.; Peng, C.; Yuan, Z.; Xie, X.; Liu, H.; Xie, Z.; Huang, S.-W.; Rao, Y.; Yao, B. Predicting Kerr Soliton Combs in Microresonators via Deep Neural Networks. *J. Light. Technol.* **2020**, *38*, 6591–6599. [CrossRef]
248. Costa, C.; Borges, L.; Penchel, R.A.; Abbade, M.L.F.; Giacoumidis, E.; Wei, J.; de Oliveira, J.A.; Santos, M.; Marconi, J.D.; Pita, J.L.; et al. Self-Phase Modulation and Inter-Polarization Cross-Phase Modulation Mitigation in Single-Channel Dp-16qam Coherent Pon Employing 4d Clustering. *SSRN Electron. J.* **2022**. [CrossRef]
249. Chen, Y.; Du, J.; Huang, Y.; Xu, K.; He, Z. Intelligent Gain Flattening in Wavelength and Space Domain for FMF Raman Amplification by Machine Learning Based Inverse Design. *Opt. Express* **2020**, *28*, 11911–11920. [CrossRef]
250. Chen, Y.; Du, J.; Huang, Y.; Xu, K.; He, Z. Intelligent Gain Flattening of FMF Raman Amplification by Machine Learning Based Inverse Design. In Proceedings of the Optical Fiber Communication Conference (OFC) 2020, San Diego, CA, USA, 8–12 March 2020; Optica Publishing Group: San Diego, CA, USA, 2020; p. T4B.1.
251. Jiang, L.; Mehedi Hassan, M.; Jiao, T.; Li, H.; Chen, Q. Rapid Detection of Chlorpyrifos Residue in Rice Using Surface-Enhanced Raman Scattering Coupled with Chemometric Algorithm. *Spectrochim. Acta Part A Mol. Biomol. Spectrosc.* **2021**, *261*, 119996. [CrossRef]
252. Li, H.; Mehedi Hassan, M.; Wang, J.; Wei, W.; Zou, M.; Ouyang, Q.; Chen, Q. Investigation of Nonlinear Relationship of Surface Enhanced Raman Scattering Signal for Robust Prediction of Thiabendazole in Apple. *Food Chem.* **2021**, *339*, 127843. [CrossRef]
253. Lussier, F.; Missirlis, D.; Spatz, J.P.; Masson, J.-F. Machine-Learning-Driven Surface-Enhanced Raman Scattering Optophysiology Reveals Multiplexed Metabolite Gradients Near Cells. *ACS Nano* **2019**, *13*, 1403–1411. [CrossRef]
254. Burzynski, N.; Yuan, Y.; Felsen, A.; Reitano, R.; Wang, Z.; Sethi, K.A.; Lu, F.; Chiu, K. Deep Learning Techniques for Unmixing of Hyperspectral Stimulated Raman Scattering Images. In *2021 IEEE International Conference on Big Data (Big Data)*; IEEE: Piscataway, NJ, USA, 2021; pp. 5862–5864.
255. Fang, Z.; Wang, W.; Lu, A.; Wu, Y.; Liu, Y.; Yan, C.; Han, C. Rapid Classification of Honey Varieties by Surface Enhanced Raman Scattering Combining with Deep Learning. In Proceedings of the 2018 Cross Strait Quad-Regional Radio Science and Wireless Technology Conference (CSQRWC), Xuzhou, China, 21–24 July 2018; IEEE: Piscataway, NJ, USA, 2018; p. 18092502.
256. Sha, P.; Dong, P.; Deng, J.; Wu, X. Rapid Identification and Quantitative Analysis of Anthrax Protective Antigen Based on Surface-Enhanced Raman Scattering and Convolutional Neural Networks. In *2021 IEEE 21st International Conference on Nanotechnology (NANO)*; IEEE: Piscataway, NJ, USA, 2021; pp. 155–158.
257. Paryanti, G.; Faig, H.; Rokach, L.; Sadot, D. A Direct Learning Approach for Neural Network Based Pre-Distortion for Coherent Nonlinear Optical Transmitter. *J. Light. Technol.* **2020**, *38*, 3883–3896. [CrossRef]
258. Lee, G.-G.C.; Haung, K.-W.; Sun, C.-K.; Liao, Y.-H. Stem Cell Detection Based on Convolutional Neural Network via Third Harmonic Generation Microscopy Images. In *2017 International Conference on Orange Technologies (ICOT)*; IEEE: Piscataway, NJ, USA, 2017; pp. 45–48.
259. Gupta, A.K.; Hsu, C.-H.; Lai, C.-S. Enhancement of the Au/ZnO-NA Plasmonic SERS Signal Using Principal Component Analysis as a Machine Learning Approach. *IEEE Photonics J.* **2020**, *12*, 20013846. [CrossRef]
260. Rajput, S.K.; Nishchal, N.K. Fresnel Domain Nonlinear Optical Image Encryption Scheme Based on Gerchberg–Saxton Phase-Retrieval Algorithm. *Appl. Opt.* **2014**, *53*, 418–425. [CrossRef] [PubMed]
261. Aşırım, Ö.E.; Yolalmaz, A.; Kuzuoğlu, M. High-Fidelity Harmonic Generation in Optical Micro-Resonators Using BFGS Algorithm. *Micromachines* **2020**, *11*, 686. [CrossRef]
262. Bresci, A.; Guizzardi, M.; Valensise, C.M.; Marangi, F.; Scotognella, F.; Cerullo, G.; Polli, D. Removal of Cross-Phase Modulation Artifacts in Ultrafast Pump–Probe Dynamics by Deep Learning. *APL Photonics* **2021**, *6*, 76104. [CrossRef]
263. Wang, L.; Gao, M.; Zhang, Y.; Cao, F.; Huang, H. Optical Phase Conjugation with Complex-Valued Deep Neural Network for WDM 64-QAM Coherent Optical Systems. *IEEE Photonics J.* **2021**, *13*, 21200412. [CrossRef]
264. Shan, M.; Cheng, Q.; Zhong, Z.; Liu, B.; Zhang, Y. Deep-Learning-Enhanced Ice Thickness Measurement Using Raman Scattering. *Opt. Express* **2020**, *28*, 48–56. [CrossRef]
265. Pereira, V.R.; Pereira, D.R.; de Melo Tavares Vieira, K.C.; Ribas, V.P.; Constantino, C.J.L.; Antunes, P.A.; Favareto, A.P.A. Sperm Quality of Rats Exposed to Difenoconazole Using Classical Parameters and Surface-Enhanced Raman Scattering: Classification Performance by Machine Learning Methods. *Environ. Sci. Pollut. Res.* **2019**, *26*, 35253–35265. [CrossRef]
266. Owaki, S.; Nakamura, M. XPM Compensation in Optical Fiber Transmission Systems Using Neural-Network-Based Digital Signal Processing. *IEICE Commun. Express* **2018**, *7*, 31–36. [CrossRef]

267. Yildiz, N.; San, S.E.; Polat, Ö. Light-Scattering Experiments in Dye-Doped Liquid Crystals Both to Determine Crystal Parameters and to Construct Consistent Neural Network Empirical Physical Formulas for Scattering Amplitudes. *Opt. Commun.* **2011**, *284*, 2173–2181. [CrossRef]
268. Owaki, S.; Nakamura, M. Compensation of Optical Nonlinear Waveform Distortion Using Neural-Network Based Digital Signal Processing. *IEICE Commun. Express* **2017**, *6*, 484–489. [CrossRef]
269. Wang, R.; Liang, F.; Lin, Z. Data-Driven Prediction of Diamond-like Infrared Nonlinear Optical Crystals with Targeting Performances. *Sci. Rep.* **2020**, *10*, 3486. [CrossRef] [PubMed]
270. Williamson, I.A.D.; Hughes, T.W.; Minkov, M.; Bartlett, B.; Pai, S.; Fan, S. Reprogrammable Electro-Optic Nonlinear Activation Functions for Optical Neural Networks. *IEEE J. Sel. Top. Quantum Electron.* **2020**, *26*, 18881115. [CrossRef]
271. Khulbe, M.; Kumar, S. Role of Nonlinear Optics in Big Data Transmission and Next Generation Computing Technologies. In *2019 9th International Conference on Cloud Computing, Data Science & Engineering (Confluence)*; IEEE: Piscataway, NJ, USA, 2019; pp. 234–238.
272. Berry, M.E.; McCabe, S.M.; Shand, N.C.; Graham, D.; Faulds, K. Depth Prediction of Nanotags in Tissue Using Surface Enhanced Spatially Offset Raman Scattering (SESORS). *Chem. Commun.* **2022**, *58*, 1756–1759. [CrossRef] [PubMed]
273. Sun, Y.; Dong, M.; Yu, M.; Xia, J.; Zhang, X.; Bai, Y.; Lu, L.; Zhu, L. Nonlinear All-Optical Diffractive Deep Neural Network with 10.6 Mm Wavelength for Image Classification. *Int. J. Opt.* **2021**, *2021*, 6667495. [CrossRef]
274. Xu, L.; Rahmani, M.; Ma, Y.; Smirnova, D.A.; Kamali, K.Z.; Deng, F.; Chiang, Y.K.; Huang, L.; Zhang, H.; Gould, S.; et al. Enhanced Light–Matter Interactions in Dielectric Nanostructures via Machine-Learning Approach. *Adv. Photonics* **2020**, *2*, 1. [CrossRef]
275. Wright, L.G.; Onodera, T.; Stein, M.M.; Wang, T.; Schachter, D.T.; Hu, Z.; McMahon, P.L. Deep Nonlinear Optical Neural Networks Using Physics-Aware Training. In *Conference on Lasers and Electro-Optics*; Kang Tomasulo, S., Ilev, I., Müller, D., Litchinitser, N., Polyakov, S., Podolskiy, V., Nunn, J., Dorrer, C., Fortier, T., Gan, Q., et al., Eds.; Optica Publishing Group: Washington, DC, USA, 2021; p. FF1A.4.
276. Miscuglio, M.; Mehrabian, A.; Hu, Z.; Azzam, S.I.; George, J.; Kildishev, A.V.; Pelton, M.; Sorger, V.J. All-Optical Nonlinear Activation Function for Photonic Neural Networks [Invited]. *Opt. Mater. Express* **2018**, *8*, 3851. [CrossRef]
277. Girija, R.; Anshula; Singh, H. Security-Enhanced Optical Nonlinear Cryptosystem Based on Modified Gerchberg–Saxton Iterative Algorithm. *Optik* **2021**, *244*, 167568. [CrossRef]
278. Singh, P.; Kumar, R.; Yadav, A.K.; Singh, K. Security Analysis and Modified Attack Algorithms for a Nonlinear Optical Cryptosystem Based on DRPE. *Opt. Lasers Eng.* **2021**, *139*, 106501. [CrossRef]
279. Ghiasuddin; Akram, M.; Adeel, M.; Khalid, M.; Tahir, M.N.; Khan, M.U.; Asghar, M.A.; Ullah, M.A.; Iqbal, M. A Combined Experimental and Computational Study of 3-Bromo-5-(2,5-Difluorophenyl) Pyridine and 3,5-Bis(Naphthalen-1-Yl)Pyridine: Insight into the Synthesis, Spectroscopic, Single Crystal XRD, Electronic, Nonlinear Optical and Biological Properties. *J. Mol. Struct.* **2018**, *1160*, 129–141. [CrossRef]
280. Agarwal, N.R.; Lucotti, A.; Tommasini, M.; Chalifoux, W.A.; Tykwinski, R.R. Nonlinear Optical Properties of Polyynes: An Experimental Prediction for Carbyne. *J. Phys. Chem. C* **2016**, *120*, 11131–11139. [CrossRef]
281. Kutz, N. Deep Learning for Control of Nonlinear Optical Systems. In *AI and Optical Data Sciences II*; Kitayama, K., Jalali, B., Eds.; SPIE: Bellingham, WA, USA, 2021; Volume 11703, p. 41.
282. Wu, J.; Li, Z.; Luo, J.; Jen, A.K.-Y. High-Performance Organic Second- and Third-Order Nonlinear Optical Materials for Ultrafast Information Processing. *J. Mater. Chem. C* **2020**, *8*, 15009–15026. [CrossRef]

MDPI
St. Alban-Anlage 66
4052 Basel
Switzerland
Tel. +41 61 683 77 34
Fax +41 61 302 89 18
www.mdpi.com

Biosensors Editorial Office
E-mail: biosensors@mdpi.com
www.mdpi.com/journal/biosensors

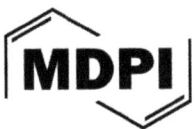

www.ingramcontent.com/pod-product-compliance
Lightning Source LLC
LaVergne TN
LVHW070737100526
838202LV00013B/1258